The Insider's Guide to the

MCAT

The Insider's Guide to the MCAT

Chirag Amin, M.D.

University of Miami School of Medicine
Class of 1996
Resident, Orthopaedic Surgery
Orlando Regional Medical Center
Orlando, Florida

Vikas Bhushan, M.D.

University of California, San Francisco, School of Medicine
Class of 1991
Diagnostic Radiologist
University of California, Los Angeles, Medical Center
Los Angeles, California

Tao Le, M.D.

University of California, San Francisco, School of Medicine
Class of 1996
Internist
Yale-New Haven Hospital
Yale University School of Medicine
New Haven, Connecticut

1999 Student Editor

Stephen Yoo

Medical Student
University of California,
Los Angeles, School of Medicine
Class of 2001

LIPPINCOTT WILLIAMS & WILKINS
Philadelphia • Baltimore • New York

Editor: Elizabeth Nieginski
Managing Editor: Darrin Kiessling
Designer: Ashley Pound Design
Typesetter: Maryland Composition
Printer: Phoenix Color

351 West Camden Street
Baltimore, Maryland 21201-2436 USA

227 East Washington Square
Philadelphia, PA 19106

Printed in the United States of America

Library of Congress Cataloging-in-Publication Data

Amin, Chirag.
The insider's guide to the MCAT / Chirag Amin, Vikas Bhushan, Tao Le.
p. cm.
ISBN 0-683-30698-7
1. Medical colleges—United States Entrance examinations Study guides. I. Bhushan, Vikas. II. Le, Tao. III. Title.
R838.5.A458 1999
610'.76—DC21 99-33185
CIP

The publishers have made every effort to trace the copyright holders for borrowed material. If they have inadvertently overlooked any, they will be pleased to make the necessary arrangements at the first opportunity.

To purchase additional copies of this book, call our customer service department at **(800) 638-3030** or fax orders to **(800) 824-7390.** International customers should call **(301) 714-2324.**

00 01 02 03
1 2 3 4 5 6 7 8 9 10

Dedication

To our teachers, who dedicated their time to providing us with knowledge and understanding.

To our colleagues and fellow premedical students, whose input, suggestions, and perspectives have been invaluable.

To our families, friends, and loved ones, who have provided us with their love and support throughout this endeavor.

Associate Contributors

Jeff Loeb
University of South Florida
School of Medicine
Class of 2001

Parag Mathur
University of California, Berkeley
Class of 1997

Hoang Nguyen
Northwestern University
School of Medicine
Class of 2000

Vipal Soni, M.D.
University of California, Los Angeles
School of Medicine
Class of 1999

contents

Foreword

Becoming a physician is viewed by many undergraduates as one of the few careers in which employment, satisfaction, and prestige remain secure. As a result, the pool of medical applicants has mushroomed over the past seven years. The number of matriculating premedical undergraduates has steadily risen and since 1990, there has been a 59% increase in the number of applicants. There are now more than three applicants for each available position in a medical school. The increased competition for admissions into medical school directly affects the number of students taking the Medical College Admissions Test (MCAT) and the need for them to perform well.

The MCAT is a formidable obstacle for most aspiring physicians. It is a stressful one-day test with 204 multiple-choice questions and two essays. The test day typically begins at 7:30 A.M. (preregistration and fingerprinting) and does not usually end until 5:30 P.M., making the MCAT not only a stressful, but also a very exhausting experience. All students applying to United States and Canadian medical schools must take the MCAT. A candidate's MCAT score and grade-point average (GPA) are the two most important factors determining medical school admission. There is a great deal of test-taking fear and anxiety surrounding the MCAT. Although most premedical students have experience with standardized tests, such as the Standardized Achievement Test (SAT) and the American College Testing assessment (ACT), the MCAT is usually their first encounter with a major multiple-choice marathon.

A candidate's MCAT score and grade-point average (GPA) are the two most important factors determining medical school admission.

When preparing for the MCAT, students tend to overwhelm themselves, which prevents them from focusing on their studying efforts and efficiently reviewing the most relevant material. Many students simply do not have the testing savvy, proper strategies, and correct advice to successfully face this strenuous experience and, thus, commonly commit the following errors:

The MCAT day is about 10 hours, making for a very stressful and tiring day.

- "Stressing out" because of an inadequate understanding of the MCAT
- Becoming overwhelmed by the length and detail of review material
- Studying material that is rarely tested on the MCAT
- Buying the wrong review books or buying too many books
- Choosing an inappropriate commercial review course
- Using study methods that are inefficient, inappropriate, or outdated

The Insider's Guide to the MCAT is a unique student-to-student guide designed to help premedical students quickly and effectively prepare for the MCAT. It includes advice on key issues, including efficient study methods, MCAT format, and score results and interpretations. It also includes compact summaries of the key topics in all four science disciplines tested on the MCAT (i.e., biology, general chemistry, physics, and organic chemistry) and key strategies on approaching the verbal reasoning and essay sections of the exam. In addition, we provide independent critical student evaluations of the major MCAT commercial review courses, review books, and sample exam books. Furthermore, we incorporate valuable test-taking advice and strategies from hundreds of students that have taken the exam, thus providing the most up-to-date information about the MCAT.

This practical guide emphasizes efficient study techniques, anxiety reduction, humor, and maximum exam performance for the time invested. In a concise manner, it presents topics, equations, and concepts that are most likely to appear in the science disciplines. Furthermore, we critically assess all the major review and exam preparation books currently on the market and recommend those to buy and those to avoid. We also provide concise summaries of the major commercial review courses.

This book is a collaborative effort from the start, compiling an abundance of strategies and insight from hundreds of students that have taken the examination. We welcome your input to further improve the book. If you have any helpful comments, strategies, high-yield facts, mnemonics, book reviews, or course reviews for the next edition, please use the forms in the How to Contribute section of this book to submit your contributions. Any student who submits material that we subsequently use will receive personal acknowledgment in the next edition of *Insider's Guide to the MCAT*.

Happy studying, and good luck!

Preface to Insider's Guide to the MCAT

This book, previously known as *Jump Start MCAT*, has been a collaborative effort from the start, which has accounted for its popularity among premedical students. Nevertheless, we believe that there is always room for improvement, and continue to look for ways to make this book even more useful to students preparing for their MCAT examination. We have updated the information on exam preparation, providing more detailed advice on exam preparation as well as an expanded description of what to expect on exam day. In response to increasing student concerns, we also expanded our sections on the verbal reasoning and writing sample sections, providing more detailed advice on how to approach these sections. Furthermore, we also updated and broadened the sections on MCAT book and course reviews, evaluating over 35 review books and providing up-to-date descriptions on the available review courses. We appreciate all of the feedback that we have received from student contributions, and encourage you to help us improve this book by giving us your feedback (see How to Contribute on page xxi to help us guide future editions of *The Insider's Guide to the MCAT*. We wish you all the best, not only on the MCAT, but also in all of your future endeavors.

Preface to Jumpstart MCAT

This book is a unique, concise review guide to help aspiring medical students prepare for the MCAT. The contributor team includes medical students who have performed exceptionally well on the current MCAT. This book provides the reader with important advice on key issues needed for MCAT success. The book is divided into five major parts:

Part I provides you with an orientation to the MCAT. Our goal is to make you more familiar with the format of the MCAT and to help you organize your preparation for the exam. Knowing the specific details pertaining to the MCAT will help you feel more comfortable with the exam.

Part II provides a concise review of the most important facts you need to know for the MCAT. We believe that if you know and understand these topics, you will have the basic knowledge needed to perform well on the MCAT.

Part III reviews the many MCAT review books currently on the market. With the help of numerous independent student evaluations, we have evaluated these books specifically for their applicability to the MCAT. We looked at numerous criteria in evaluating these review books, including the quality and accuracy of the questions and explanations, readability, length, quality and number of visual aids (i.e., tables, diagrams), and cost. We hope our reviews make your search for resources easy and quick.

Part IV focuses on the commercial MCAT review courses that are available to students. We have summarized the key features of each review course, including information about cost, and hours of classroom instruction. Although we do not recommend a review course for every student preparing for the MCAT, students who want a more structured study environment and learn better from lectures may benefit from this information.

Finally, **Part V** briefly discusses the medical school application process. We provide insight on various steps in the application process, including advice on writing your personal statement, soliciting letters of recommendation, and the medical school interview. We provide you with guidance, from a student perspective, about what to expect and prepare for after taking the MCAT.

We hope you find this book useful and that it makes preparing for the MCAT easier for you. We greatly appreciate any comments, suggestions, or criticisms that you may have (see How to Contribute on page xxi). We look forward to receiving your input for future editions. Best of luck on the MCAT!

Acknowledgments

This book would not have been possible without the encouragement and support of many people. We gratefully acknowledge the thoughtful comments, corrections, and suggestions of the numerous premedical students, medical students, and faculty who have supported the authors in developing this book. Special thanks to the Staff at Williams & Wilkins—Elizabeth Nieginski, Darrin Kiessling, Julie Scardiglia, Tim Satterfield, Kevin Thibodeau, and Christopher O'Callaghan—for their helpfulness and understanding. Also, we would like to thank especially Yi-Meng Yen, for his expert assistance with the diagrams and illustrations in this book. We are especially grateful to Ashley Pound, who crafted the interior and exterior design, contributing to the book's unique personality. Other individuals who provided assistance and support include Andrea Fellows, Jonathan Kirsch, Gianni Le, Kelly Ray, Marc Mickiewicz, and Vik Panchal. All of these individuals enthusiastically contributed to this work and have our sincere appreciation.

Chirag Amin
Vikas Bhushan
Tao Le

How to Contribute

The Insider's Guide to the MCAT was created from the contributions and experiences of many students who successfully completed the MCAT. We invite you to participate in this process. Please send us your suggestions for mnemonics, diagrams, and test strategies as well as personal ratings and comments on review books that you used. The preferred way to submit corrections or suggestions is via electronic mail addressed to:

Chiragamin@aol.com
Vbhushan@aol.com
Taotle@aol.com

For MCAT news, updates, and corrections, visit our Internet Website at:

http://www.s2smed.com

Otherwise, please send entries, neatly written, typed, or on disk (Microsoft Word) to The Insider's Guide to the MCAT, 1015 Gayley Ave., #1113, Los Angeles, CA 90024. You can also use the contribution forms on the following pages.

Contribution Form

Name: ______________________________

School/Affiliation: ______________________________

Address: ______________________________

____

Telephone: ______________________________

Cool tips, mnemonics, strategies, and corrections

Did you take a commercial MCAT review course? If so, which one? What was your overall assessment? Please comment on the quality of the review material, the classroom instruction, price, and the other resources at the review centers. Would you take the course again?

What student-to-student advice would you give someone preparing for the MCAT?

How else would you improve *The Insider's Guide to the MCAT*? Any other comments or suggestions? What did you like most about the book?

What aspects of the MCAT exam (e.g., concepts, topics, strategies) did you experience that you felt were not thoroughly covered in this book?

Attach additional sheets if necessary. Thanks for your help!

(fold here)

Return Address

____

____

____

Postage required

Attn: Contributions
The Insider's Guide to the MCAT
1015 Gayley Ave., #1113
Los Angeles, CA 90024

(fold here)

Book Reviews

Name: ______________________________

School/Affiliation: ______________________________

Address: ______________________________

____

Telephone: ______________________________

We need your feedback to help us rate and evaluate MCAT books for future students. Please comment on the MCAT books that you used below. Rate the books with a letter grade (e.g., A^+, B, C^-).

Title/Author/Publisher: ______________________________

Grade: __________ Time requirement: __________

Pros: ______________________________

____

Cons: ______________________________

____

Title/Author/Publisher: ______________________________

Grade: __________ Time requirement: __________

Pros: ______________________________

____

Cons: ______________________________

____

Title/Author/Publisher: ______________________________

Grade: __________ Time requirement: __________

Pros: ______________________________

____

Cons: ______________________________

____

Title/Author/Publisher: ______________________________

Grade: __________ Time requirement: __________

Pros: ______________________________

____

Cons: ______________________________

____

Photocopy this form if necessary. Thanks for your help!

(fold here)

Return Address

____

____

____

Postage required

Attn: Contributions
The Insider's Guide to the MCAT
1015 Gayley Ave., #1113
Los Angeles, CA 90024

(fold here)

PART I

exam preparation

A Stop Worrying!

THIS BOOK IS intended to make your Medical College Admissions Test (MCAT) studying and preparation easier, more efficient, and less stressful. By helping you understand more about the MCAT, we will help you get the most out of your exam preparation. You are already familiar with taking science courses that require you to memorize large amounts of information in a short period of time. In addition, you have already taken standardized examinations such as the Scholastic Aptitude Test (SAT), the American College Testing Program (ACT), and various achievement tests. When preparing for the MCAT, however, you may become overwhelmed, which prevents you from focusing on your study efforts and the most relevant material. Typical errors that students make when approaching the MCAT include:

- "Stressing out" due to an inadequate understanding of the MCAT
- Starting to study too late
- Studying material that is rarely covered by the MCAT
- Not buying the right review books or buying too many books
- Leaping into a review course before looking
- Using study methods that are inefficient, inappropriate, or outdated
- Not understanding how the American Association of Medical College (AAMC) scores the MCAT or how MCAT scores affect an applicant's chances for admission

This book contains advice on how to avoid these common mistakes, thus helping you get the most out of your studying. First, however, you must understand the format and content of the MCAT.

1 WHAT IS THE MCAT?

The MCAT is a 1-day, 10-hour test that includes three multiple-choice sections and two essays. The MCAT test day usually begins at 7:30 A.M. with preregistration and fingerprinting and ends at about 5.30 P.M. after all the test booklets are collected and accounted for. It is taken by all students applying to United States and Canadian medical schools, as well as by many applying to osteopathic and chiropractic schools. The exam is given only in the United States and Canada. The exam is administered twice a year, once in April and once in August. Approximately 58,000 students took the MCAT in 1998, a number which has risen considerably over the past several years. In general, a medical school candidate's grade-point average, MCAT scores, and interview are the most important factors influencing medical school admission committees that make acceptance decisions.

MCAT scores and GPA are the two most important factors in your application.

The number of students applying to medical school is increasing, whereas the percentage of applicants accepted into medical school is declining.

2 HOW DO I SIGN UP FOR THE MCAT?

The MCAT is administered and scored by the Educational Testing Service under the guidance of the Association of American Medical Colleges (AAMC). In 1997, the cost of the examination was $160. A fee reduction is available for eligible individuals, lowering the cost of the MCAT examination to $55; see "Is the MCAT Expensive?" (Part I A 3) for details. Current registration packets include an application (registration) card together with all current MCAT testing information. The packets should be available each February at your college's premedical advisory offices, as well as at local commercial test preparation centers. You can also get the packet by mail by phoning or writing:

MCAT Program Office
P.O. Box 4056
Iowa City, IA 52243
(319) 337-1357

Register early to get your favorite site.

You must register for the MCAT at least 6 weeks before the examination date. However, you should register to take the MCAT as soon as possible; if you register late, you may not get the testing site you want. More than one premedical student has had to rent a car and hotel room to take the MCAT at some out-of-the-way site. You should visit different testing sites near your residence or college, especially if your college is not an MCAT site. If the test-taking environment is important to you, we recommend that before registering, you familiarize yourself with the lecture hall, seating arrangements, cafeteria, and so forth.

3 IS THE MCAT EXPENSIVE?

You may qualify for an MCAT fee reduction.

Consult our review (Parts III and IV) for advice about the best books and courses for your money.

Yes and no. In terms of the $40,000 to $100,000 you might have spent on your undergraduate education, the cost of the MCAT and the medical school application process is a drop in the bucket. On the other hand, preparing thoroughly for the MCAT ends up costing more in money and time than most students initially estimate. You will spend $160 to register for the MCAT, $100 to $300 on review books, and possibly another $700 to $1000 on a review course. For this reason, **invest your time and money carefully in review books and courses.** Also, have realistic expectations about review books and commercial review courses. What you get out of a specific book or course will depend on you—your motivation, the amount of time you spend studying, and what resources are available to you. Don't expect to buy your way to a good score. Consult our review (Parts III and IV) for advice about the best books and courses for your money. If you can demonstrate financial need, you may apply for the $55 MCAT reduced registration fee [a form is included with the MCAT application, or you can request an MCAT fee reduction form by calling AAMC student services at (202)828-0600]. Some review courses also offer a discount for students who are receiving financial aid; contact course administrators for details.

You should also keep in mind that the application process for medical schools gets more expensive from here on. You will be expected to pay $15 to $30 for each school you check off on your American Medical Colleges Admission Service (AMCAS) application, as well as $50 to $100 for each secondary application and each non-AMCAS application. Again, the same fee reduction or waiver process exists for these application fees; consult the AMCAS application for additional information. Furthermore, students are expected to pay for travel (plane, hotel, car) expenses associated with medical school interviews (unless you apply to certain combined graduate-degree programs). Never mind that medical school can cost upward of $150,000 for the 4 years.

4 WHEN SHOULD I TAKE THE MCAT?

If you are planning to apply to medical schools during your senior year, take the MCAT in either August or April of your junior year: **the year before you apply to medical school** (Figure 1-1). The advantage of the August date is that it could give you a school-free summer in which to focus solely on preparing for the MCAT. If you opt to take the test in April, you will allow yourself more time to finish requisite and supplementary course work for the MCAT, but you may have less time for MCAT preparation—depending on your academic course load. Other students taking the MCAT in April are also taking courses at this time, however; you are not at a disadvantage. Consider taking a light spring-semester course load.

In any case, avoid taking the test prematurely. *Do not take the MCAT until you have finished all the requisite course work* (see Part I E 1). You can take the April MCAT while finishing one or two (not three) required science courses, but you will have to cover the later material in these courses on your own before taking the MCAT. In addition, some medical schools prefer that all their applicants' MCAT scores be from the same time period so they can accurately compare applicants (most schools will accept MCAT scores within 2–3 years of applying; consult the AAMC *1999–2000 Medical School Admissions Requirements* for details).

January	
February	
March	Deadline for registering for the April MCAT (6 weeks before test date)
April	April MCAT (usually mid-April)
May	April MCAT score reports sent out (6 weeks after test date)
June	AMCAS applications accepted (June 15)
July	Deadline for registering for the August MCAT (6 weeks before test date)
August	Early decision application deadline (August 1)
	August MCAT (usually mid-August)
September	
October	August MCAT score reports sent out (6 weeks after test date)
November	AMCAS application deadline
December	

Figure 1-1. Premedical MCAT flowchart and timeline.

Timing the MCAT is critical.

More important, avoid taking the MCAT in the fall of the year that you plan to apply to medical school (i.e., August of your senior year). Most medical schools interview and select candidates for admission on a rolling basis, meaning that they begin interviewing and accepting students with scores from previous MCAT sessions before the AAMC releases the August MCAT scores to the medical schools. Far too many qualified medical students have been rejected or put on a waiting list by all the medical schools to which they applied—because they postponed taking the MCAT.

5 WHAT SHOULD I BUY RIGHT AWAY?

Purchasing these three publications is a must!

Even before you register for the MCAT, you should order the three sets of publications made available by the AAMC. The first set contains the *MCAT Student Manual* and *MCAT Practice Test 1,* and it costs approximately $20. The second set of publications contains *MCAT Practice Items* and *MCAT Practice Test 2* (which is the actual MCAT examination that was administered in April 1991) and also costs approximately $20. *MCAT Practice Test 3* is the latest offering from the AAMC, and costs approximately $20. These publications offer the only real MCAT questions available for your test preparation. For a more detailed description of these and other currently available MCAT materials, please consult Part III, MCAT Review Books, beginning on page 183.

The fourth book for your shelves is a copy of the current *Medical School Admission Requirements,* another publication written by the AAMC, which gives admissions information and application deadlines for all medical schools in the United States and Canada. This publication also contains useful information for minority applicants as well as for high school students who plan to apply to combined college and medical school programs. All these books can be found in most undergraduate bookstores, or they can be purchased by writing or calling:

Membership and Publication Orders
Association of American Medical Colleges
2450 N. Street, NW
Washington, DC 20037-1129
(202) 828-0416

B What Is the Format of the MCAT?

THE MCAT HAS four major sections: verbal reasoning, physical sciences, writing sample, and biological sciences. All sections are multiple choice except the essay section, and they contain both passage-based and discrete multiple-choice questions. Each multiple-choice question has four choices. In the three sections, you are allotted an average of 78 seconds per question. The writing sample section contains two essays that are to be completed in 60 minutes (Figure 1-2).

1 VERBAL REASONING

The verbal reasoning section includes 8 to 11 passages on various subjects from the humanities (e.g., literature and history), the social sciences (e.g., sociology and anthropol-

7:30 A.M. Preregistration & Fingerprinting

MCAT Test Day

Registration & Seating	
Verbal Reasoning	*65 questions in 85 minutes*
Break	
Physical Sciences	*77 questions in 100 minutes*
Lunch	
Writing Sample	*2 essays in 60 minutes*
Break	
Biological Sciences	*77 questions in 100 minutes*

5:30 P.M. End of Test Day

Figure 1-2. Format of MCAT administration.

ogy), and the natural sciences (e.g., astronomy, geology, and paleontology). Each passage is followed by 6 to 10 related questions. Therefore, this section mainly tests your ability to understand each passage, to evaluate the material within that passage, and to use this material to answer the questions posed.

2 PHYSICAL SCIENCES

The physical sciences section tests your ability to understand and apply concepts from physics (50%) and inorganic chemistry (50%). Therefore, this section mainly tests your ability to understand and evaluate the material within each passage, then use this information to answer the questions posed. Approximately 62 of the 77 questions refer to 10 to 11 passages. You are expected to answer these questions using both the information you read in the passage and your general knowledge of physics and inorganic chemistry; many passages include graphs and tables that you are expected to interpret and apply. Each passage is followed by 5 to 10 questions. The remaining questions—approximately 15—are not based on the written passages, and are designed to evaluate your conceptual knowledge of physics and inorganic chemistry.

3 WRITING SAMPLE

See Part II B for high-yield facts that will help you master the essay.

The writing sample section of the MCAT requires that you write two independent essays. You are given one-half hour (timed separately) for each essay question, during which time you are expected to write a well-organized, persuasive, legible, and error-free essay developed around a central idea. You are not expected to have any specific knowledge of the essay topic. Instead, for each essay, the AAMC will present you with a statement, and you are expected to do the following:

- Explain what the statement means.
- Describe a specific situation in which the statement does **not** hold true.
- Discuss what you think determines when the statement holds true and when it does not.

4 BIOLOGICAL SCIENCES

Unlike the physical sciences section in which physics and general chemistry weigh equally, the biological sciences section contains more biology (65%) than organic chemistry (35%).

The biological sciences section tests your ability to understand and apply concepts from biology (65%) and organic chemistry (35%). Approximately 62 of the 77 questions are based on 10 to 11 passages, with each passage followed by 5 to 10 questions. (The remaining questions—approximately 15—are not based on passages, and are designed to evaluate your conceptual knowledge of biology and organic chemistry.) You are expected to answer these questions using both the information in the passage and your general knowledge of biology and organic chemistry; in addition, many passages include graphs and tables that you are expected to interpret and apply.

C Scoring

1 HOW IS THE MCAT SCORED?

***There is no penalty for guessing.** Do not leave any answers blank!*

In each section except the writing sample, your raw score is based on the number of questions you answer correctly. *There is no penalty for guessing.* Fill in all answer spaces. Your raw score is then converted to a scaled score between 1 and 15, with 1 being the lowest and 15 the highest. The only scores you receive will be between a 1 and 15 for each multiple choice section and a letter score for the essay portion of the examination. The AAMC will not tell you how many questions you answered correctly or incorrectly. However, the AAMC will provide the percentile of your scaled score. The percentile explains what fraction of students achieved a comparable or a lower score than you.

Although premedical students often perceive some sections (e.g., physical sciences) as tougher than others, the AAMC scales the distribution of scores to a standard distribution, with a mean of 8.0 and a standard deviation of 2.5 for each section. This figure is determined by adjusting the raw-score to scaled-score conversion scales (Figure 1-3). In addition, each examination administration uses a slightly different conversion scale, sometimes resulting in no scores in the 14 to 15 or 1 to 2 range on a particular section. This effect occurs more often with the verbal reasoning scores than with the biological science or physical science scores.

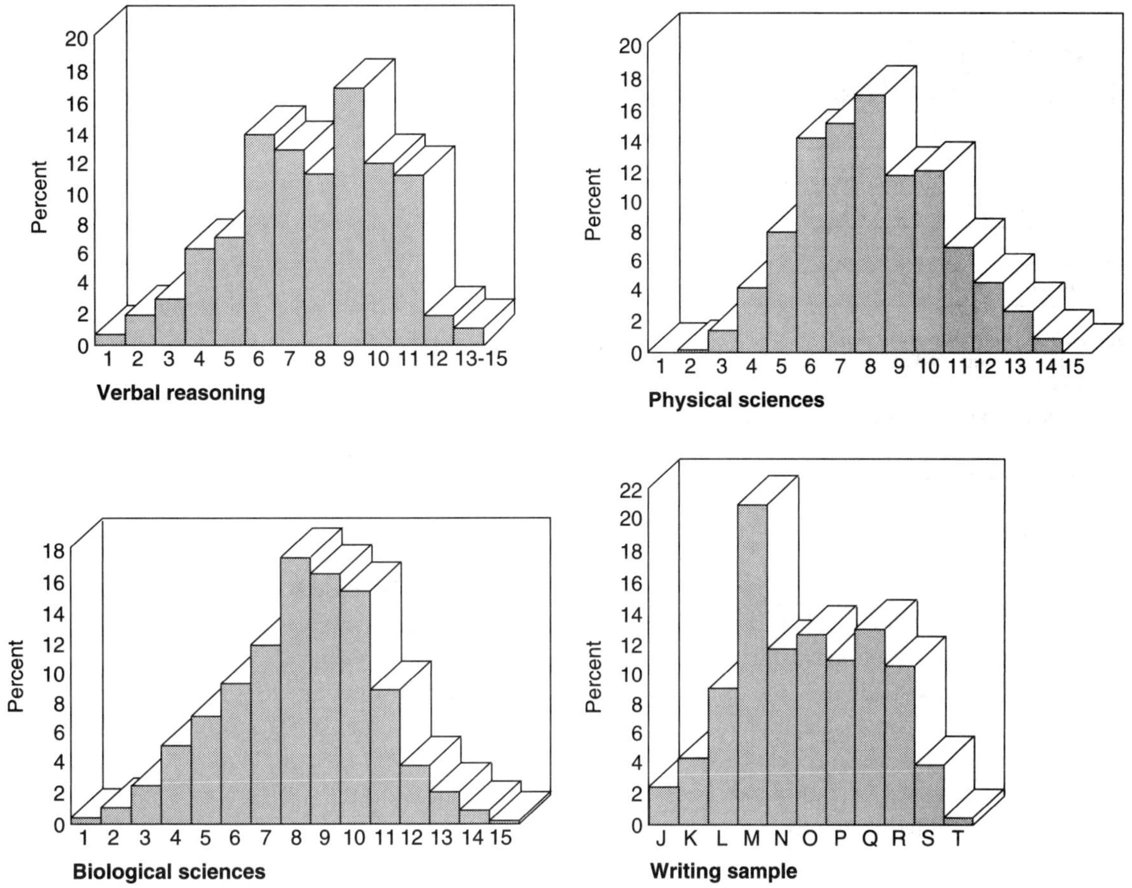

Figure 1-3.
Distribution of MCAT scores (combined April and August 1995). *Percent* = percent achieving scores.

The writing sample section of the MCAT is scored differently from the other three sections.

The writing samples are scored on the basis of their overall quality with no separate evaluations on organization, content, grammar, coherence, fluency, or other essay-writing criteria. Each essay is evaluated by two readers. After reading an essay, each reader independently assigns it a score based on a scale of 1 (lowest) to 6 (highest). The final essay score averages the two readers' scores. If these scores vary by more than one point, a third reader evaluates the essay in question to determine the final score. The final essay scores for both essays are then combined and converted into a letter score ranging from J (lowest—equivalent to a total of 2 points) to T (highest—equivalent to a total of 12 points).

To help you understand how the MCAT is scored and how scores are distributed, a sample score report with distribution information for the combined April and August 1995 MCAT administrations is included as Figure 1-4. Look at the score distribution in Figure 1-3; notice how many people score within 1 standard deviation of the mean (8 ± 2.5).

2 WHO GETS THE SCORES?

Although medical school admission committees do look at other factors, your grade-point average (GPA; both science and overall), your MCAT score, and your interviews are the most important factors determining whether you will be admitted to medical school. In their efforts to sift through the large number of candidates who apply to med-

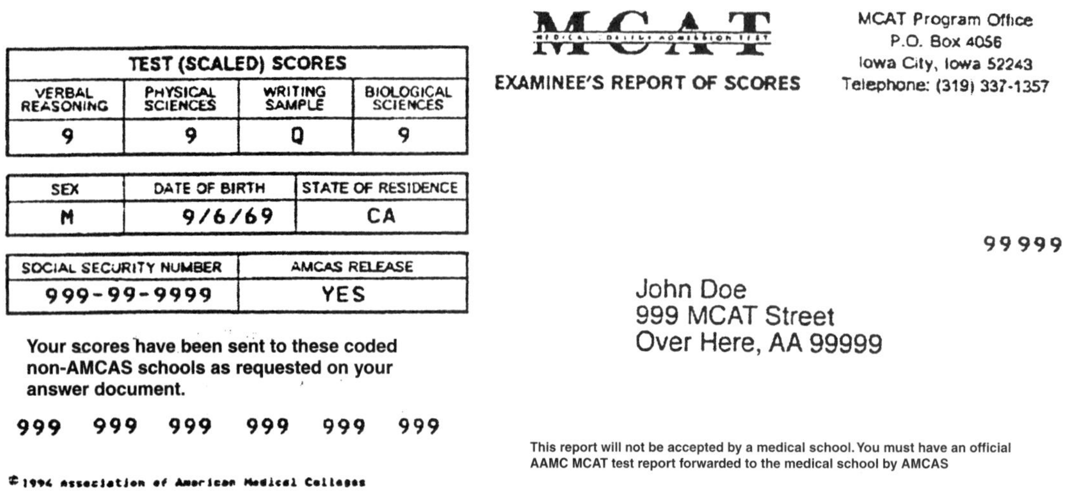

MCAT

EXAMINEE'S REPORT OF SCORES

MCAT Program Office
P.O. Box 4056
Iowa City, Iowa 52243
Telephone: (319) 337-1357

TEST (SCALED) SCORES			
VERBAL REASONING	PHYSICAL SCIENCES	WRITING SAMPLE	BIOLOGICAL SCIENCES
9	9	Q	9

SEX	DATE OF BIRTH	STATE OF RESIDENCE
M	9/6/69	CA

SOCIAL SECURITY NUMBER	AMCAS RELEASE
999-99-9999	YES

99999

John Doe
999 MCAT Street
Over Here, AA 99999

Your scores have been sent to these coded non-AMCAS schools as requested on your answer document.

999 999 999 999 999 999

This report will not be accepted by a medical school. You must have an official AAMC MCAT test report forwarded to the medical school by AMCAS

©1994 Association of American Medical Colleges

Figure 1-4.
Sample MCAT score report.

ical school each year, some schools use a "formula" based on student grades and MCAT scores to determine which candidates will be interviewed.

Given this formula, grades and MCAT scores **can** offset each other. The formula usually uses a sliding scale; that is, a high GPA can compensate for low MCAT scores. Conversely, if you have lower grades, extremely high MCAT scores can dramatically improve your chances in the medical school admissions process. Nevertheless, the most successful applicants possess both high grades and good MCAT scores, so you should work hard on both.

Some schools use "cutoffs"; that is, they require a specific minimum score on the MCAT, GPA, or both before inviting you for an interview. As a result, the remainder of your application often cannot offset low grades or low MCAT scores, no matter how many hours you volunteered in the emergency room or how well you performed in intramural sports.

3 WHAT DO I NEED TO SCORE ON THE MCAT?

When you begin preparing for the MCAT, you must set realistic numerical goals. The MCAT is the only objective measure by which the medical school admission committees can compare students from different schools; therefore, the test is especially pivotal if you come from a lesser known or smaller school. In fact, for many students the MCAT score is the most vital component of the medical school application because it reflects a student's most recent academic performance. It is usually taken as a sign of academic progress or, on the down side, regression. For example, getting a C, then B+, and then a 13 in physical sciences may be perceived as continuing improvement, whereas an A– and B+ followed by a 6 may be perceived as a negative trend.

Before studying for the MCAT, set rough numerical goals for yourself on each section. First, see Table 1-1, which lists the available average MCAT scores and grades for the 1996 entering classes from the 126 medical schools in the United States. The data come from several sources, including the *1998–99 Medical School Admissions Requirements,* published by the AAMC. (Disclaimer: The scores and GPA information listed in Table 1-1 should be used only as a general guideline. To obtain the most current GPA information and average MCAT scores for a particular medical school, contact the medical school's admissions department.) If you really want to go to a particular medical school and your grades are somewhat lower than the mean GPA associated with that

TABLE 1-1. GPA/MCAT average scores for American medical schools

School	Science GPA	Non Science GPA	Overall GPA	Biological Sciences	Physical Sciences	Verbal Reasoning	Mean Score	% Matriculated In-State Applicants
ALABAMA								
Alabama			3.56	9.9	9.7	9.8	9.8	84.0
Alabama, South			3.60	9.9	9.6	9.8	9.95	92.0
ARIZONA								
Arizona			3.55	8.6	9.3	9.4	100.0	100.0
ARKANSAS								
Arkansas			3.52	9.1	8.9	9.5	9.2	99.0
CALIFORNIA								
Stanford			3.60	11.0	11.0	10.0	10.7	50.0
Loma Linda			3.63	9.8	9.5	9.6	9.83	57.2
California, U of								
Davis			3.40	11.9	11.9	11.9	11.9	97.0
Irvine	3.6		3.63	10.7	10.4	9.2	10.1	100.0
Los Angeles (UCLA)	3.75	3.64	3.74	12.0	11.0	11.0	11.3	93.0
San Diego			3.66	11.0	11.4	10.4	10.9	99.0
San Francisco		3.75	3.74	12.0	11.0	11.0	11.3	75.0
California, Southern			3.50	10.7	10.5	10.0	10.4	83.0
COLORADO								
Colorado			3.60	9.9	9.9	9.9	9.9	81.0
CONNECTICUT								
Connecticut			3.55	10.0	10.0	10.0	10.0	90.0
Yale			3.60	91.5	11.2	10.7	11.1	9.0
DISTRICT OF COLUMBIA								
George Washington			3.40	10.0	10.0	10.0	10.0	1.9
Georgetown	3.58		3.51	10.0	10.0	10.0	10.0	0.8
Howard			3.10	8.2	8.0	7.6	7.9	3.6
FLORIDA								
Florida			3.71	9.4	9.0	9.1	9.16	95.0
Miami			3.65	10.0	9.4	10.0	9.8	97.0
Florida, South	3.70	3.70	3.70	10.2	10.2	9.7	10.0	100.0
GEORGIA								
Medical College of								98.9
Mercer								100.0
Morehouse								71.0
Emory			3.69	10.4	10.4	10.0	10.3	48.3
HAWAII								
Hawaii			3.55	10.15	10.23	8.83	9.7	93.0
ILLINOIS								
Illinois, U of								95.3
Illinois, Southern								100.0
Chicago—Pritzker	3.52		3.53	10.5	10.2	10.2	10.3	45.2
Northwestern			3.56				75th percentile	35.0
U Health Sci Chicago			3.30					40.3
Loyola—Stritch			3.5					50.0
Rush								86.7

Continued

TABLE 1-1. GPA/MCAT average scores for American medical schools—Cont.

School	Science GPA	Non Science GPA	Overall GPA	Biological Sciences	Physical Sciences	Verbal Reasoning	Mean Score	% Matriculated In-State Applicants
INDIANA								
Indiana			3.69	9.8	9.6	9.7	9.6	96.0
IOWA								
Iowa	3.60		3.60	9–10	9–10	9–10	9–10	80.0
KANSAS								
Kansas							60th percentile	89.2
KENTUCKY								
Kentucky			3.55					90.5
Louisville			3.60					90.5
LOUISIANA								
Louisiana State								
New Orleans	3.40							100.0
Shreveport	3.40		3.50					100.0
Tulane			3.50					14.9
MARYLAND								
Maryland			3.56				9.0	87.5
Johns Hopkins								15.1
Uniformed Services, Health Sciences			3.51				10.2	N/A
MASSACHUSETTS								
Massachusetts	3.50							100.0
Harvard			3.70	11.5	11.7	10.7	11.3	40.2
Boston								37.0
Tufts								28.2
MICHIGAN								
Michigan, U of			3.60					55.2
Michigan State								87.9
Wayne State			3.50					95.7
MINNESOTA								
Minnesota, U of								
Duluth			3.54	9.4	8.9	9.1	9.13	94.0
Minneapolis			3.59					92.6
Mayo			3.70	10+	10+	10+	10+	19.0
MISSISSIPPI								
Mississippi			3.48					100.0
MISSOURI								
Missouri, U of								
Columbia	3.60		3.70					99.0
Kansas City								69.7
Saint Louis	3.69		3.70	10.8	10.0	10.3	10.63	31.6
Washington	3.75	3.78	3.76	11.9	12.1	11.1	11.7	9.0
NEBRASKA								
Nebraska			3.76					97.5
Creighton	3.50		3.60					20.7

TABLE 1-1. GPA/MCAT average scores for American medical schools—Cont.

School	Science GPA	Non Science GPA	Overall GPA	Biological Sciences	Physical Sciences	Verbal Reasoning	Mean Score	% Matriculated In-State Applicants
NEVADA								
Nevada	3.50	3.60	3.60	9.7	9.2	9.1	9.3	90.3
NEW HAMPSHIRE								
Dartmouth								7.2
NEW JERSEY								
UMDNJ—New Jersey Medical School			3.44					92.3
UMDNJ—Robert Wood Johnson			3.54					87.0
NEW MEXICO								
New Mexico			3.45				8.79	94.5
NEW YORK								
SUNY								
Brooklyn								99.0
Buffalo			3.65				10.4	99.3
Stony Brook			3.53	11.0	11.0	10.0	10.6	98.0
Syracuse								93.1
Columbia								20.8
Cornell	3.58			10.6	10.6	10.6	10.6	48.2
New York University								48.1
Rochester			3.60				10.0	38.3
Albany			3.40					39.4
Albert Einstein								47.7
Mount Sinai			3.52				10.2	52.7
New York Medical								29.2
NORTH CAROLINA								
UNC Chapel Hill								87.5
East Carolina			3.50	8.4	8.1	8.6	8.12	100.0
Duke								32.0
Bowman Gray of Wake Forest								54.6
NORTH DAKOTA								
North Dakota	3.58		3.61	9.1	8.9	9.1	9.0	75.4
OHIO								
Cincinnati								83.4
Medical College of	3.38		3.48	9.24	9.17	9.13	9.18	84.2
Northeastern (NEOUCOM)								100.0
Ohio State			3.50					79.5
Wright State								90.0
Case Western Reserve			3.50				10.0	60.8
OKLAHOMA								
Oklahoma			3.57				9.44	95.0
OREGON								
Oregon Health Sciences			3.60					56.25

TABLE 1-1. GPA/MCAT average scores for American medical schools—Cont.

School	Science GPA	Non Science GPA	Overall GPA	Biological Sciences	Physical Sciences	Verbal Reasoning	Mean Score	% Matriculated In-State Applicants
PENNSYLVANIA								
Penn State			3.65					42.8
Temple	3.40						10.0	64.7
Pittsburgh			3.61				10.7	62.3
Pennsylvania, U of			3.60				10–11	28.6
Thomas Jefferson	3.50						9.9	43.9
Medical College of								50.4
RHODE ISLAND								
Brown								10.3
SOUTH CAROLINA								
Medical University								91.1
South Carolina, U of								91.7
SOUTH DAKOTA								
South Dakota	3.51	3.65	3.57	8.8	8.2	8.3		98.0
TENNESSEE								
Tennessee State, East			3.30	8.9	8.9	9.7	9.17	90.0
Tennessee, Memphis			3.50	10.0	9.0	9.0	9.3	92.7
Vanderbilt			3.75				11.2	9.6
Meharry								20.0
TEXAS								
Baylor			3.70	11.0	11.0	11.0	11.0	75.6
Texas, U of								
Houston			3.54					98.5
San Antonio			3.51					92.5
Dallas (Southwestern)								90.0
Galveston			3.50					94.0
Texas A & M			3.64				9.3	99.4
Texas Tech			3.59					97.5
UTAH								
Utah								75.0
VERMONT								
Vermont			3.40				8.9	41.9
VIRGINIA								
Virginia, U of			3.57				10.3	65.5
Medical College of			3.42				9.9	69.2
Eastern Virginia								61.1
WASHINGTON								
Washington			3.54	10.4	10.0	10.0	10.1	92.2
WEST VIRGINIA								
Marshall			3.40					93.75
West Virginia			3.61	9.3	8.7	9.1	9.0	95.5
WISCONSIN								
Medical College of								48.0
Wisconsin								83.2
OUTSIDE THE U.S.								
Ponce			3.31					77.0
Puerto Rico	3.50		3.59	8.0	7.0	6.0	6.7	97.4
U Central del Caribe			3.12					79.7

school, aim to score above their published MCAT mean. According to the *1998–99 Medical School Admissions Requirements*, published by the AAMC, for the 1996–97 entering medical school class, the mean cumulative GPA was 3.54. Also, keep in mind that the published means include minority students; you should consider the data in Table 1-2 when evaluating your GPA and MCAT scores.

From reviewing Table 1-1, you can generalize: If you want to get into a highly competitive public or private medical school, plan on obtaining MCAT scores of at least 11 to 12 on each section while maintaining a GPA of at least 3.8. On the other hand, if you are interested in attending one of the less competitive public schools, you may get by with MCAT scores of 9, 10, or higher. In the case of the less competitive private schools, you probably need to obtain scores of 9 to 11, or higher. In general, the lower limits of MCAT scores and GPAs in applicants accepted into medical school are 9s in each section and 3.0 respectively. However, because many of the highly competitive schools do not release their GPA/MCAT information, you should not rely on published score reports alone. Furthermore, out-of-state students should consider not applying to medical schools that have not accepted any out-of-state applicants (e.g., UC Davis, Mercer, LSU-Shreveport). Perhaps the best advice is to speak to senior premedical students from your undergraduate college about their experiences to get a better understanding of admissions standards.

If you want to get into a highly competitive public or private medical school, plan on obtaining MCAT scores of at least 11 to 12 on each section while maintaining a GPA of at least 3.8.

Because many of the highly competitive schools do not release their GPA/MCAT information, you should not rely on published score reports alone.

Few schools give their average scores on the essay (writing sample) section, thereby making it even harder to judge what essay score you need to get into medical school. In general, the essay section is not weighed as heavily as the other three sections. However, you should still take this section seriously (see Part I B 3, C 1); a below-average score on this section will harm your chances for gaining admission into medical school. In addition, medical schools can (and occasionally do) request copies of applicants' essays.

The essay section gets less weight than the other three sections.

To help refine your MCAT goals, take a diagnostic MCAT test (one with a 1 to 15 scale) at least 2 months before the actual MCAT administration. You can use your practice scores to gauge your workload for the following months.

- If you miss your target on all sections, do not despair; many people improve dramatically after intensive preparation. You should, however, plan on spending the bulk of your time in the following months preparing for the MCAT.
- If your performance is uneven and if you score more than 1 to 2 points below your goal on a particular section, plan on spending a lot of time on that particular area.
- If you hit the bull's-eye, raise your expectations—the higher your score, the better your chances of being admitted to the school of your choice.

4 SHOULD I RETAKE THE MCAT?

If your MCAT scores do not meet your expectations and you are willing to invest many more months studying, retaking the exam is an option. Do not be intimidated or discouraged by your first set of scores. Remember that the MCAT is a 1-day examination, and **anyone** can have a bad day. If your scores are inconsistent with your college grades (see Table 1-1), or with your practice scores, you definitely should consider retaking the exam.

Before you decide to try again, however, be aware that medical schools will weigh your second score more strongly than your first, which means that you **can** redeem yourself with a markedly better MCAT performance the second time around. Thus, you want

AAMC research shows that people who retake the MCAT improve approximately 1 point overall without additional preparation.

If you decide to retake the test, use the experience you gained from your first MCAT test.

Your goal in retaking the MCAT should be to increase your total score by at least 2 points.

to ensure that you can at least match your first set of scores, if not improve them. In fact, medical schools assume that students who retake the MCAT will do better the second time; **AAMC research shows that people who retake the MCAT improve approximately 1 point overall without additional preparation**. Your goal in retaking the MCAT should be to increase your total score by at least 2 points.

In addition, when you retake the MCAT, you are usually not as enthusiastic or motivated as you were the first time around. Therefore, obtaining the same level of MCAT proficiency or a higher level may involve considerably more effort and time. Use the experience gained from your first MCAT test to improve your level of preparedness the next time around.

5 SHOULD I APPLY TO MEDICAL SCHOOL EVEN IF I HAVE WEAK SCORES?

If you do poorly on the MCAT and you think that retaking the exam will not help, consider that some premed students with an 8 or less do get into medical schools in spite of their MCAT scores. Many medical schools use a "formula" or a cutoff based on a numerical combination of GPAs and MCATs, so a good GPA may compensate for weaker MCAT scores.

If your GPA is also borderline, you have two choices.

a. Improve your GPA as rapidly as possible.

Consider taking a number of easier classes, or classes without grade competition until you mail your application. You can even consider taking "graded independent study" or community-college courses to improve your GPA. Consult your adviser and successful premeds from your school.

b. Your file needs something that makes your application distinctive or exceptional.

For example, you could perform extraordinary volunteer work or community service, participate in a ground-breaking research experience, or become an all-American sports star.

6 SHOULD I RELEASE MY SCORES? IF SO, WHEN?

When you register to take the MCAT, you may elect to have your scores withheld. If you choose this option, you are the only one who will receive a copy of the scores. If you decide not to release your scores, you can request additional score reports to be sent to the medical schools that you request, for an additional fee for each score report, by writing to the address below. However, the AAMC does not offer a fee waiver for additional score reports, a policy that applies to all examinees. The disadvantages of this option are that you give up your six free medical school reports and incur a 2-month delay in reporting your scores to medical schools. If you are taking the test late (say, in the fall of your senior year), this option should be dismissed.

Additional Score Reports
Section for Student Services
Association of American Medical Colleges
2501 M Street, N.W., Suite 1
Washington, DC 20037–1300

D Minority and Foreign Students

1 WHAT IF I AM A MEMBER OF A MINORITY GROUP?

Many American medical schools have aggressive recruitment policies for underrepresented minorities. The AAMC defines "underrepresented minorities" as African Americans, Native Americans (American Indians and Alaskan natives), Mexican Americans, and mainland Puerto Ricans. If you belong to one of these minorities, your GPA and MCAT scores might be slightly less important than discussed previously (Table 1-2). Other factors such as community service may be just as important. Consult the AAMC *1999–2000 Medical School Admissions Requirements* for details.

TABLE 1-2. Profile of 1995 applicants accepted by medical schools

Variable	African American	Mainland Puerto Rican	Mexican American	Native American	Commonwealth Puerto Rican	Other Hispanic	White	Asian
Sci GPA	2.92	3.03	3.01	3.10	3.07	3.28	3.45	3.57
Non Sci	3.31	3.30	3.35	3.37	3.49	3.48	3.57	3.59
Cum GPA	3.09	3.15	3.16	3.22	3.26	3.38	3.5	3.51
VR	7.4	7.9	8.3	8.5	5.7	9.1	9.6	9.2
PS	6.9	7.6	7.8	7.4	6.7	8.7	9.4	10.1
BS	7.2	7.9	8.3	8.0	7.1	8.9	9.5	9.9
WS	O	O	O	O	N	O	O	O

2 WHAT IF I AM A FOREIGN STUDENT?

Most American medical schools require that foreign students attend college in the United States for at least 1 year—and even then, foreign students are not eligible for most financial aid (and sometimes must place their entire tuition in an escrow account before matriculating). Although foreign students often have difficulty gaining acceptance into American medical schools, it can be done. If you are a foreign student, you must perform extremely well on the MCAT (especially on the verbal reasoning and essay sections) and maintain your GPA. The best advice may come from talking with the few successful foreign applicants each year. Use your contacts to track them down.

E Course Work

1 WHAT COURSES DO I NEED FOR THE MCAT?

Make sure that, at a minimum, you have completed all of the required course work before you take the MCAT.

Focus on specific MCAT subject material while taking your premed courses.

The course work of the well-prepared MCAT student is similar to (but not the same as) that required for medical school admission (Table 1-3).

To prepare for the MCAT, you should take at least 1 year of biology with laboratory, including at least one semester of cellular/molecular biology and one semester of organismic/evolutionary biology. In addition, you should take 1 year of inorganic chemistry with laboratory, although you can get away with an accelerated one-semester course in inorganic chemistry if you had college-level or advanced placement chemistry in high school. You should also have at least one semester of organic chemistry with laboratory; the second semester of organic chemistry is usually required for medical school admission but is not necessary for the MCAT biological sciences section. Finally, 1 year of physics (preferably with laboratory) is necessary for the MCAT. **There is no calculus-based physics on the exam.**

Some schools offer special premed versions of the previously mentioned science courses, many of which focus on medical/biological applications of chemistry, physics, and math. These courses are an excellent idea, especially if your main interest in such subjects stems from having to take the MCAT and wanting to go to medical school. If you take the more rigorous classes, be prepared for the workload, and be aware that much of what you learn will be more advanced than the concepts you will use when taking the MCAT. Pay specific attention to subject material tested frequently on the MCAT.

Most schools also offer or require a semester of English composition or expository writing. You should take this course; not only is it required for most medical schools, but also it will help you refine your writing skills for the essay section of the MCAT. Finally, for the verbal reasoning section, you should read journal articles and books, both scientific and nonscientific, to bolster your reading speed and comprehension.

Supplemental course work is useful but not crucial for MCAT success. If you have the time, take a class in vertebrate or human physiology, because many of the passages, graphs, and tables in the biological sciences section are standard fare in a good physiology course. A course in biochemistry can also enhance your MCAT preparation, by familiarizing you with concepts that appear frequently on the MCAT (acids and bases,

TABLE 1-3. Undergraduate courses for MCAT preparation

Necessary	Supplementary	Optional
1 year biology: cellular/molecular biology organismic/evolutionary biology	Expository writing Cell biology	Upper level mathematics Ecology
1 year inorganic chemistry	Second semester organic chemistry	Upper level physics
1 semester organic chemistry	Human physiology	Human anatomy
1 year noncalculus-based physics	Biochemistry	Physical chemistry

metabolism, enzymes, and hormones). Finally, a course in speed reading, reading comprehension, and test-taking can help with the entire exam, especially if you are a slow reader and have a hard time finishing tests.

2 WHAT IF I'VE ALREADY GRADUATED FROM COLLEGE?

If you graduated from college without the necessary courses or with low grades in your science course work, a postbaccalaureate program may be right for you. These programs are designed for people with college degrees who need further course work before applying to medical school. Such programs normally offer the basic premedical requirements as well as supplemental advanced science courses. Students are expected to maintain a minimum grade-point average. If you fulfill their requirements, those who sponsor these programs will usually help you apply to medical school by writing letters of recommendation, reviewing your application, and in some cases preparing you for the MCAT (if not, consider taking a review course). In addition, some of these programs are specifically geared for underrepresented minorities and disadvantaged students.

Consider a postbaccalaureate program if you need a more intensive review of the physical and biological sciences.

If you enroll in one of these programs, expect to spend the bulk of your time studying for your classes. Since these programs typically last up to 2 years (and especially since many postbaccalaureate students are older), students are often tempted to take the MCAT early in their postbaccalaureate training, to accelerate the process of entering medical school. Unless your performance on the sample exams is awe inspiring, wait until you have finished **all** the necessary course work before taking the MCAT, even if it means waiting an extra year before going to medical school. In addition, consider taking advanced courses in physiology and biochemistry to further your MCAT preparation.

Finish all of the necessary coursework before taking the MCAT.

If you wish to continue your education while studying for the MCAT on your own, one good option is a Master's in Public Health (MPH) program. This type of program will broaden your perspective on medicine, and admission committees often consider an additional degree a favorable asset. Besides, this degree is respectable to add to an MD (i.e., MD, MPH), as opposed to doing research and getting a master's degree in science that you will rarely mention in the future. Getting a PhD is entirely different (and a lengthy) process.

F When Should I Start Preparing for the MCAT?

PREP TIME FOR THE MCAT varies among individuals. Following is a timeline that you can use in the weeks, months, and years before taking the MCAT.

1 YEAR BEFORE

The AAMC claims that "the scientific competency you will be expected to demonstrate on the MCAT is derived from basic principles and concepts in biology, general chemistry, organic chemistry, and physics." Therefore, first and foremost you should finish all of the required course work during the years leading up to the MCAT. Also consider supplemental course work like physiology and biochemistry to boost your MCAT preparation. Try to study MCAT material in parallel with your preparation for these courses—a strategy that should improve your grades along with your MCAT scores.

If you have one or more years before you plan to take the MCAT, you should also consider taking certain advanced science courses (see Part I E 1). Such courses can help you better understand basic scientific concepts by discussing them in more complicated contexts. Again, if you take the MCAT in April, plan a light spring semester to gain more time then to study for the MCAT.

Know your strengths and weaknesses in terms of the MCAT.

Before your urgent preparation for the MCAT begins, you should know your strengths and weaknesses in the material tested on the exam. Essentially, you should use this time to learn the basic sciences and other relevant material well the first time so you can minimize review time in the weeks before the MCAT; or if you are weak in the verbal reasoning or writing sample section, you can practice writing essays. Many schools offer writing tutorial courses on a pass/fail basis.

The MCAT stresses reading comprehension, not just a fund of knowledge. Read both scientific and nonscientific topics in the years before the exam. Read a variety of expository and opinion articles found in periodicals such as *Newsweek, Time, Scientific American, Journal of the American Medical Association,* and the *New England Journal of Medicine.* These articles will not only help you with the verbal reasoning section but also improve your ability to interpret and apply passages in the science sections. If you are a slow reader, consider taking a speed reading course. It will also help you with your medical school interviews; interviewers love well-informed and well-balanced candidates.

2 MONTH BEFORE

In the months preceding the test administration, register for the MCAT (see Part I A 2) and get the AAMC practice materials and student manual. Before registering for the MCAT, talk to people who have already taken the test to find out about test sites. Try for a favorable environment; the smaller the room and the fewer the number of students in that room, the more efficiently proctors can administer the test (and hence, the shorter the test). In addition, large desks help you organize your test materials, and spread-out seating provides an environment with fewer distractions. As mentioned earlier, if the testing environment is key for you, visit local testing sites, choose the site you like best, and register for the MCAT as soon as possible.

Plan to "peak" the day of the MCAT.

You should be studying seriously for the exam several months before the test date.

You should be studying seriously for the exam several months before the test date. At this time you should also decide about a commercial review course and buy the latest editions of MCAT review books. If you are bothered by family and friends who ask about your MCAT preparation and goals, do not tell them you are taking the MCAT (or do not tell them when you are taking it). You should also consider that preparing for the MCAT is like preparing for a race; you should peak the day of the MCAT. Accordingly, the months before the exam are a buildup to the "big day." Start by taking a few practice tests to identify your strengths and weaknesses before designing your preparation schedule. Then prepare a timeline that sets deadlines for the completion of certain topics and dates for practice tests. For the physical sciences and biological sciences sections, combine content review with practice tests, and for the verbal reasoning and essay sections, work through as many practice passages and questions as possible. If you doubt your ability to organize your exam preparation, or you need help with the subject matter, research and enroll in a reputable review course at least 2 months before the exam. Remember that you want to peak the day of the MCAT.

3 THREE WEEKS BEFORE

Building up your endurance is essential to MCAT success.

At this point, you should be completing your subject-by-subject review. For the next 2 weeks, you should concentrate on taking practice tests under simulated MCAT conditions. Have a friend time the sections for you, and start the test at 9 A.M. to get used to the time of day the MCAT is administered. If you finish a section early, **do not go on to the next section until time is up.** Building up your endurance is essential to MCAT success. Also, do not look at the answers to the test until you complete the entire practice test.

Most important, after each test, you should go through the answers and carefully analyze your mistakes. Keep a list of topics with which you have trouble, and consult science textbooks for additional information on these subjects.

4 ONE WEEK BEFORE

If you have already put in a lot of preparation time and are meeting your goals on the sample tests, take it fairly easy the last week before the MCAT. Do a full-length practice test under proctored conditions 1 week before the test date. If you are in a review course, the instructors will usually administer one MCAT under simulated testing conditions.

During the week, you should focus on going through practice passages, not on learning new material. The idea is to develop more test-taking stamina than you will need on the exam day. If you are really fanatical about the test, and you have little or no concurrent course work, you can try the following schedule:

- Early morning—practice verbal passages.
- Late morning—practice physical science passages.
- Noon—break for lunch.
- Early afternoon—write one or two essays.
- Late afternoon—practice biology passages.

If possible, try to adhere to the same basic daily schedule (start time and breaks) you will use on the test day. Try to wake up at the same time you plan to arise on the test day, and go to sleep at the same time you plan to go to bed the night before the exam. Remember that sleep deprivation has cumulative effects; a good night's sleep on the Thursday night before the test is as important as a good night's sleep on the Friday night before the test. If it is convenient, go to the test center and do these practice passages there. Each evening, you may also want to spend an hour going over the list of subjects that give you trouble. Analyze your "stupid" errors, and plan how to avoid them on the test day.

5 ONE DAY BEFORE

Relax.

If you have an established pattern that worked for previous examinations, keep it on this final day before the MCAT. Of greatest importance is to relax. Stress over the test is perfectly normal, but do not let it unnerve you. If you feel stressed, find something to keep your mind off the test; for example, go see a movie. Try not to study the day before the exam. If you must study, do not study new material; simply scan high-yield facts like those in this book. The night before the exam, set out five or six # 2 pencils and a few black pens, registration materials, two picture IDs, and a nonbeeping timer. You may also want to make lunch and snacks the night before to avoid food hassles the day of the exam.

G Day of the Exam

Arrive at the test center early.

TAKING THE EXAM is stressful enough. Plan the day in advance to avoid stress about anything else. A wake-up call helps. Eat a nutritious breakfast. Protein may enhance logical thinking capabilities; eat something more substantial than sugared cereal. Plan to arrive at the test center no later than 7:30 A.M. If you are using public transportation, have everything rehearsed, and allot sufficient time for delays.

If you get to the test center early and have free time, try to stay away from study material. Instead, read something light, such as newspapers, magazine articles, or maybe even practice passages. If you decide to do practice passages, however, do not answer the questions or look up their answers; the idea is to get into the right frame of mind for the verbal reasoning section and avoid using test time for warming up. This free time is also opportune for a trip to the bathroom.

1 ADMINISTRATIVE MECHANICS AND WHAT TO EXPECT ON THE TEST DAY

Before you get a seat assignment, the administrators will fingerprint you (think of it as prison for a day). Next the administrators give you an answer booklet for all the test sections, as well as endless standardized forms to fill out. Think of this stage as another test, this one a test in patience. Expect to spend up to an hour for fingerprinting, seating, and filling out administrative information in the answer booklet. At the beginning of every section, the administrators will hand out a question booklet for that section. At the end of every section, the administrators will collect the question booklet and the answer sheet, which you will tear out of the answer booklet. At this point, they will also check the name on your picture ID against the name on the answer sheet. Every time the proctors let you leave the room for a break or for lunch, they will ask to see your card on your return. All this distributing and collecting of materials prolong the length of the MCAT from 6 to almost 10 hours. **Do not expect to finish early or even on time**.

a. Morning Session

The test day is not the time to experiment with new techniques. For example, wear earplugs or use a nonbeeping timer only if these techniques have previously worked for you.

You should make full use of the 10-minute break after the verbal reasoning section. Visit the restroom even if you don't feel the urge. If you want a snack, stay away from candy bars. Snacks with complex carbohydrates (such as fruits and granola bars) provide the right amount of energy to pace yourself through the day.

b. Lunch

Lunch is your chance to regroup and replenish depleted energy supplies. Avoid talking about the test at this time, because the stress of this discussion can adversely affect your performance on the rest of the test. Do not take a nap after lunch. Bring your lunch to avoid depending on the cafeteria services or being subject to the unfortunate mishaps that can be associated with leaving the testing site. Avoid heavy or spicy foods.

c. Afternoon Session

During the second 10-minute break after the essay, go for a short walk or stretch. Now is the time to indulge in candy bars or other sweets. Research shows that a drop in subjective alertness is normal during the middle of the afternoon, although many students catch their "second wind" in the middle of the biological sciences section. If this happens to you, check your early answers for careless mistakes. Finally, if you finish the biological sciences section early, use the extra time to check your answers.

2 AFTER THE EXAM

As soon as you finish the MCAT, go out and celebrate. Remember that you have just finished one of the longest and most difficult exams you will ever face. And do not fret about your mistakes; the exam is over; no worrying or rethinking is going to change your score. If you are very concerned that you did poorly, you may want to debrief by analyzing the areas that gave you trouble and making notes on what to study if you retake the exam. Then, put these notes aside until the scores come out. Remember that the MCAT alone does not determine your success in applying to medical school and that these scores are not correlated with your degree of success or failure in medical school or in your medical career.

Do not fret about your mistakes; the exam is over; no worrying or rethinking is going to change your score.

You can expect score reports in the mail within 6 to 8 weeks.

PART II

high-yield mcat facts

A Verbal Reasoning

1 INTRODUCTION

The verbal section of the MCAT has become increasingly important in the past few years. Statistics have shown that the level of performance on the verbal section has a high correlation to how well a medical student will perform on the United States Medical Licensing Exam (USMLE—i.e., the boards). As a result, medical schools have made the verbal score an increasingly important factor when considering admission of applicants to their respective shcools. It is very commonplace these days to hear of medical schools making the verbal score one of their distinguishing factors.

You cannot study specific content material for the verbal reasoning section.

This makes it even more necessary than before to do well on the verbal section. The one very difficult aspect about this section is that there is less room for error on the verbal section than there is on the other respective sections of the MCAT. The reason for a curve that does not allow much error is that so many people make so few mistakes. With so many people achieving perfect or close to perfect scores, the top of the curve (the higher scores) is harder to reach. Do not be dismayed! Even though there is less room for error, it is our belief that the verbal section is the easiest of all the sections to study for. There is no need to memorize data or facts as is needed in the biological sciences section. Also there is no need to be able to figure out formulas as is needed in the physical sciences section. What is needed is familiarity with the types of questions on the verbal section, an ability to comprehend passages at a fast pace, and an ability to make inferences and apply the facts given in a passage to other situations. This all comes down to PRACTICE. The key to the verbal section is practice.

The key to doing well on the verbal section is practice!!!

In the following section we will review different techniques to approaching verbal passages that will improve your verbal score. No matter how much you read about these techniques, however, you will never improve your verbal score unless you practice. You will not become familiar with what types of questions the MCAT asks unless you take multiple tests and see firsthand what the MCAT is testing. You will not be able to complete the verbal section on time unless you train your mind to read and comprehend at a rate that is faster than normal. You will not know how to skim the passages for only the facts that are needed to answer the questions unless you practice. You need to train your mind as an athlete trains his or her body for competition. Practice, practice, practice. They were onto something when the cliché practice makes perfect was coined. What was true back then, still holds true today. Practice.

2 TIME ALLOTMENT

The verbal section presents 65 multiple-choice questions and passages in an allotted time of 85 minutes. This gives you an average of 1.3 minutes per question (not a lot of time). In addition, you must read the 8 to 11 passages on which the questions are based, which means that you have even less time available to answer each question. A very good standard to go by is to allow a little over 1 minute per question, a figure that includes the time to read the appropriate passage. According to this rule of thumb, for a seven question passage, you have 8 minutes to read the passage, then read and answer the questions. If you follow this time management strategy, you will have approximately 10 extra minutes for checking your answers after you finish the section or for finishing a difficult passage. Use the 8 minutes for 7 questions rule as a guideline to pace yourself both when you practice and when you take the actual test.

Try to keep the pace of spending approximately one minute per question.

3 GENERAL PRINCIPLES AND STRATEGY

Well now that we are motivated to practice, what and how should we be practicing? After all, if you practice with techniques you are not comfortable with or methods that are giving you the wrong answer, will it really help? Of course not. Practice with a methodical system and in a way that facilitates learning and familiarity with the MCAT. So if we were to recoin the cliché, perfect practice makes perfect.

Find the approach that works best for you, and stick with it!

Now not every student will prepare for the verbal section in the same way. Each and every person has their own way and method of reading and comprehending.There exists such a variety of ways in which students like to approach the verbal section. As long as the methods are perfect for you, that is all that matters. Remember, you are taking the test, not everyone else. Therefore, the only thing that matters is if you are achieving the scores you want. Many of the techniques and study methods that are listed below are proven techniques that will help you to improve your score. Not all techniques and methods, however, are for everyone. Try all of the suggestions, but if some of them do not work for you, do not push it. It is my belief, however, that you will find that the strategies listed below will be very helpful and give you insight on how to train for the verbal section. Again, training is key, and as we systematically break down each part of the verbal section that needs to be mastered in order to do well, you will find your confidence growing and your scores improving.

The biggest and most common problem that students have is reading the actual passage in such a short period of time. Often these passages are not simple excerpts from science books or easy-to-read novels, but contain content that is difficult to understand. If you are like many other premedical students who suffer from this dilemma, you need to train yourself to be able to read the passages in a sufficient and efficient amount of time in order to leave yourself time to answer the questions. The faster you are able to read and comprehend the passage, the more time there is to answer the questions and the more your confidence will grow.

You will never be able to read the verbal passages in the MCAT at a consistent and efficient rate unless you are used to reading that type of material. The first step in training yourself is to become adjusted to the type of literature you will encounter in the MCAT. Once in a while you will come across verbal passages that are scientific in nature. For most premedical students, this will not be a problem since you are studying so much science for the other sections of the MCAT. The majority of the verbal section, however, comes from material that is largely unfamiliar to most students. You need to become familiar with these types of complex, intelligent, and subjective pieces of literature. Make it a daily habit to read material from different sources in order to become accustomed to reading and comprehending literature from different sources. Listed below are some good sources for practice reading for the MCAT.

Broaden your reading scope to become more efficient with non-scientific passages.

Reader's Digest
Atlantic Monthly
The Economist
The New York Times
New Yorker
Scientific American

As you make it a daily or even weekly habit, these types of passages and articles will become easier for you to read. With something such as this, do not expect improvement immediately. This type of strategy requires time and commitment. Consistency is the key.

Remember, when you are reading these articles, you are trying to train yourself to read faster with a greater level of comprehension. It is nice to be able to read these magazines over Sunday morning coffee and bagels, but your ultimate goal is to become familiar enough with these MCAT-like pieces of literature that reading articles from these magazines will become second nature to you. If you are having problems at first, read for understanding. Make sure that you are able to read an article and understand the facts that are being presented. After you have reached a level of comfort in reading these articles at your own pace, begin to time yourself. Give yourself a certain amount of time to finish each article. As your rate of reading improves (without any compromise in your understanding), allot progressively shorter amounts of time to finish articles. Familiarity will increase your speed and level of understanding. That is our ultimate goal—to be able to come back to the verbal section and read the passages in a short enough time that you will be able to answer all the questions for the appropriate passage within the allotted time.

Read for understanding, then work on improving your reading speed.

Below we have listed in stepwise fashion how to train yourself for reading the verbal passages in the given time.

Read pieces of literature to familiarize yourself with MCAT-like passages. Ensure that you are comprehending the article. This entails that at the minimum you are able to understand the following about the article:

Tone of the author's voice
Main idea of the passage
Inferences that can be made
The type of person the author is likely to be
Information recall

Keep these concepts in mind as you are reading the passages.

Begin to time yourself so that you speed up your reading. Be sure to practice "skimming the passage," and looking for these things as you read along. Once you feel comfortable with your reading speed and level of comprehension, practice a lot on MCAT passages.

4 MENTAL PREPARATION

Attitude is often a forgotten subject when students are preparing for an exam. Confidence is of the utmost importance for the MCAT, especially for the verbal section. Your attitude going into and during the exam WILL affect how you perform. The more confidence that you have, the better off you are for the exam. Now there exists a difference between arrogance and confidence. Do not think that you are the next Pulitzer Prize winner, but be able to have the mindset that you know that you can do well on this section.

Attitude is important for a second reason. The verbal section is the first section of the MCAT. That's right! So at 8:00 A.M. in your test center, when you open the exam to begin, the first section you will encounter is the verbal section. Therefore, how you feel about the verbal section will affect your performance on the other sections of the MCAT. You do not want to be in a position where you are mulling over how you did in the verbal section as you are trying to figure out how inertia affects the movement of a rock rolling down a hill. When you develop the confidence to know that you can do well on the verbal section, it will show on the exam. No matter how hard the verbal section may have been, your attitude is that you have prepared for this section and are confident that you will do well. This will allow you to carry that attitude into the following sections and will improve your scores on those sections as well.

Keeping a positive attitude during the verbal reasoning section will give you momentum for the rest of the MCAT examination.

Of course, confidence does not come from nowhere. Therefore, it is that much more necessary to ensure that you prepare diligently for this section. Many people think that because the verbal section is not a "hard core science," preparation can only do so much. Let us dismiss this notion right now. You can never over-prepare for anything on the MCAT. We must be redundant again and emphasize practice. The more you practice, the better your scores will become, and the more confidence you will gain. Confidence only comes with practice.

5 APPROACHES TO VERBAL REASONING PASSAGES

There are a number of different ways you can approach the passages in the verbal reasoning section. Many people have different styles and accordingly, one certain way of approaching this section works best for them. We have described below the different ways that you can approach the verbal reasoning section. Our advice is to try all of them and see which one works best for you. The important thing is to feel comfortable with that particular methodology and to be able to finish on time. If you can accomplish those two things, that method should work well for you.

Allow yourself only 2 minutes per passage.

Read first, questions second: Critically read each passage in less than 2 minutes and then answer the questions. If you decide to use this approach, find ways to improve your reading comprehension and your efficiency in answering questions. Some test takers find it helpful to spend 10 to 15 seconds (no longer) scanning the passage before reading the entire selection. In this way, you can quickly identify the central thesis of the passage, the main ideas of each paragraph, and the direction or slant of the passage before you begin reading. Some people find that this technique reduces time spent reading and locating the answers to the questions within the passage.

Skimming the questions first may help you focus on what to look for in each passage.

Skim questions, read passage, answer questions: Read the questions first, read the passage, and then answer the questions. Some people find that knowing the questions gives them a good idea of what to look for in the passage, which saves time during the reading process. However, a majority of students find that this technique ultimately wastes more time. It is unlikely that you will remember all the questions while you are reading the passage, so you will have to read the questions again, anyway. Determine whether this technique saves you time when doing verbal reasoning passages; if not, stick with the first option. If this option does work for you, it can be very effective.

Mark key phrases so you can quickly refer to them.

Mark key phrases: Other students prefer to mark the passage as they read, underlining or circling important ideas as they are presented. Briefly jot down in the margins one or two phrases summarizing each paragraph. It may also help to circle specific words that indicate a change of thought or idea (e.g., however, although). By glancing at your notations, you can quickly find relevant information to help answer the questions. If this "landmark" technique improves comprehension and helps locate answers without slowing your progress or interrupting your train of thought, it is recommended. Beware: it is easy to go overboard. Nevertheless, with practice, annotations serve as a "conceptual map" that help you quickly locate the answers to the questions within the passage.

6 TYPES OF QUESTIONS THAT APPEAR IN THE VERBAL SECTION

After you have mastered the technique of reading the passages in such a short amount of time, the next step is to become familiar with the types of questions that are presented on the MCAT. The MCAT is a very consistent test. By the time you have finished your studying for the verbal section of the MCAT, you should be able to predict what types of questions will show up on the exam. There exist a few different types of questions for the MCAT. We will list and explain each type of genre below. Apply the information below by practicing with sample exams. Try to become adjusted to the different types of questions that are asked. Many questions could be asking the same thing, but in a different manner. For instance, one question may ask you what the tone of the author's voice is. Another question may ask you to determine how the author feels about the subject. Both questions are essentially the same question. They both want to know what are the author's feelings on the subject matter. If you are able to recognize how the author is feeling, any question in this type of genre can be answered correctly. As you become familiar with the types of questions, you will be able to discern what to look for as you read the passage. Pretty soon it will be natural for you to notice the author's tone of voice or feelings as implied by his or her vocabulary. However, I must emphasize again that this familiarity and recognition come only by practice and analysis.

There are many different types of questions. Identifying what type of question is being asked will help you tremendously to answer correctly.

> **Main idea:** This type of question is asking you to see if you know what the passage is all about.

The main idea question can come worded in many different ways. The most obvious course is to directly ask you, "What is the main idea of the passage?" However, there are other questions that are basically asking the same thing.

If you were to give a summary of the passage...
The main theme of the passage is...
Of the following, the author is most interested in...

These types of passages can oftentimes be perceived as easy, but in reality are the hardest ones to answer. Most people think too superficially about these types of questions and are distracted by the language or style of the passage. A good technique to help you with this type of question is to make notes in the margins of the passage about the main ideas in each paragraph. Summarize the main points of each paragraph and look for a structured argument, or the flow of ideas that are being presented. This will help you to outline the main points of the passage, making it easier to see what the main idea is. This technique will also help you organize your thoughts about the passage, helping you to answer other questions.

Try to summarize in your head the main points of each paragraph

> **Tone of the passage:** This type of question is asking you to perceive how the author feels about the subject. These questions may also be asked many different ways.

The author's attitude toward the subject was...
The author seems to feel that...
What is the tone of the author's voice?

Look for key phrases, transitions, and adjectives to help determine the author's tone.

Students have two big problems with this type of question. The first is that students second-guess themselves. After an answer is formulated, students start to change their answer because they really are not sure in the first place what the tone of the author is. Usually your first instinct is correct. Unless evidence is obvious against your first pick (and it almost never is), try not to change it.

The second problem students have with this type of question is that they introduce their own feelings into the passage. This is especially true if the topic is a touchy one. Remember, no matter how strongly you feel about the subject matter, and no matter how controversial the topic may be, the MCAT is not asking for YOUR feelings. The MCAT is asking you to determine what the AUTHOR is feeling. Try to leave out all bias for or against the topic matter.

A good exericise is to take passages from different magazines and look for adjectives. Associate good or bad feelings with how the word is being used in the context of the passage. Try to read through a passage by concentrating on the different descriptive words that are being used. The best way to tell the tone of an author's voice is to examine the vocabulary that is being used. Familiarizing yourself with various adjectives and in what context they are being used will help you identify the tone of the author's voice.

Make annotations that will help you locate specific details in the passage.

Recall: This is probably the simplest of all types of questions that appear on the verbal section. These questions ask you to remember the facts that were presented in the passage. The answer choice will not be worded exactly as it was in the passage. There will probably be some, if not significant, rewording or paraphrasing of the facts. The best way to attack these types of questions is to actually go back to the passage and reread the section that presented the relevant information. This is where making notes in the margins comes in handy. If you have notes in the margins on what each paragraph is about, it becomes much easier and faster to locate the appropriate facts to answer the question. Again, we emphasize that most of the time the answer will not be word for word from the passage. Do not look for a duplicate within the passage. The opposite is also true for these types of questions. Do not look for an answer that is overly complex or complicated. Most of the time, these factual recall questions are fairly straightforward and only take a little bit of insight into the passage to come up with the correct answer. Another good strategy that works for some is to actually skim the questions before you read the passage. That way you are able to identify the recall questions beforehand and can concentrate on looking for specific pieces of information in the passage.

Use logical reasoning in combination with specific facts found in the passage to answer these questions.

Deduction: Deduction questions will ask you to answer questions about items that are not necessarily dealth with directly in the passage, but can be implied or inferred. These types of questions will also ask you to apply the information that is presented in the passage to a new or different situation. The answer to these types of questions CANNOT be found in the passage. You must utilize your skills of reasoning and detection in order to figure out what is the correct answer. Do not assume you can find the right answer. You must *come up* with the right answer. While you are drawing your conclusions to try to answer the questions, make sure that your assumptions are based on the facts, statements, and opinions that are presented in the passage. Many students insert facts that may be related to the passage but came from a source other than the passage itself. The passage is the one and only source of information you can use to deduce the answer, no matter how much you may already know about the subject matter.

These four types of questions are the common types of questions that you will see on the MCAT. There are other types of questions that may arise, and by no means is this list exhaustive. The types of questions given here, however, are very common and should be at the top of your list of things to familiarize yourself with for the MCAT. You must train your mind to become accustomed to noticing these things as it is reading the passage. A good exercise is to read a magazine or newspaper, and try to determine all of the above as you are reading. As you pick up your copy, try to figure out the tone of the author's voice. Notice what adjectives are being used. Without looking at the title, determine what the main point of the passage is. Again, practice makes perfect. The more you get your mind thinking and observing these things, the easier it will be to notice them on MCAT passages and the easier the questions will seem.

7 RUNNING OUT OF TIME

If you are running out of time (i.e., if you have 5 minutes or less) and you have passages left to read, start answering questions without reading the passage. Remember that the AAMC does not have a guessing penalty, and that they do not require students to choose an inflammatory, extreme, or improperly biased answer. Therefore, eliminate answers that state, "Native Americans were much more primitive than the colonists who replaced them" or "Doctors make way too much money." Cross out unreasonable answers, and then **take a guess for every question**.

Stay on pace!

Do not leave any answer circles blank—there is no guessing penalty.

Following are two ways to avoid running out of time. First, when a particular passage gives you a lot trouble, go to the next passage and return to the troubling passage at the end (but don't forget it). Second, fill in the answer sheet after each passage. Far too many students tell horror stories of botching entire sections by planning to fill in the entire answer sheet at the end of the section and then running out of time. Some test takers prefer not to fill out the answer booklet every single time they answer a question; instead, they mark the question booklet with the correct answer and then fill in all the correct answers ("batch fill-in") after each passage.

8 PARTING WORDS

Remember, practice is the key to the verbal section. That is, practice done correctly. The MCAT is a standardized test that requires a person to become adjusted to. If you do not familiarize yourself with the type of test the MCAT is, you will never be successful. Continue to train yourself for the verbal section. It is rare that you will see quick development, since the skills you are trying to improve take a long time to develop. Keep at it, being consistent with your system of studying, and you will see improvement. Practice, practice, practice.

B Writing Sample

1 INTRODUCTION

There are three simple tasks to the writing sample that can be mastered in a short amount of time.

This portion of the MCAT is the most unique. It is tested and graded in a different manner than the rest. Many people think that the writing sample has the least importance of all the sections of the MCAT. Therefore, many people tend to disregard it and don't do well. What a foolishg notion! The writing part of the MCAT is the simplest and easiest part to do well on. There are three simple tasks (explanation of statement, counterexplanation of statement, and settlement) that can be practiced and mastered in a short amount of time. Within a small amount of investment of time every week, you will be able to attain a great writing score that can only strengthen your application to medical school. Therefore, we should strive to do well on ALL sections of the MCAT. As we did in the verbal section, we will break down the writing sample. We need to key in on the differences in format and grading, and approach this section with those things in mind.

2 SCORING

Grading follows a holistic rather than an analytic approach

The writing sample of the MCAT is the only portion of the exam that is not tested in the multiple-choice format. Therefore, grading this portion of the exam becomes much more difficult than the rest of the MCAT. What does this mean for the average pre-medical student who is taking the MCAT? The essays that you write for this section of the MCAT are graded holistically. That means the reader is not looking at the minute details. Rather, the reader is trying to form an overall impression of how well you write from a large picture point of view. Anywhere from 30,000–60,000 students take the MCAT for each administration. To ensure that this many essays are graded in a reasonable amount of time (read $$$), readers spend no more than about 90–120 seconds evaluating each essay (yes, a mere one to two minutes per essay). As the student, you need to use this information to your advantage. There are certain implications to this style of grading that, if taken into account, will improve your strategy in approaching this section of the exam. These implications will be listed and covered in the following section.

3 WRITING STRATEGIES

a. Originality

Take for instance, if you are writing an essay for an English class, the professor will examine every allusion and personification. The professor is supposed to spend quality time reading your essay. This, however, is the MCAT. Can you imagine reading over 500 essay? What a long and, sorry to say, boring task. These graders will become bored, aggravated, and tired by the time they reach your essay; they have been sitting in the same room reviewing essay after essay, minute after minute, for hours on end. In addition, they have probably read essays similar to yours many more times than you can imagine. None of the graders can maintain a high level of interest after reading so many student essays on the same topic. What does this mean for you? Well put yourself in the graders position. Originality is probably the first thought that comes to your mind. Yes, originality is definitely needed. But when there are 50,000 students taking the MCAT, where is there room for originality? Even if you are original, readers may not notice because they are keeping such a torrid pace of reading. So then, what matters more than originality?

Make your essay stand out from the crowd—be original!

b. Readability

More important than originality is to make their job of reading your essay easier. Yes, that's right. Do not search for the perfect allusion or allegory; just make their job easy. Of course if some thoughts of literary genius overcome you at the exam, by all means write it down. For the most part, stay away from complicated allusions and hard-to-read text. This may be great for your English 101 class, but for the MCAT that approach will backfire on you. This does not mean that you cannot use complex sentence structure or big SAT-like words. If you can incorporate them into the essay, that is great. It will show them that you are a well-educated and intelligent person, deserving of a high mark. If these writing tools, however, make the essay hard to read, then it becomes a problem. Big words and complex sentence structure can still be easy to read. I think we get the picture. Remember, keep it simple. The next question to ask is how? Well, remember the two F's: first impression and follow the instructions.

First impressions

First, focus on how your essay looks at the superficial level. As a student, you probably learned the old adage, "quality over quantity." Well, for the MCAT, temporarily forget what you have learned. This approach is well suited when you have all night to write an essay that is due the next day ☺, but the essay section is under strict time control. A lengthy essay (at least 2½ pages long) makes a good impression; it implies that you are fluent and comfortable with the English language. If it's too short, the graders may assume the worst.

First impressions are the most importrant.

Second, avoid errors. Accept the fact that your essay will not be all A+ rhetoric, because it comes with the territory. Do not, however, use this as an excuse to make mistakes. **If you do happen to make a mistake, draw a neat single line through it. Place parentheses around it and keep going.** (This method is the "medicolegally correct" way to fix errors in patient charts). Some students have even used erasable ink. The main objective, however, is to be neat. If you have messy handwriting, it is imperative that you improve. Work diligently to improve your handwriting so that it is legible. I don't need to say that the neater a paper looks, the better the first impression. The excuse that medical doctors have poor handwriting carries no weight here, especially since graders are not medical doctors. Think with common sense here.

Cross out mistakes neatly.

Neatness does count (indirectly)!

c. Formatting

There are many other areas that can improve the first impression you give on your essays. Listed below are some other simple suggestions. There may be more you can think of. That's great. Be sure to incorporate them.

- **Follow the margins:** Do not have uneven margins on the left-hand side of the paper. A nice, straight, and even edge will give the impression of order and neatness.
- **Double space:** This advice is given with a certain stipulation. Only double space if you know you will not run out of room. Double spacing gives off a less

Easy readability will get your essay noticed and can improve your score.

crowded impression and makes the essay much easier to read. Remember that your job is to make the essay easy to read!

- **Indent your paragraphs:** We will talk about dividing the paragraphs into an organized information structure in the next few pages. Each new paragraph from a superficial point of view, however, should have an obvious new beginning with an indentation. Some people like to skip lines, but we advise against this. Indentation makes the separation of paragraphs more obvious. If there is anyplace where separation needs to be obvious, it is in your paragraphs. The reason being that paragraphs will mark the beginning of a new point. Remember again, easy to read!

d. Content

Follow the instructions

Your essay will be destined for failure if you do not follow the directions!

You have taken care of the superficial view of the essay. Now it looks professional and gives the impression that you are fluent, organized, and neat with your writing. Now you need to make sure that what you say in the essay is what they are looking for! The essay may give the impression that you know what you are talking about, but the readers can still read (given it is only for about 2 minutes). Therefore, it is essential that you have good content. Content is not the content that you are looking for in an English class. That kind of content is concerned with depth of knowledge and insight. Although you do have to provide a certain depth of knowledge and insight on the MCAT, the main thing you need to accomplish is to follow the instructions. There are three tasks that need to be defined, and if these tasks are written about in a complete manner, you will receive high marks. Most people find that they barely have enough time to finish an essay in thirty minutes, let alone sit there and think about the topics for a while to come up with some deep philosophical insight into the topic. Remember how much time these readers spend on each essay? **Answer the questions. That is what the MCAT is asking for.** So let us define the three tasks the MCAT wants on the essay and how to do them well.

Writing sample tasks

Make sure you address each task in a clear and concise manner.

Task #1—Explanation of statement: The first task that you are assigned is to explain the statement. In whatever way possible, you need to tell the reader what is meant by the statement you are given. This includes your interpretation. A very good tool to use here is to provide an example. There is no better way to illustrate what you are talking about than to provide a picture to the reader of what is being said. Remember, be as clear as possible. It is essential to articulate youself well in this paragraph. The reason being that every other point in the essay is founded on the assumptions and interpretations you make in this paragraph. As we will talk about in the next point, the second paragraph should be your counterexplanation. Giving and describing a situation where the thesis is not true. In order to write an effective counterexample, you need to clarify your original point effectively. The clearer you make the original thesis, the easier the rest of the essay will be.

Use examples to help convey the point you are trying to make.

Task #2—Counterexplanation of statement: As stated earlier, the purpose of the second task is to describe when the thesis or statement given is not true. This is also effectively communicated with examples. One note: Do not get so carried away with thinking about examples that you forget to actually write about the task! Remember to accomplish what the MCAT tells you to do. However, do try to use examples because it makes the reading more interesting, conveys good comparison and association skills, and makes it easier to write longer essays. One spin-off that works very well in the MCAT is to use current events as an example. This means that you will have to have read up on the daily news, which not many premedical students make time for! If, however, you are following our advice in training yourself for the verbal section, you will be up-to-date on current events and examples should come easier. For those of you who are more comfortable with writing and examples seem to come easier, we suggest that you write **two** counterexamples. One being a current one and the other a classical or quintessential example. This will illustrate even more to the reader of your fluency, literary technique, and culture! Do not think you are required to give two counterexamples. If you give one good one, you are accomplishing the task the MCAT is giving to you. Be happy!

Quotations can add eloquence to your essay.

Task #3—Settlement: Now that you have explained the thesis and the antithesis, you have created a conflict. The only thing left to do is to resolve or settle the conflict. The two former tasks could be accomplished via objective measures, to a certain degree. You are making certain assumptions when you explain the thesis and antithesis, but you could not change the statement. Both tasks should have been fairly mechanical. The third task, however, is where your interpretations turn into implications. You must evaluate which option is the more suitable one. As stated, this includes considering the long-term ramifications and justifying why the thesis is good or bad. You will not be graded for your opinion. Everyone is expected to have one. What you will be graded on is whether or not you have supported your argument well. Does this make sense? Again, we emphasize clarity and neatness!

Try to convey a logical and rational line of thinking.

Again, your objective is to fulfill the three tasks well. If you are able to do this, you will score well on the writing section of the MCAT. It is not as easy as it looks. The hardest part for many is finding examples. It is good practice to take statements from tests and to try to think of examples and counterexamples within a 5-minute time limit. Whether your example is sufficient or great, remember to accomplish the three tasks.

The first and last sentences of a paragraph are the most important.

4 PACE YOURSELF

Timing is one, if not the most important factor in this section. Most students find that 30 minutes is just not enough time to write an effective essay with good examples. They feel "rushed" and are mostly never satisfied with their essays. Of course, this happens because the students enter unprepared and untrained for this section. Timing is the key. Many different situations can arise where you become flustered or encounter "writer's block." The natural response at this time is to panic. Only experience will allow the test taker to handle this type of panic properly. Experience with timing is one of those major factors. As you practice writing essays, you should have a timeline that you have developed. A good suggestion is to take 5–7 minutes in the beginning to make an outline and think of examples. You want to jot down a structured outline that shows your answer to all three tasks that are listed above. After that is completed, the next step is to write the actual essay. By the actual MCAT, you should have practiced enough tests in

Having a good outline and examples will save you time and make the essay writing a lot easier.

order to write effectively and fluently with speed. You should not spend more than 10 minutes trying to think of an outline and examples. That is even pushing it a little. With practice you should have a feel for how long you have. Make sure you leave about 3 minutes at the end to look for spelling, grammar, and other mistakes. Again, crossing out a mistake and correcting it looks better than leaving it to be seen.

Suggested time line:

Outline and Examples	Essay Writing	Proofreading
7 minutes	20 minutes	3 minutes

These time suggestions are not to be held as if the law. They are, however, very practical suggestions that make sense. Feel free to play around a minute or two from each section. Some of you may be faster writers but need more time to formulate. Some may want more time to proofread. But remember, never at any time compromise your ability to accomplish the three tasks. An added bonus is to be able to add all the suggestions above in the 30 minutes.

5 MORE WRITING STRATEGIES

STRATEGY

- Be politically correct.
- Forget slang.
- Avoid repeating yourself in the essay (this concept may seem obvious, but is harder than you think, especially when only 5 minutes remain and you develop writer's block).
- Analyze rather than overexplain the topic.
- Write the essay as if you were writing an article for a newspaper. You want a sensational headline (first sentence) and closing line (last sentence) that leaves them thinking (puts the question in a new light).
- Favorite essay topics on the MCAT include the environment, politics, and philosophy. Familiarity with these topics is helpful as is understanding basic principles and fundamentals in these areas.
- Use a number of descriptive "action" words as well as imagery without going overboard to capture the reader's attention.

6 PARTING WORDS OF ADVICE

Practice!!!

I think we are beginning to see a recurring theme throughout this book. Practice is the key to doing well in all of the sections. Almost no one on the first try can write in a manner accomplishing all of these suggestions. Writing is especially tough because the grading is subjective. You may often feel that you are making no progress. The important thing here is to find someone who can look over your essays and tell you if you are accomplishing these tasks. The essay needs to make a first impression, be readable, accomplish the assigned tasks, and finished within the allotted time. Only with practice can you accomplish this.

7 SAMPLE ESSSAYS WITH CRITIQUES

We have enclosed examples of essays to show you what we are talking about.

This is not the perfect essay, but it will effectively show you what to look for, and give you a good idea of what a decent essay looks like.

Topic: Scientists should use creative inspirations rather than careful planning as a best solution to their problems.

Essay:

Many scientists believe that creative inspiration, rather than careful planning results in the best solution to a problem. Creative inspiration refers to using one's imagination to inspire oneself to unique solutions that may be unorthodox. Careful planning refers to solving a problem in a very well thought out manner that is cautious and wary of all the pitfalls and problems that may occur as the experiment proceeds. An example of creative inspiration can be seen in Albert Einstein's theory of relativity. The theory of relativity was not something that could have been conceived without Einstein using his imagination. This topic is so far from the intuitive, that careful planning is an unlikely source of his thoughts.

Other scientists believe that careful planning, rather than creative inspiration results in the best solution to a problem. In the field of pharmacology, scientists must use careful planning to find a solution to a problem. When making a drug, scientists must be careful in the synthesis to ensure that toxicity will not ensure if the patient uses the drug. Any type of contamination could result in severe undesirable side effects. Synthesizing drugs to be used by patients should not be the time to become creative and try different chemicals out. The potential to cause damage is very high. This type of procedure requires very careful planning.

The two separate statements in this sentence are not necessarily mutually exclusive. As a matter of fact, there are many if not most instances in which a scientist must use creative inspiration and careful planning to find a solution to a problem. The nature of scientific problems and discovery is to venture into the unknown. The whole purpose of performing scientific research is to show the world what has yet to be discovered. It is a natural conclusion that it requires creative inspiration to be able to think of solutions that have yet to be solved. Only inspiration can lead a scientist to an unknown solution. If, however, careful planning is left out, the solution will never be discovered. The scientific method, by which all science is done, is by nature a very exact and precise method. This is due to the requirement that the experiment needs to be reproducible. If the experiment is done in a careless manner, the results are not valid because they cannot be reproduced. Therefore, it takes creative inspiration to think of possible solutions, but careful planning to test to see if those solutions are viable. For example, Erwin Schroedinger discovered quantum mechanics by using creative inspiration as well as careful planning. Quantum mechanics was a very different way of thinking from previous scientific fields. Inherent to the field of quantum mechanics are many careful calculations and many steps of deduction and problem solving that require careful planning. When finding a solution to a problem, the best results come from careful planning and creative inspiration.

Comments: If we were grading this essay on a curve, it would have received a score of 4.5 out of 6.0. We cannot comment on first impressions because the essay has been typed out. It is of good length, but a little too short for the first two paragraphs. The student did accomplish the three tasks that were assigned to him. This type of essay is considered a compare and contrast type essay that requires the student to discuss which type of method is better, or if both are valid. The first task was answered in a very standard way; the student defined the words that needed to be defined. This method is a little too methodical. It would be good to put more transitions in-between the definitions so the reader does not open the essay by feeling that the question was answered from a dictionary. One good thing that this student does is give many examples. Incorporating examples this early in the essay is never a bad idea. One criticism is to make sure that your example is fully explained. The word "intuitive" could be explained in more detail as it is not fully understood what is meant here.

The counterexample task is also accomplished. This part of the essay is also a little short. The example is good, but it would not hurt to use two examples here. An example that is a current event would definitely be a plus. If this student were to add a current event where a person suffered from the misuse or toxicity of a certain drug as an example, that would be good. Again, if the paragraphs seem too short, you may give the impression you do not have enough to say.

The closing paragraph is the strongest point of this essay. This is what allows the student to receive the score he did. The student does a very good job of explaining how the two are not mutually exclusive, but are in reality, partners. He explained the very nature of science and how the statement applied to it. That is, afterall, what the essay is essentially talking about. Again, the student gives an example that provides a good mental picture to solidify the argument.

The logic in this essay is sound. The wording, however, could use some work. This is especially true for the first two paragraphs. If the student can expand on the first two so that they flow better, this would definitely be a good essay.

The following is an example of a bad essay.

Topic: Politicians should vote according to their constituents' beliefs and not their own.

Essay:

Politicians have been caught in the debate of whether they should vote according to their beliefs or to worry about whether their constituents agree with those beliefs. To worry about whether one politician's constituents agree with those beliefs is to follow the standard of the political party regardless of one's personal beliefs. Many politicians vote according to their beliefs. If a politician wants to raise taxes, he should vote in favor to raise taxes, even if this differs from the decision of the political party. In the novel My Own Beliefs by Marrell Hlousek, a lesson is taught that one can not be happy following the ideas of others. In the novel, a man finds happiness by following his own beliefs, regardless of the people around him.

However, another group believes politicians should vote according to his constituents, regardless of personal beliefs. Many believe that a politician should represent a certain political party and therefore should vote on what his constituents agree with. In the novel Mr. President by George Husak, a person becomes President simply by telling the public what they want to hear. This satire shows that a politician is able to follow his constituent's beliefs and disregard personal beliefs.

There are circumstances that a politician should vote according to his belief and sometimes should take into account the beliefs of his constituents. Politicians should vote according to their beliefs; however, when a debate lies within a political party, a politician should listen to the beliefs of the constituents. A politician should take both sides of the political party into account and determine a conclusion according to his own beliefs.

Comments: This essay would receive a score of 2.0 out of 6.0. This essay is an example of what you do not want to do. The first criticism that immediately comes to mind is that this student did not adequately answer all three tasks. The first task is insufficiently defined. There is too much repetition of facts and no real explanation of what the statement means. The author makes an incorrect assumption in that he thinks the constituents believe the same things the political party does. Also, the author makes an opinion by stating what the politician should do instead of objectively explaining the statement.

The second task is not completed in any better fashion. Again, the wrong assumptions is made that the political party and the politician's constituents are the same. He gives one example that is not relevant because it only explains how a politician gets elected, not what a politician should do once in office.

Finally, there is no resolution to the statement in the third task. There is too much ambiguity and it is much too hard for the grader to try to figure out what the student is trying to say with the limited amount of time he will spend grading the essay.

This essay did not complete the tasks—the length was too short and there were no good examples given.

Now that you see an example of a good but not perfect essay and a bad essay, it should give you an idea of what is expected. There were weak and strong points to these essays, and it should help you to visualize what is needed for a quality score. The next thing to do is practice. Listed below are practice topics for you to use to practice for the writing section. Good luck!

8 PRACTICE WRITING SAMPLE TOPICS

Practice your MCAT writing sample skills with the following topics:

- Politicians should always vote with their beliefs.
- The only justifiable reason for war is if you are attacked yourself.
- Medicine should be available to everyone, no matter what the cost to society.
- The President has a responsibility to society to live a moral life.
- Morality is defined by social culture.

C Introduction to the Physical Sciences

The physical sciences section is difficult and thorough. Study hard and try to excel on this section of the MCAT.

AFTER FINISHING the verbal reasoning section, most students feel the effects of time pressure, but begin to relax during the first 15-minute break. Unfortunately, the physical sciences section comes next and hits the unprepared student like a sledgehammer. For many MCAT test takers, the physical sciences section is the most difficult section of the exam. In fact, the AAMC uses a more generous conversion curve for the physical sciences than it does for the other sections, meaning that you can get more questions wrong before your score goes down. In any case, the majority of medical schools admit students with slightly lower average physical sciences scores than their biological sciences and verbal reasoning scores, which means that most students get many physical sciences questions wrong. However, this dark cloud has a silver lining. You can do very well in relation to the other applicants without getting all of the questions right as long as you know how to prepare and practice for the physical sciences section.

Most students have difficulty finishing this section within the time allotted. Work quickly and efficiently.

In the physical sciences section, you must answer 77 questions within 100 minutes. Just as with the verbal reasoning section, you have 1.3 minutes per question. Once again, spend 1.25 minutes on each question (which will leave you a little extra time for answering hard questions and for checking your answers). Do not get bogged down on any one question or passage. Skip a passage that gives you a lot of trouble, and go back to it at the end. You can "batch fill-in" the answer sheet, but never go to the next passage without filling in the answers from the previous one. The MCAT has no guessing penalty, so answer every question, even those nasty electromagnetism ones!

Practice doing simple calculations in your head or by hand.

The AAMC states that the physical sciences section is evenly divided between inorganic chemistry and physics. When preparing for inorganic chemistry, focus on important chemical concepts, not on small details. Do not worry about memorizing the boiling point of ethanol; instead, understand why liquids boil and how boiling points change with intermolecular attraction and molecular weight. Instead of memorizing the gas laws, understand why the volume of a gas increases when you heat it at constant pressure. If you study inorganic chemistry concepts instead of memorizing fact after fact, you will do better on this section of the exam. Finally, practice doing simple calculations in your head or by hand, because you cannot use a calculator on the day of the test (your parents had to do it this way).

Practice quick calculations. You must be comfortable in estimating and performing calculations with numbers in scientific notation.

With the possible exception of organic chemistry, most premedical students fear the physics questions more than the questions from any of the other scientific disciplines. Do not fear this section; once again, concentrate on concepts, not on memorizing equations. The physics tested on the MCAT is not that difficult; a lot of it (especially mechanics) can be understood using common sense, especially gravity and kinematics. Know Newton's laws cold; they contain the most important principles of mechanics. Electricity and magnetism are a little more difficult; but once again, if you stress qualitative concepts, you will do fine. The passages will include many of the necessary details for answering the multiple-choice questions.

BEWARE

The questions and answers interspersed among the high-yield facts are strictly for understanding and content reinforcement, and they are very valuable for this purpose. However, they do not reflect the content, format, or difficulty of questions that appear on the actual MCAT exam.

D Physics

1 KINEMATICS

Kinematics is the study of objects in motion with respect to space and time. In particular, kinematics is used when calculating parameters for the motion of an object, such as its velocity, acceleration, and distances traveled over a given period of time.

STRATEGY

To do well on the physical sciences section of the MCAT, you must know the following very basic, very important equations cold. Practice doing problems with these formulas until they are second nature. You do not need to know calculus for the MCAT, so you can focus on these simple non–calculus-based formulas and ace the MCAT kinematics questions.

$$x = x_0 + v_0 t + \frac{1}{2} at^2$$

$$v = v_0 + at$$

$$v^2 = v_0^2 + 2as$$

a = acceleration (m/s^2)
s = distance traveled (m)
t = time (sec)
v = current velocity (m/s)
x_0 = initial position (m)
v_0 = initial velocity (m/s)
x = current position (m)

In addition, always estimate before you calculate your answer. For instance, assume that g = 10 m/s^2. Scan the answer choices to see how precise they expect your calculations to be.

QUESTION

A car has a constant acceleration, going from rest to 20 m/s in 5 seconds. How far does the car travel in that time?

ANSWER

First, calculate the acceleration of the car.

$$v = v_0 + at$$

$$20 = 0 + a \times 5$$

$$a = 4 \text{ m/s}^2$$

Then find the distance traveled.

$$x = x_0 + v_0 t + \frac{1}{2} at^2$$

$$x = 0 + 0 \times 5 + \frac{1}{2} \times 4 \times 5^2$$

$$x = 50 \text{ meters}$$

or

$$v^2 = v_0^2 \quad 2as$$

$$20^2 = 0^2 + 2 \times 4 \times s$$

$$400 = 8s$$

$$s = \mathbf{50\ meters}$$

QUESTION

The velocity of a particle is plotted over time as shown.

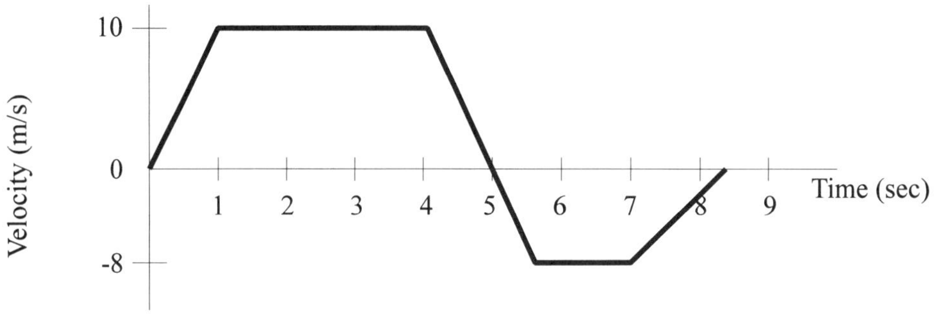

(a) How fast is the particle accelerating between 4 and 6 seconds?
(b) How far does the particle travel in the first 5 seconds?
(c) What is the net distance that the particle travels between 4 and 6 seconds?

ANSWER

To answer these graphic-interpretation problems, you must understand how to extract the necessary information from them. In general, the slope of a graph is equal to the change along the y-axis divided by the change along the x-axis.

In this situation:

$$slope = \frac{\Delta v}{\Delta t} = a$$

(a) The slope of the line between t = 4 and t = 6 seconds is:

$$\frac{-8 - 10}{6 - 4} = \mathbf{-9\ m/s^2}$$

(i.e., acceleration is less than zero because the object is decelerating)

(b) To find the distance [i.e., the area under the curve (AUC)], either split this area into two triangles and a rectangle or remember the formula for the area of a trapezoid. For simplicity, solve for the area of a trapezoid.

$$Area = \frac{B + b}{2} h$$

B = length of the base of the trapezoid
b = length of the top of the trapezoid
h = height of the trapezoid

$$x\,(0 \rightarrow 5) = AUC\,(0 \rightarrow 5) = \frac{5 + 3}{2} \times 10 = \mathbf{40\ meters}$$

(c) This question is similar to the one in (b):

$$\text{Net } x = AUC\,(4 \rightarrow 5) + AUC\,(5 \rightarrow 6) = 5 + (-6) = \mathbf{-1\ meter}$$

TEST CORRELATION

The physical sciences section on the MCAT contains many kinematics questions, both discrete and passage-based. Sometimes these questions are framed in terms of sound or light (e.g., How far or how fast has this sound/light wave traveled?), and you must use these kinematics equations in combination with the sound and light equations (see Part II D 9).

2 PROJECTILES

Projectile motion is the movement of an object in space with respect to its path of motion in both the vertical direction (y) and the horizontal direction (x). The path of motion, known as its trajectory, is always parabolic when gravity is involved. At the highest point of the projectile's trajectory, the velocity in the vertical direction (v_y) is zero. The velocity in the horizontal direction (v_x) remains constant throughout the projectile's trajectory. **You can maximize the distance traveled by a projectile by firing it at a 45-degree angle.**

$$v_x = v_0 \cos(\theta)$$
$$v_y = v_0 \sin(\theta)$$

v_x = velocity in the horizontal direction (m/s)
v_y = velocity in the vertical direction (m/s)
v_0 = initial speed of the object (m/s)
θ = angle between the vector v_0 and the horizontal plane

The x-component of velocity is used to find the total distance traveled. The y-component of velocity is used to find out how long the projectile was in the air.

STRATEGY

Divide and Conquer. With this strategy, you separate the initial velocity vector of the projectile into horizontal and vertical components and treat these values as separate entities (Table 2-1). "Plug and chug" these values into the appropriate kinematics equation.

TABLE 2-1. Calculation of velocity and displacement

Horizontal	Vertical
$v_x = v_{xo}$	$v_y = v_{yo} + gt$
$x = v_{xo}t$	$v_y^2 = v_{yo}^2 + 2gy$
$v_{xo} = v_o\cos\theta$	$y = v_{yo}t + {}^1/_2 gt^2$
	$v_{yo} = v_o\sin\theta$

g = acceleration due to gravity; *t* = time; *v* = velocity; *x* = horizontal displacement; *y* = vertical displacement. (Reprinted with permission from Roth, D: *MCAT Essentials*, Baltimore, Williams & Wilkins, 1998, p 118.)

BEWARE

When calculating the total horizontal distance traveled by the projectile, simply multiply the horizontal component of the velocity (v_x) by the total time of the projectile in flight. However, when determining the total time in flight of the projectile that was fired from the ground, the answer is twice the time it takes the projectile to reach zero velocity, which occurs at the peak. Moreover, because gravity acts as a negative acceleration when the projectile is ascending, you must use $-10\ m/s^2$ for g.

TEST CORRELATION

Projectiles are a very popular topic in the physical sciences section because they can be specifically discussed in a passage, followed by many kinematics and force questions. A passage might dramatize a rocket launch, a cannon firing, or even a ball being thrown into the air. Given the great variety of real-life applications that can be explained by projectiles, you should practice solving problems dealing with projectiles until you develop speed and accuracy.

QUESTION

A person standing at the edge of a 200-meter cliff throws a 10-kg ball off the edge of the cliff at a 30° angle with respect to the horizontal. The ball was thrown off the cliff with an initial velocity of 20 m/s.

(a) What is the total time that the ball was in flight?
(b) How far did the ball travel horizontally?
(c) What was the maximum height that the ball attained off the ground?

ANSWER

The best way to solve projectile problems is to "divide and conquer" by separating the horizontal (x) and vertical (y) components of the projectile. We can begin by drawing a simple diagram of the projectile:

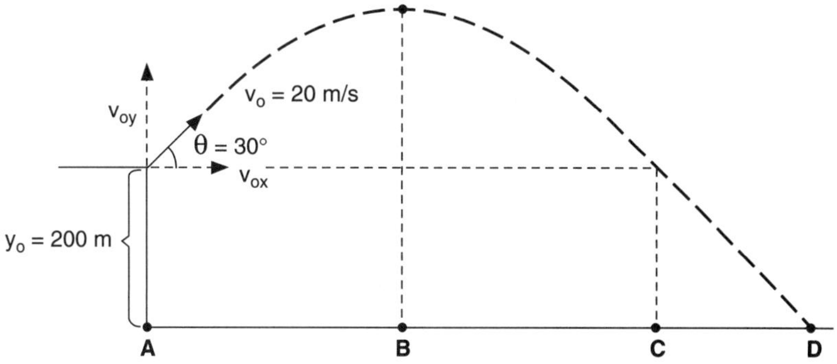

Point **A** = starting point of projectile
Point **B** = peak height of projectile
Point **C** = point where projectile returns to height of cliff
Point **D** = ending point of projectile

$v_{oy} = v_o \sin\theta = 20 (\sin 30°) = 10$ m/s $\qquad \sin 30° = 0.5$

$v_{ox} = v_o \cos\theta = 20 (\cos 30°) \approx 17$ m/s $\qquad \cos 30° = \frac{\sqrt{3}}{2} \approx .85$

(a) Total time in flight = time $(A \rightarrow B)$ + time $(B \rightarrow C)$ + time $(C \rightarrow D)$, where time $(A \rightarrow B)$ = time $(B \rightarrow C)$

Use the formula:

$$v = v_0 + at$$

$$v_{peak\ height} = v_{0y} - g\,[\text{time } (A \rightarrow B)]$$

$$0 = 10 \text{ m/s} - 10 \text{ m/s}^2\,[\text{time } (A \rightarrow B)]$$

Time $(A \rightarrow B)$ = time $(B \rightarrow C)$ = 1 sec

To find time (B → D), use the formula:

$$x = x_0 + v_0 t + \tfrac{1}{2} at^2$$

$$y_{\text{ground}} = y_0 - \tfrac{1}{2} gt^2$$

$$0 = 205 - (\tfrac{1}{2})\,(10)\,[\text{time } (C \rightarrow D)]^2$$

$$\text{Time } (B \rightarrow D) = \sqrt{41} \approx 6 \text{ sec}$$

Therefore, time in flight = time $(A \rightarrow B)$ + time $(B \rightarrow D)$

= 1 sec + 6 sec = **7 sec**

(b) Because the ball was thrown at an initial velocity of 20 m/s with no component of horizontal acceleration,

$$\text{Horizontal distance traveled} = (v_{0x})\,(\text{total time in flight})$$

$$= 17\ \text{m/s} \times 7\ \text{sec} = \mathbf{119\ m}$$

(c) Maximum height can be determined using the following formula:

$$y_{max} = y_0 + \left| \frac{(v_{0y})^2}{2g} \right|$$

$$y_{max} = 200 + \left| \frac{10^2}{2(-10)} \right| = \mathbf{205\ m}$$

3 FORCES AND NEWTON'S LAWS

a. Newton's First Law

An object in motion tends to stay in motion (in the absence of friction), as an object at rest tends to remain at rest.

MNEMONIC

This is the law of physical inertia (as opposed to mental inertia, of which the most compelling example is the student who avoids studying).

b. Newton's Second Law

Force equals mass multiplied by acceleration:

$$F = ma$$

F = force (newtons, N, or kg·m/s^2)
m = mass (kg)
a = acceleration (m/s^2)

Another form of Newton's law follows:

$$\tau = I \times \alpha$$

τ = torque
I = moment of inertia
α = angular acceleration

MNEMONIC

Because the moment of inertia is a difficult topic for many students to grasp, think of torque as analogous to force (τ = F × radius) in the way that inertia is analogous to mass.

c. Newton's Third Law

For every force (action), there is an equal and opposite force (reaction).

MNEMONIC

This law explains why a gun kicks back when you fire it. It kicks back due to conservation of momentum (p).

d. Centripetal force

is the inward force of an object as it moves in a circular path around a point. Without centripetal force, the object would move along a straight-line tangent to its circular path.

$$F = ma$$

and

$$a_c = \frac{v^2}{r}$$

Therefore,

$$F_c = m \times \frac{v^2}{r}$$

a_c = centripetal acceleration (m/s^2)
F_c = centripetal force (N)
m = mass of object (kg)
r = radius of the circular path (m)
v = velocity of object (m/s)

MNEMONIC

This equation explains why the velocity of a car decreases rapidly as you round a turn even if your foot is on the gas pedal (unless you floor it). Turning means that you change the direction of velocity by using force, which slows down your car through friction. Similarly, if you twirl a yo-yo around your head sideways, you must pull inward on the string to keep the yo-yo orbiting at a constant speed (the way the sun keeps the earth in orbit).

e. Force of Gravity

Newton's law of gravitation states that every mass or particle in the universe is attracted to every other mass or particle by a force that is **directly** related to the masses

Gravitational force is inversely related to the square of the distance between two objects, so doubling the distance between two objects would reduce gravitational force to one-fourth of its initial value.

of the objects and **inversely** related to the square of the distance between the objects. This force is called gravitational force.

$$F_g = G\frac{m_1 m_2}{r^2}$$

F_g = gravitational force (N)
m_1, m_2 = mass of each object (kg)
r = distance between the two objects (m)
G = universal gravitational constant (7×10^{-11} N·m^2/kg^2)

On the surface of the earth, m_1 is the mass of the earth (constant) and r is the radius of the earth (also fairly constant). Thus, when dealing with gravitational problems that take place on earth, the simplified form of the equation may be used:

$$F_g = mg$$

F_g = gravitational force (N)
m = mass of object (kg)
g = gravitational constant (9.8 m/s^2) = $\frac{Gm_1}{r}$

MNEMONIC

Note the similarity between this equation and the equation for electricity and magnetism (F = qE), or Coulomb's law. Electricity and magnetism are difficult topics for many students to grasp; it may help to think of mass as similar to charge and force being similar to electric field strength multiplied by charge.

STRATEGY

When you are solving problems dealing with forces, draw a **free-body diagram** of all the forces acting on the object.

4 INCLINED PLANES

a. Forces on an Incline

On an inclined plane, the acceleration of the object going down the inclined plane is not equal to the acceleration due to gravity. Instead, you must take into account the angle of the inclined plane:

$$F = mg\sin(\theta) = ma$$
$$a = g\sin(\theta)$$

F = force on the object (N)
g = gravitational constant (9.8 m/s^2)
a - acceleration (m/s^2)
m = mass of the object (kg)
θ = angle between the inclined plane and the horizontal axis

b. Friction

Working against gravitational force is a frictional force (f) that opposes the motion of the object going down the inclined plane. The force of friction always acts directly opposite to the direction of motion.

You can see, then, why it is easier to push an object up a smooth inclined plane as opposed to lifting an object off the ground; the angle decreases the component of gravitational force opposing the plane of motion, and the smooth inclined plane has a small coefficient of friction (μ). Look at the following equation and Figure 2-1.

$$\begin{aligned} f &= \mu mg \cos(\theta) \\ &= \mu F_N \end{aligned}$$

f = frictional force (N)
m = mass of object (kg)
θ = angle between the inclined plane and the horizontal axis

μ = coefficient of friction
g = gravitational constant (9.8 m/s^2)
F_N = normal force acting on the object (N)
F_g = gravitational force acting on the object (N)

Note the forces acting on the object; for example, gravitational force, normal force, and frictional force.

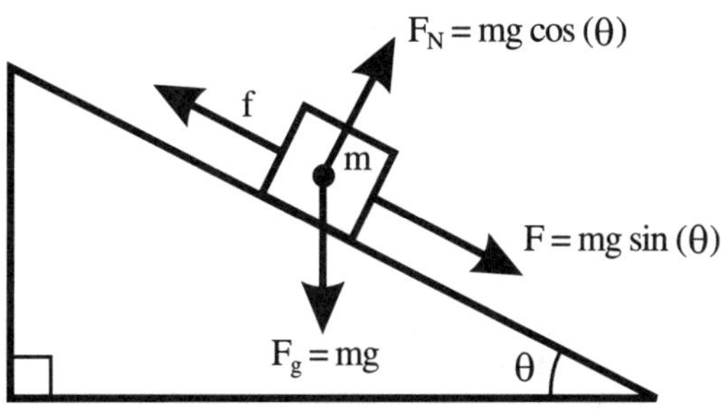

Figure 2-1.
Object on an inclined plane: Free-body diagram.

5 SPRINGS, HOOKE'S LAW, AND SIMPLE HARMONIC MOTION

a. Pendulums and Springs

are two examples of systems that exhibit simple harmonic motion (Figure 2-2). A pendulum consists of a mass suspended by a string, with the upper end of the string fixed to a point. A spring system consists of a mass affixed to the end of a spring, with the upper end of the spring fixed to a point.

Note that the period of a simple pendulum does not vary with the mass of the pendulum or with the height of its swing; **the only variable that affects the period is the length of the pendulum.**

Hooke's law describes the force exerted on a mass at the end of a spring when the spring is displaced from its position of rest.

$$F = -kx$$

F = force (N)
k = spring constant (N/m)
x = displacement (m)

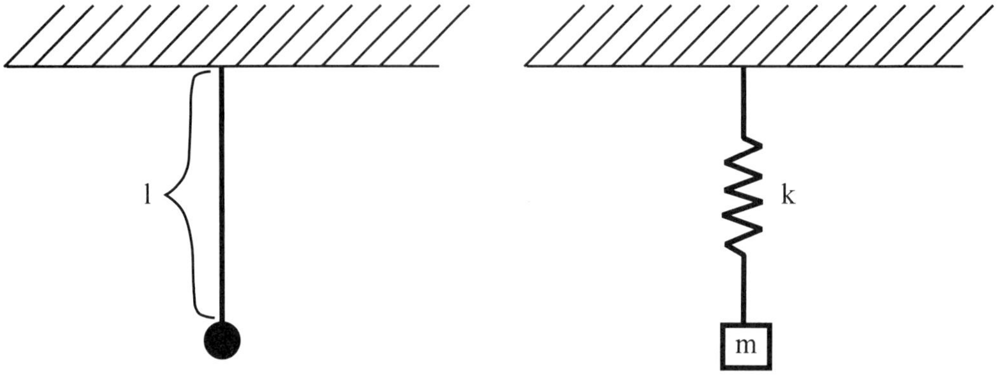

Figure 2-2.
A simple pendulum and a mass–spring system. l = Length of the pendulum string (m); m = mass of the object (kg); k = spring force constant (N/m).

b. Potential Energy of a Spring

When a spring is elongated or shortened through displacement, the spring stores an elastic potential energy. Through subsequent movement, this potential energy can be converted to kinetic energy. The total energy of the spring system is:

$$E = \frac{k}{2}x^2$$

E = total energy (N·m)
k = spring constant (N/m)
x = displacement (m)

c. Period of a Simple Pendulum

The period of motion of a simple pendulum is the time it takes for the mass to undergo one full cycle of motion:

$$T = 2\pi\sqrt{\frac{l}{g}}$$

T = period of motion (s)
l = length of pendulum (m)
g = gravitational constant (9.8 m/s^2)

d. Period of a Simple Harmonic Oscillator

The period of a simple harmonic oscillator (such as a spring system) is the time required for the spring to complete one cycle.

$$T = 2\pi\sqrt{\frac{m}{k}}$$

T = period of motion (s)
m = mass at the end of the spring (kg)
k = spring constant (N/m)

QUESTION

For a simple pendulum
(a) At which point does the greatest velocity occur?
(b) If the length of the string is doubled, what happens to the period of the pendulum?
(c) If the mass at the end of the pendulum is doubled, what happens to the period of the pendulum?

ANSWER

(a) The pendulum accelerates until it reaches its vertical orientation; therefore, its velocity is greatest when it is vertically oriented.
(b) Given that

$$T = 2\pi\sqrt{\frac{l}{g}}$$

If

$$l' = 2l, \text{ then } T' = T\sqrt{2}$$

(c) Trick question! (Yes, you will find them on the MCAT.) Notice that m (mass) is not part of the preceding equation. The period of oscillation for the pendulum does not change.

6 WORK AND ENERGY

a. Force

Strictly defined, force is what causes an object (mass) to accelerate in a particular direction. As discussed earlier, Newton's second law states that force equals mass times acceleration, or F = ma.

b. Work

is defined as the product of the force exerted on an object times the distance that the object is displaced by that force. If you hold a weight over your head, you are not doing work (although it may feel as though you are) because work is done only when a mass is moved over a certain distance by applying a force (e.g., dragging an object up an inclined plane or weight-lifting). Work is measured in newton-meters (N·m) or joules (J). Note that 1 J = 1 N·m.

$$W = F \times d$$

w = work (J)
F = force (N)
d = distance (m)

c. Kinetic energy

is the energy associated with the movement of an object.

$$KE = \frac{1}{2}mv^2$$

KE = kinetic energy (J)
m = mass (kg)
v = velocity (m/s)

d. Potential energy

is the energy that is stored in a system and can be converted into motion or work. The following equation describes the potential energy of a mass with respect to gravity.

$$PE = mgh$$

PE = potential energy (J)
m = mass (kg)
g = gravitational constant (9.8 m/s^2)
h = height (m)

STRATEGY

> By understanding the units on which physics concepts are based, you will understand and solve physics problems better than by just memorizing formulas. Try to approximate before you calculate your answer. Assume that g (gravitational acceleration) is approximately 10 m/s^2.

e. Conservation of Energy

The total energy of a kinematic/kinetic system is always constant in the absence of relativistic effects (the Einstein stuff—not on the MCAT).

$$PE + KE = \text{constant}$$

f. Power

is the rate at which work takes place on a particular object during a given unit of time. The standard unit of power is the watt, which equals a joule/sec.

$$P = \frac{W}{t} = F \times v$$

P = power (watts)
W = work (J)
t = time (s)
F = force (N)
v = velocity (m/s)

QUESTION

> A 10-kg object is dropped off a 20-m building. Given negligible air resistance, what is the speed of the object just before it hits the ground?

ANSWER

Because air resistance is negligible, assume conservation of energy. First, note two things. At the top, the object is not in motion and kinetic energy = 0 because v = 0. However, at the top, potential energy = mgh. At the bottom, potential energy = 0 because h = 0. Therefore, according to conservation of energy:

$$KE_{bottom} = PE_{top}$$

$$\frac{1}{2}mv^2 = mgh$$

$$v = \sqrt{2gh} = \sqrt{2 \times 10 \times 20} = \mathbf{20\ m/s}$$

Note that mass appears on both sides of the equation, so it cancels out.

TEST CORRELATION

Remember that the MCAT is multiple choice. Do not waste time with excessive precision in calculations. Sometimes scanning the answers can help you decide how accurate a calculation is needed.

7 COLLISIONS: MOMENTUM AND ENERGY

a. Momentum

is the movement of an object (or mass) with a given velocity. It is measured in kg·m/s.

$$p = mv$$

p = momentum (kg·m/s)
m = mass (kg)
v = velocity (m/s)

Due to **conservation of momentum**, the final momentum of an isolated system is equal to the initial total momentum of that system.

$$\sum p_{before} = \sum p_{after}$$

In elastic collisions (e.g., when two billiard balls collide), both momentum and energy are conserved. In a perfectly elastic collision, the objects bounce off each other without any deformations in shape or structure and without any of the energy given off as heat.

In completely inelastic collisions, momentum, but not energy, is conserved. Some energy is given off as heat or is used to deform the shape or structure of the colliding objects (e.g., plasticine balls colliding and deforming).

In inelastic collisions, two bodies "stick to each other" after the collision. (You can duplicate this action by forming two balls of silly putty and making them collide.) Remember, momentum is always conserved, but energy is conserved only in a perfectly elastic collision.

b. Impulse

The impulse of a force on a mass is the change in momentum of that mass or the force applied to that mass over a given period of time.

$$i = F\Delta t = \Delta p = m\Delta v$$

i = impulse (kg·m/s)	F = force (N)
Δp = change in momentum (kg·m/s)	Δt = duration (s)
m = mass of object (kg)	Δv = change in velocity (m/s)

BEWARE

Remember that velocity and momentum are both vectors that have both a speed and a directional component. Therefore, always assign a specific direction as positive and the opposite direction as negative.

QUESTION

Two balls hit each other in a head-on collision. Before the collision, ball A, which has a mass of 2 kg, was moving north at a speed of 5 m/s, whereas ball B, which weighs 4 kg, was moving south at 3 m/s. After the collision, ball B is moving north at 1 m/s.

(a) What are the speed and direction of ball A after the collision?

(b) Is this collision elastic or inelastic?

ANSWER

In these types of problems, take into account the direction in which the balls are moving. You can arbitrarily decide that a particle traveling north has a positive velocity whereas a particle traveling south has a negative velocity.

(a) Conservation of momentum

$$\sum mv_{before} = \sum mv_{after}$$

$$(2 \text{ kg})(+5 \text{ m/s}) + (4 \text{ kg})(-3 \text{ m/s}) = (2 \text{ kg})(x \text{ m/s}) + (4 \text{ kg})(+1 \text{ m/s})$$

$$-2 = 2x + 4$$

$$x = -3 \text{ m/s}$$

Therefore, after the collision, ball A is moving south at **3 m/s.**

(b) To determine whether the collision is elastic, you need to know whether energy has been conserved:

$$\sum \frac{mv^2}{2}_{before} = ?\sum \frac{mv^2}{2}_{after}$$

$$(2 \text{ kg})(5 \text{ m/s})^2 + (4 \text{ kg})(-3 \text{ m/s})^2 = ?\ (2 \text{ kg})(-3 \text{ m/s})^2 + (4 \text{ kg})(+1 \text{ m/s})^2$$

$$86 \neq 22.$$

Energy is not conserved; therefore, this was an **inelastic** collision.

TEST CORRELATION

Momentum is frequently tested through hypothetical situations with billiard balls and collisions. Understanding of impulse is frequently tested on the MCAT in passages that involve car accidents. Because there are many motor vehicle accidents each year, collisions are a "trendy" topic that can be expected to appear on the MCAT.

8 TORQUE AND EQUILIBRIUM

a. Torque

is the tendency of a force to rotate an object about an axis (Figure 2-3). Torque (τ) is measured in N·m. Notice that the units are the same as those used for energy, but torque and energy are not the same.

$$\tau = F \times r$$

τ = torque (N·m)
F = force (N)
r = radius (m)

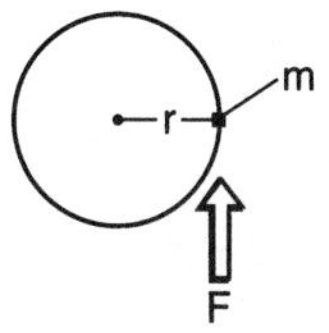

Figure 2-3. Torque. F = applied force; m = mass; r = the moment arm. (Reprinted with permission from Roth, D: *MCAT Essentials*, Baltimore, Williams & Wilkins, 1998, p 145.)

MNEMONIC

This equation explains why a larger crowbar can pry things open more easily than its smaller counterpart can because the larger one (greater r) has more torque for a given force.

b. Equilibrium

In this state, the following is true:

$$\sum F = 0$$

$$\sum \tau = 0$$

QUESTION

A 2-kg uniform meter stick has a fulcrum at the 40-cm mark. A 5-kg mass rests on the 10-cm mark. A 3-kg mass rests on the 60-cm mark.

Where must a 4-kg mass rest to achieve equilibrium?

ANSWER

To solve this problem, draw the picture and **assign distances relative to the position of the fulcrum.** Remember that a uniform mass has its center of mass at its center (i.e., the meter stick acts as a mass that rests at the 50-cm mark).

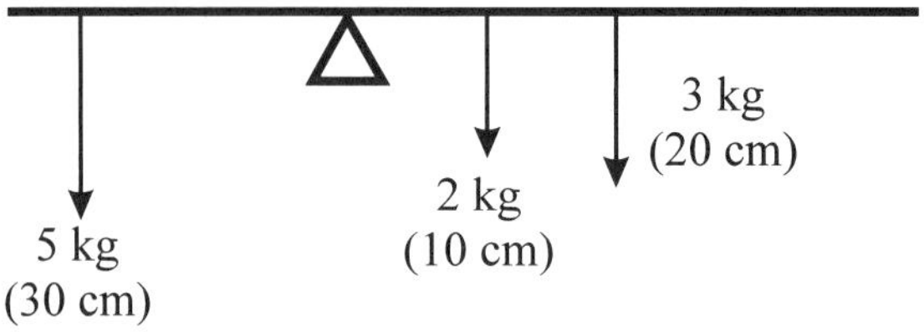

From this picture, you can set up your equation. It doesn't matter on which side you put your unknown 4-kg mass. If you put the mass on the wrong side, your answer (distance) is simply a negative number instead of a positive number.

Equilibrium

$$\sum \tau_{counterclockwise} = \sum \tau_{clockwise}$$
$$(5\text{ kg})(30\text{ cm}) + (4\text{ kg})(x\text{ cm}) = (2\text{ kg})(10\text{ cm}) + (3\text{ kg})(20\text{ cm})$$
$$150 + 4x = 80$$
$$x = -17.5\text{ cm}$$

Therefore, the 4-kg object should be 17.5 cm to the **right** of the fulcrum.

$$\text{Position of the mass} = \text{Fulcrum} + \text{Distance from the fulcrum}$$
$$= 40\text{ cm} + 17.5\text{ cm} = \mathbf{57.5\text{ cm}}$$

9 SOUND AND LIGHT

a. Wavelength

is the distance required to complete one full cycle of a wave.

b. Frequency

is the rate at which cycles occur, or the number of cycles per unit of time. Frequency is measured in hertz (Hz = cycles per second).

Sound and light have constant velocities under constant conditions. Sound and light waves with high frequencies have short wavelengths and high energies. Sound and light waves with low frequencies have longer wavelengths and lower energies.

$$v = f \cdot \lambda$$

v = velocity (m/s)
f = frequency (Hz)
λ = wavelength (m)

STRATEGY

Visible light waves usually have wavelengths that are hundreds of nanometers (nm $= 10^{-9}$ m). Sound waves typically have wavelengths of several meters. Knowing these facts may help you eliminate bogus answer choices that appear on the MCAT.

c. Sound Intensity

The intensity of a sound wave is the rate at which the energy flows through a given area, or the power of the sound wave per unit area. Sound intensity is determined by the amplitude of the sound wave. Volume is often measured in decibels (dB).

Because sound intensity is inversely proportional to the square of the distance from the source, decreasing the distance from the source by one-half increases the intensity of the sound fourfold.

$$V = 10 \log \left(\frac{I}{I_0}\right) \qquad \Delta V = 10 \log \frac{I_{new}}{I_{old}}$$

V = volume of sound (dB)
I = intensity of the sound at a given point (W/m^2)
I_0 = threshold of hearing (10^{-12} W/m^2)

I_{new} = new sound intensity (W/m^2)
I_{old} = original sound intensity (W/m^2)

QUESTION

A person turns up the radio from 20 dB to 40 dB. By how many fold has the intensity of the sound increased?

ANSWER

Using the preceding equation:

$$\Delta V = 10 \log \left(\frac{I_{new}}{I_{old}}\right)$$

$$40 - 20 = 10 \log \left(\frac{I_{new}}{I_{old}}\right)$$

$$2 = \log \left(\frac{I_{new}}{I_{old}}\right)$$

$$\frac{I_{new}}{I_{old}} = \textbf{100-fold}$$

STRATEGY

In chemistry, pH also works on a log scale. Therefore, you should understand the 100-fold difference in hydrogen ion concentration between a pH 2 and a pH 4 solution.

TEST CORRELATION

Waves are basic to many physics topics (e.g., sound, light, and kinematics ; therefore, questions involving the formula v = fλ are popular on the MCAT. In fact, this equation appears on the MCAT so often that we have dubbed v = fλ "MCAT's favorite formula." You should be able to link concepts of waves to sound, light, and kinematics. Expect to use the formula v = fλ and to see at least one question (maybe even a whole passage) involving waves.

QUESTION

A laser that emits a 500-nm beam of light passes from air (n = 1) through a tank of water (n = 1.33) that has a diameter of 25 m.

(a) What is the velocity of the light wave as it passes through the tank of water?

(b) What is the frequency of the light wave?

(c) By what percentage is the original speed of the light wave reduced as it passes from air to water?

(d) How long does it take the light wave to traverse the tank of water?

ANSWER

(a) $v_{H_2O} = c/n$

$v_{H_2O} = 3 \times 10^8/1.33 \approx \mathbf{2.25 \times 10^8\ m/s}$

(b) $v = f\lambda_{air}$

$f = v_{air}/\lambda_{air} = 3 \times 10^8/500 \times 10^{-9} = \mathbf{6 \times 10^{14}\ Hz}$

(c) $\Delta v = \dfrac{n_{air}}{n_{H_2O}} = \dfrac{1}{1.33} = 0.75 \qquad 1 - 0.75 = 0.25$

Therefore, the speed of the wave decreased by **25%.**

(d) $x = v_0 t$

$25 = 2.25 \times 10^8\ (t)$

$t = \dfrac{25}{2.25 \times 10^8} \approx \mathbf{1 \times 10^{-7}\ sec}$

ANSWER

10 OPTICS

a. Reflection

occurs when light rays traveling in a given medium encounter a second medium and travel back from the boundary between the two media. The angle of the reflected ray always equals the angle of the incident ray.

$$\theta_{incident} = \theta_{reflected}$$

b. Refraction

When light rays traveling in a given medium encounter a second medium and travel into it, they bend (refract) at the boundary between the two media. *Snell's law* concerns the angle of the refracted ray.

Snell's law. Light changes its direction of propagation at an interface between two media (e.g., air and glass, as in Figure 2-4). The angle of refraction of a beam of light (θ_r) depends on its angle of incidence (θ_i) at this surface, as follows:

$$n_r \sin(\theta_r) = n_i \sin(\theta_i)$$

n_r, n_i = indices of refraction of the refractive and incident media
θ_r, θ_i = angle of the refracted and incident rays with respect to a plane **perpendicular to the reflecting surface** (see Figure 2-4).

Critical angle is the angle of incidence (θ_i) for which the angle of refraction (θ_r) is 90°.

$$\sin(\theta_{critical}) = \frac{n_r}{n_i}$$

$\theta_{critical}$ = critical angle
n_r, n_i = indices of refraction of the refractive and incident media

$$n_1 \sin\theta_1 = n_2 \sin\theta_2 \qquad \sin\theta_C = 1/n_2$$

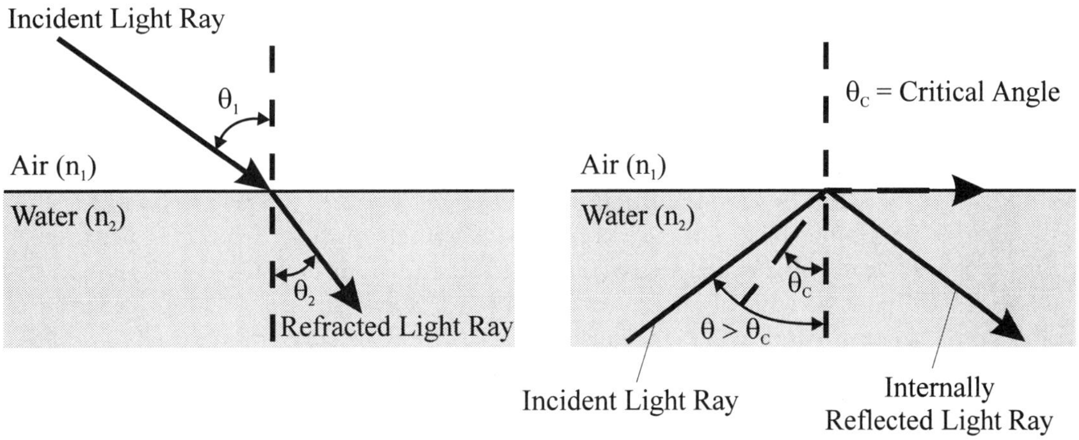

Figure 2-4.
Refraction and reflection.

A critical angle exists only when light is traveling from a more optically dense medium to a less optically dense medium. If the angle of incidence is higher than the critical angle, no refraction occurs. The ray of light instead experiences total internal reflection, which is how diamonds sparkle.

You should be aware of how the properties of light waves change when light passes into a more dense medium (e.g., $n_{glass} = 1.5$) from a less dense medium (e.g., $n_{air} = 1$). When light waves pass into a medium with a higher index of refraction (i.e., a more dense medium):

1. velocity decreases because $n = c/v$ (velocity is inversely proportional to the index of refraction).
2. frequency of the wave remains unchanged.
3. the energy of the wave remains unchanged, and this wave energy is directly proportional to the wave frequency $E = hf = hc/\lambda$.
4. wavelength decreases (i.e., **"blue shift"** occurs because velocity decreases and frequency remains unchanged, via $v = f\lambda$).
5. the angle of the ray of light relative to the normal is smaller (the beam bends back toward the normal as in the preceding diagram, per Snell's law).

MNEMONIC

Therefore, when a light wave passes from a less dense to a more dense medium, it gets **slower and bluer.**

When the homework you're doing gets more and more dense, you get the "blues" and are slow to get things done.

c. Lensmaker's Equation

If you know the distance of an object (d_o) from a lens of known focal length (f), the following equation lets you calculate the position (d_i) of the image formed from the lens:

$$\frac{1}{f} = \frac{1}{d_o} + \frac{1}{d_i} = \frac{2}{r}$$

f = focal length of lens (m)
d_o = distance of the object from the lens (m)
d_i = distance of the image from the lens (m)
r = radius of curvature of the lens (m)

STRATEGY

For both a lens and a mirror, a positive image distance d_i is characteristic of a real image (the image formed is composed of light that is really present). A negative d_i represents a virtual image (the image observed is **not** formed from real light). A positive focal-length value occurs only in a converging lens or mirror, whereas a negative focal length is consistent with a diverging lens or mirror (Figure 2-5). For a diverging lens, the image is always virtual, erect, and smaller (Figure 2-6 and Table 2-2). Lenses and mirrors bend light rays in opposite ways. A convex lens and a concave mirror are both converging ($f > 0$), whereas a concave lens and a convex mirror are both diverging ($f < 0$).

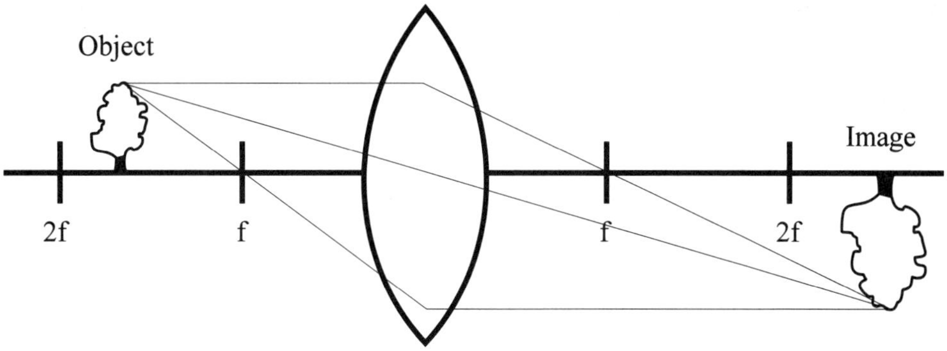

An object placed between the focal distance and the radius of curvature (2f) of a converging lens will form a real image that is inverted and larger than the object.

Figure 2-5.
A converging lens.

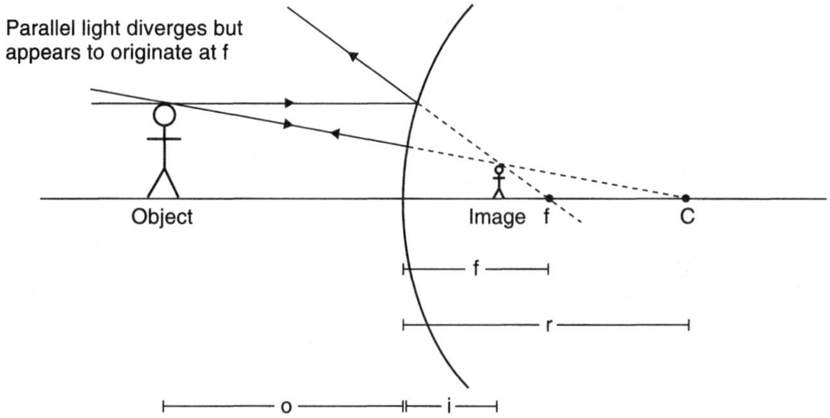

Figure 2-6.
Convex mirror. (Reprinted with permission from Roth, D: *MCAT Essentials*, Baltimore, Williams & Wilkins, 1998, p 41.)

TABLE 2-2. Image using converging and diverging lenses

Condition	Converging Lens Image	Diverging Lens Image
$d_O < f$	Virtual, erect, larger	Virtual, erect, smaller
$f < d_O < 2f$	Real, inverted, larger	Virtual, erect, smaller
$d_O = 2f$	Real, inverted, same size	Virtual, erect, smaller
$d_O > 2f$	Real, inverted, smaller	Virtual, erect, smaller

1. **Magnification.** The relative height of an image compared to its object is the same as the ratio of their distances from the lens.

$$M = \frac{-d_i}{d_o} = \frac{h_i}{h_o}$$

M = magnification ratio
d_i = distance of image (m)
d_o = distance of object (always positive, m)
h_i = height of image (m)
h_o = height of object (m)

HIGH-YIELD MCAT FACTS

Physics

BEWARE

If the magnification ratio (M) is positive, the image is erect. If M is negative, the image is inverted.

2. **Diopter** is a unit of refractory power in which the focal distance of the lens is in meters. Diopters (not focal lengths) are additive.

$$D = \frac{1}{f}$$

D = diopter (m^{-1})
f = focal length (m)

For example, a converging lens with a focal length of +20 cm (0.2 m) is a +5 diopter lens.

$$+5 \text{ diopters} = \frac{1}{0.2 \text{ m}}$$

11 SOUND

Sound must travel through a medium; it does **not** travel in a vacuum. Therefore, one cannot hear an explosion in outer space (one of the many flaws in movies about outer space).

Sound is transmitted by the vibration of particles within the medium (which is why your room shakes if you crank up the bass on your stereo). The higher the density of the medium, the greater the speed of sound. Pitch is determined by, and proportional to, the frequency of the sound wave. Intensity is determined by the amplitude of the sound wave (Figure 2-7).

a. Beats and Beat Frequency

The superposition of two waves of slightly different wavelengths and frequencies gives rise to beats. Specific beats are observed as oscillations of the amplitude of the entire pattern. The beat frequency is:

$$f_{beat} = |f_1 - f_2|$$

f_{beat} = beat frequency (Hz)
f_1, f_2 = frequencies of overlapping waves (Hz)

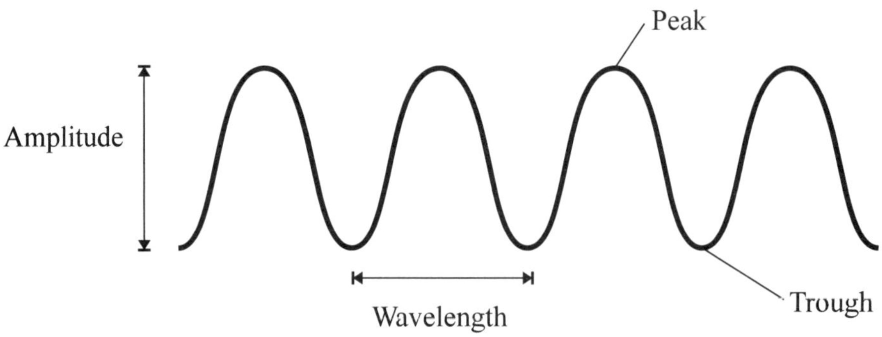

Figure 2-7.
A sound wave.

QUESTION

When two sounds are different, one 330 Hz and the other 320 Hz, what is the beat frequency?

(a) 10 Hz

(b) 650 Hz

(c) 5 Hz

(d) 20 Hz

(e) 0 Hz

ANSWER

The correct answer is (a). Recall that:

$$f_{beat} = |f_1 - f_2|$$
$$= |\,330\text{ Hz} - 320\text{ Hz}\,| = \mathbf{10\ Hz}$$

QUESTION

If a piano key is hit simultaneously with a 400-Hz note on a nearby xylophone, a beat with a frequency of 15 Hz is produced. What is the frequency of the piano key?

I. 385 Hz

II. 400 Hz

III. 415 Hz

(a) I only

(b) II only

(c) III only

(d) I and III only

(e) Cannot be determined from information given

ANSWER

The correct answer is (d). Plugging the answers into the preceding equation shows that I and III would produce a beat with a frequency of 15 Hz, whereas II would not produce a beat at all.

b. Doppler Effect

The Doppler effect describes the change in sound frequency that results from motion of the source relative to a sound detector.

$$f' = f\,\frac{v \pm v_d}{v \mp v_s}$$

f' = new frequency (Hz)

f = original frequency (Hz)

v_s = velocity of sound source (m/s)

v_d = velocity of sound detector (m/s)

QUESTION

If a car is accelerating as it comes toward you with its horn honking, does the sound of the horn:

(a) increase in pitch

(b) decrease in pitch

(c) decrease in volume

(d) increase in volume

(e) increase in pitch and volume

ANSWER

The correct answer is (e). You know from experience that a horn sounds louder when a car approaches at rapid speed (because intensity is inversely proportional to the square of the distance from the source). The pitch of the horn increases to a higher note, just as pitch increases when you hear a police car blaring its siren as it moves toward you. As the car (or police car) moves past you, the pitch decreases rapidly—the Doppler effect.

Standing waves and closed or open nodes. The amplitude of the wave at the closed end of a pipe, for a standing wave, is always zero (node). The amplitude of a standing wave at the open end of a pipe is always maximal (antinode). When a pipe is closed at one end, the standing wave created has a maximum wavelength of four times the length of the pipe. A pipe with both ends open or closed can support a standing wave whose maximal wavelength is two times the length of the pipe (Figures 2-8 and 2-9).

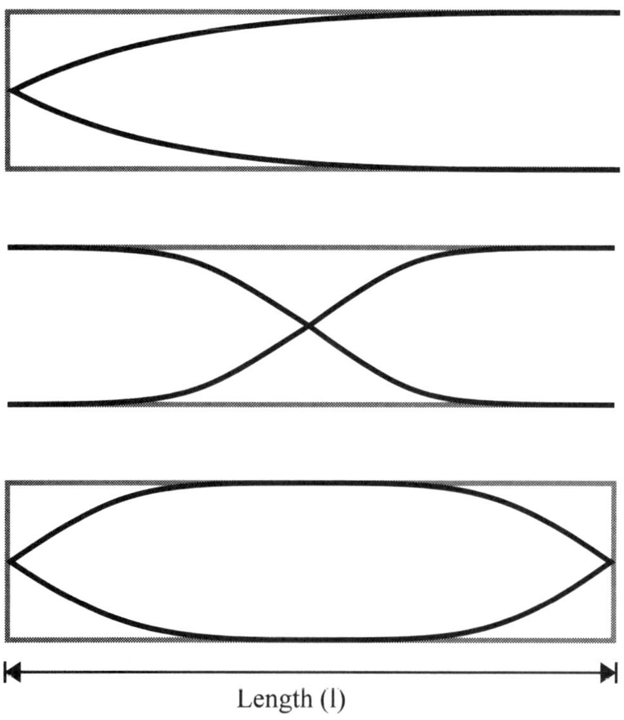

Pipe closed at one end:

$$\text{wavelength} = \frac{4(l)}{n}$$

where n = 1, 3, 5, 7, ...

Pipe with both ends closed or open:

$$\text{wavelength} = \frac{2(l)}{n}$$

where n = 1, 2, 3, 4, ...

Figure 2-8.
Standing waves in pipes.

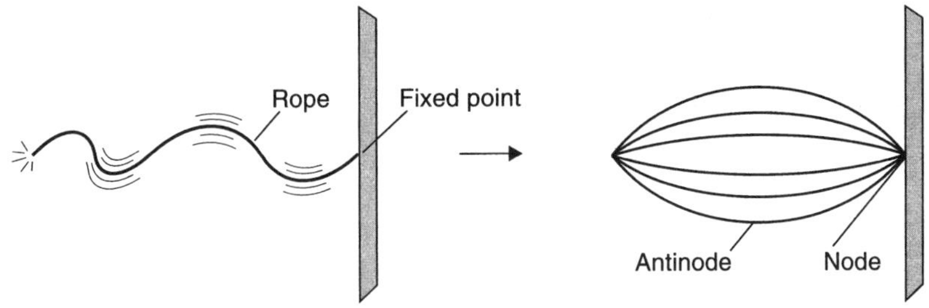

Figure 2-9.
Standing wave. (Reprinted with permission from Roth, D: *MCAT Essentials*, Baltimore, Williams & Wilkins, 1998, p 138.)

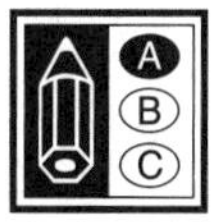

Doppler echocardiography (an imaging technique akin to sonar that uses ultrasound waves to view heart structures) is a recent advance in medical technology. The writers of the MCAT may pose questions about the Doppler effect to be sure that you understand this emerging technology.

12 FLUIDS AND HEAT TRANSFER

a. Fluid Flow

The two types of fluid flow are laminar and turbulent.

1. **Laminar flow** occurs when a liquid flows at a steady rate, and all of the flow is generally in one direction.
2. **Turbulent flow** occurs when the liquid moves in all directions and there is a loss of energy caused by the movement. In this instance, some of the flow equations, mainly Bernoulli's equation, do not apply.

Laminar flow occurs in the middle of a pipe or blood vessel, whereas turbulent flow occurs more often at the periphery of a pipe or a blood vessel.

b. Pressure Changes

1. **Pressure** is force per unit area:

$$P = \frac{F}{A}$$

P = pressure (pascals [Pa = N/m^2])
F = force (newtons, N)
A = area (m^2)

A pressure difference can be described in terms of the fluid flow rate and the resistance to flow:

$$\Delta P = \Phi \cdot R$$

ΔP = change in pressure
Φ = flow
R = resistance

HIGH-YIELD MCAT FACTS
Physics

BEWARE

You must understand the concept of resistance. It applies not only to pressure, but also to circuits, which you can see in Ohm's law, where V = IR (see Part II D 14 a). Voltage is analogous to pressure gradient; current is analogous to flow.

2. **Poiseuille's law** describes the resistance to flow of a fluid through a pipe. It states that resistance (R) is directly proportional to the viscosity (η) of the fluid and inversely proportional to the fourth power of the radius (r) of the tube or vessel of length (L) in which it flows.

$$R = \frac{8\eta L}{r^4}$$

R = resistance η = viscosity
L = length r = radius

Fluid velocity is inversely proportional to the cross-sectional area of the pipe or blood vessel.

3. **Continuity Equation.** For steady flow, which means that the same amount of fluid that enters an area will leave that area, the speed of flow along a small group of associated streamlines decreases with increasing cross-sectional area.

$$A_1 v_1 = A_2 v_2$$

A_1, A_2 = cross-sectional area of the entering and leaving streamline bundle
v_1, v_2 = flow velocity in the entering and exiting streamline bundle

TEST CORRELATION

Fluid dynamics are a trendy MCAT topic because they apply to blood circulation and organ perfusion.

4. **Bernoulli's Equation.** For a given streamline, the sum of the pressure, the potential energy density, and the kinetic energy density is a constant.

$$P + \rho gh + \tfrac{1}{2}\rho v^2 = \text{constant}$$

P = pressure ρ = density
g = gravitational constant h = height
v = flow velocity

Clearly, then, if an element of fluid increases its height along a stream, either its velocity or pressure must decrease.

QUESTION

The diameter of the brand new water gun for your sprinkler is one-third the diameter of the hose. If water flows through the hose at 10 m/s, how rapidly does the water flow out of the water gun?

ANSWER

The cross-sectional area of the hose is nine times the area of the water gun (the area of a circle is proportional to the square of the radius). According to the continuity equation:

$$A_{hose} \times v_{hose} = A_{gun} \times v_{gun}$$

Because $A_{\text{hose}} = 9A_{\text{gun}}$, $9A_{\text{gun}} \times v_{\text{hose}} = A_{\text{gun}} \times v_{\text{gun}}$; therefore, $v_{\text{gun}} = 9 \times v_{\text{hose}}$. Hence, the velocity of the water flowing out of the water gun is 9 (10 m/s) = 90 m/s.

QUESTION

An atherosclerotic plaque occludes a blood vessel and decreases the radius of the vessel to half its original size. How much would pressure need to increase to maintain the same amount of blood flow in the vessel?

ANSWER

Poiseuille's law shows that resistance is inversely proportional to r^4.

$$\Delta P = FR = F\frac{8\eta L}{r^4}$$

By reducing r to its original size, R and thus ΔP increase by 2^4 (i.e., by 16). The same amount of flow would thus require 16 times the original pressure, a situation that could easily lead to a heart attack or stroke.

c. Heat Transfer

The three mechanisms of heat transfer are conduction, convection, and radiation.

1. **Conduction.** Heat transfer occurs through the direct contact of two objects.
2. **Convection.** Heat transfer occurs through the random motion of particles in the heated material.
3. **Radiation.** Heat transfer occurs through the emission of electromagnetic waves.

13 ELECTROSTATICS AND ELECTROMAGNETISM

a. Electric Fields

A gravitational field is associated with mass, and an electric field is associated with charge. An electric field (E) exerts a force on a charged particle (q) as follows:

$$F = qE$$

F = force (N)
q = charge (coulombs)
E = electric field strength (volts/m, V/m)

b. Voltage

is the potential energy per unit charge. The voltage difference is often defined operationally as the work (W) necessary to move a charge (q) from one position to another.

$$V = \frac{W}{q}$$

Many people find electromagnetism more challenging than mechanics; using the analogies that follow, you can tackle electrostatics and electromagnetism in the same way that you solve kinematics equations.

MNEMONIC

> Think of charge (q) as analogous to mass (m), and an electric field (E) as analogous to the acceleration (a). Then, the equation F = qE is analogous to F = ma, and the equation $F = kq_1q_2/r^2$ is analogous to $F = Gm_1m_2/r^2$.

14 ELECTRICITY, CIRCUITS, RESISTANCE, AND CAPACITANCE

a. Ohm's Law

The electrical potential between two points depends on the current and the resistance to current flow.

$$V = IR$$

V = voltage (volts, V)
I = current (amperes, amp = coul/sec)
R = resistance (ohms, Ω)

b. Power

As discussed in the kinematics section, power is the work expended per unit time (power = work/time). The electrical expression for power is:

$$P = IV = I^2R = \frac{V^2}{R}$$

P = power (watts, W)
V = voltage (volts, V)
I = current (amperes, amp = coul/sec)
R = resistance (ohms, Ω)

c. Resistance

The resistance to current flow increases with wire length and decreases with wire cross-sectional area.

$$R = \frac{\rho_0 L}{A}$$

R = resistance (ohms, Ω)
L = wire length (m)
ρ_0 = resistivity (property of material of the wire)
A = cross-sectional area of the wire (m^2)

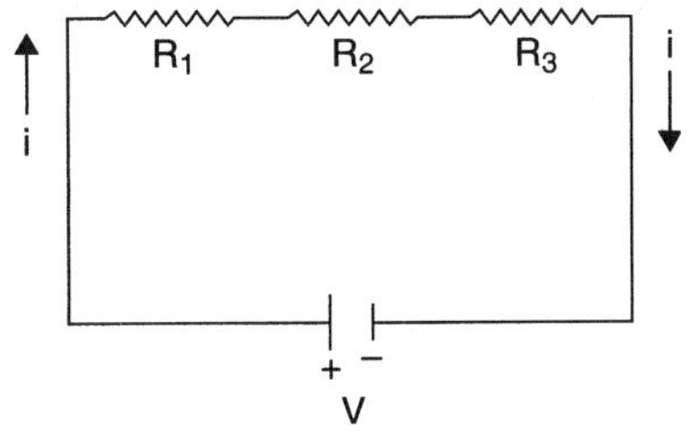

Figure 2-10. Series circuit. *i* = current; *R* = net resistance; *V* = voltage. (Reprinted with permission from Roth, D: *MCAT Essentials*, Baltimore, Williams & Wilkins, 1998, p 132.)

d. Resistance of a Circuit

Deriving an equivalent resistance of a circuit to represent complex clusters of resistors is a good first step in tackling a circuit problem.

1. **Resistors in series.** (Figure 2-10) In this situation, several resistors are strewn along a single path of wire. Resistors in series have the same current going across each resistor. The resistance (R_{eq}) of a set of resistors in series is the sum of the component resistors:

$$R_{eq} = R_1 + R_2 + R_3$$

> This example of resistance is the famous scenario of the cheap Christmas lights. The current must flow through all of the resistors (lights), so shutting off one light opens the entire circuit and causes all the lights to go off.

MNEMONIC

2. **Resistors in parallel.** (Figure 2-11) In this situation, several parallel paths of wire, each with its own resistor, travel downstream and later merge. Resistors in parallel have the same voltage going across each resistor. The equivalent resistance (R_{eq}) of a set of resistors aligned in parallel is determined by:

$$\frac{1}{R_{eq}} = \frac{1}{R_1} + \frac{1}{R_2} + \frac{1}{R_3}$$

> When Christmas lights are arranged in parallel and you shut off one light, the voltage through each bulb stays the same, but the total current decreases. Thus, the remaining lights are unaffected.

MNEMONIC

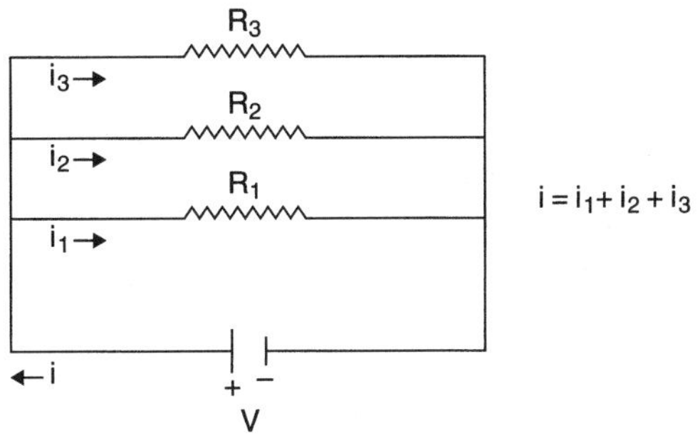

Figure 2-11. Parallel circuit. (Reprinted with permission from Roth, D: *MCAT Essentials*, Baltimore, Williams & Wilkins, 1998, p 109.)

QUESTION

In the following circuit, what is the current going through the 6Ω resistor?

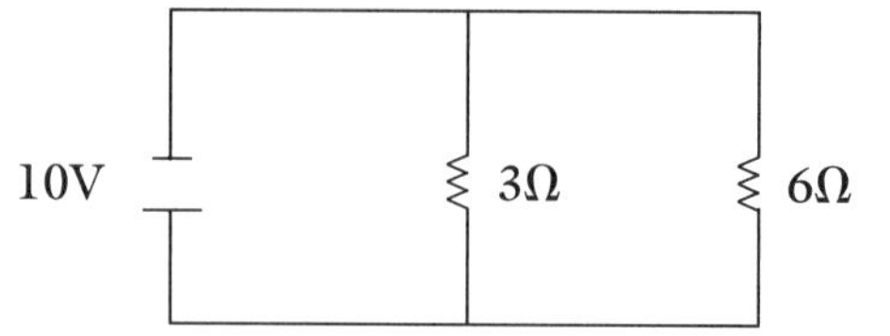

ANSWER

Since resistors arranged in parallel have the same voltage going across each resistor, the answer can be easily calculated using Ohm's Law:

$$V = IR$$

Rearranging the variables you get:

$$I = \frac{V}{R} = \frac{10}{6} = \mathbf{1.25\ amps}$$

e. Capacitance

Two plates of area (A) and separation distance (d) define a capacitor(Figure 2-12). Capacitance can be thought of as a measure of the storage of charge per volt. **Dielectrics,** which increase ε_0 relative to air, decrease the effective distance (d) between the plates of the capacitor, thereby causing:

- Increase of capacitance
- Decrease of voltage across the capacitor

$$C = \varepsilon_0 \frac{A}{d}$$

C = capacitance (farads, F)
A = plate area
ε_0 = dielectric constant of the medium between the two plates
d = distance separating the plates

The capacitance is related to the charge (q) and the voltage (V) of a circuit as follows:

$$q = CV$$

q = charge (coulombs)
C = capacitance
V = voltage

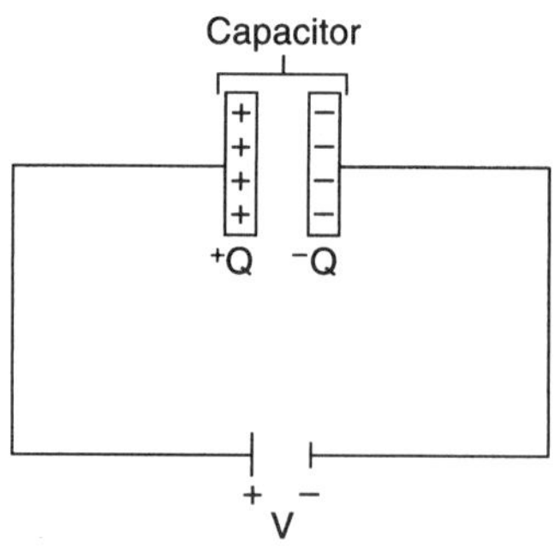

Figure 2-12.
Capacitor. (Reprinted with permission from Roth, D: *MCAT Essentials*, Baltimore, Williams & Wilkins, 1998, p 28.)

f. Voltage Across a Capacitor

The voltage (V) across a capacitor equals the electric field (E) across the capacitor times the distance (d) between the plates:

$$V = Ed$$

g. Capacitance of a Circuit

Like equivalent resistance, equivalent capacitance is a useful concept.

1. **Capacitors in series.** The equivalent capacitance of a set of capacitors placed in series along a single path of wire is calculated as follows:

$$\frac{1}{C_{eq}} = \frac{1}{C_1} + \frac{1}{C_2} + \frac{1}{C_3}$$

2. **Capacitors in parallel.** The equivalent capacitance derived for capacitors placed on parallel paths in a circuit is the sum of the contributing capacitances.

$$C_{eq} = C_1 + C_2 + C_3$$

Capacitors **in series** have the **same charge** (q) going across each capacitor; capacitors in **parallel** have the **same voltage** (V) going across each capacitor.

QUESTION

What is the resistance of a 100-watt lightbulb that is plugged into a 120-volt DC circuit?

ANSWER

To find the answer, use the equation:

$$P = \frac{V^2}{R}$$

P = power (watts, W)
V = voltage (volts, V)
R = resistance (ohms, Ω)

Rearranging the equation:

$$R = \frac{V^2}{P} = \frac{120^2}{100} = \mathbf{144\ \Omega}$$

15 RIGHT-HAND RULE

The magnitude and direction of the magnetic force (F) on a wire of length (L) depend on the magnitude and direction of the magnetic field (B) and the length of the wire (Figure 2-13).

$$F = ILB\sin(\theta)$$

F = force (N)
I = current (amp)
L = length of wire (m)
B = strength of the magnetic field (gauss)
θ = angle between vector B and wire

The right-hand rule has many versions. You may have learned a different one. Nevertheless, you should use the version given here, so you won't be confused.

The direction of the force, current, or magnetic field can be predicted if you know the other two directions and use the right-hand rule.

- Place your index finger in the direction of motion of a positively charged particle (i.e., point it in the opposite direction if the particle is an electron).
- Place digits 3–5 in the direction of the magnetic field.
- Your thumb points in the direction of the force.

QUESTION

If an electron particle is traveling to the right as it enters a magnetic field that is moving as shown, what is the direction of the force that acts on the electron when it enters the magnetic field?

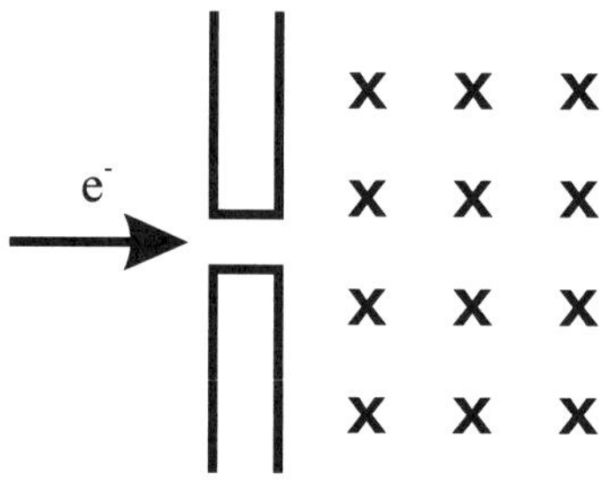

ANSWER

Using the right-hand rule, the index finger points to the left because this example deals with an electron (negative charge). Other fingers are pointing into the page. Your thumb (i.e., the force) should be pointing **down**.

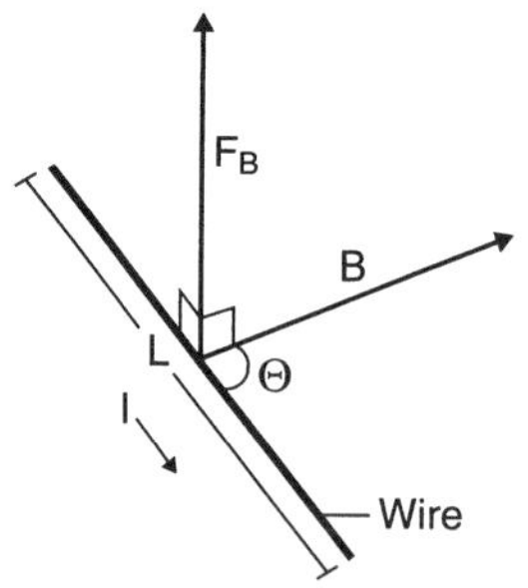

Figure 2-13. Magnetic force. (Reprinted with permission from Roth, D: *MCAT Essentials*, Baltimore, Williams & Wilkins, 1998, p 90.)

16 ELECTROMAGNETIC ENERGY

Electromagnetic waves (with constant speed $c = 3 \times 10^8$ m/s) include a vast range of frequencies, from radio waves at the lower end to gamma rays at the higher end of the spectrum (Figure 2-14). The energy of these waves is directly proportional to their frequency (f) and inversely proportional to their wavelength (λ).

$$E = hf = h\frac{c}{\lambda}$$

E = energy of light (J)
f = frequency (Hz)
λ = wavelength of light (m)

h = Planck's constant
c = speed of light (m/s)

Remember,

$$E = mc^2$$

E = energy
m = mass
c = speed of light

Based on the preceding equations, the higher the frequency is, the higher the energy; so gamma rays can be more dangerous to human tissue than x-rays.

MNEMONIC

In the visible spectrum, **ROY G. BIV** describes the order of colors from **low to high frequency,** and from **long to short wavelengths.**

R Red
O Orange
Y Yellow
G Green
B Blue
I Indigo
V Violet

White light is a continuous spectrum of all colored wavelengths. Thus, an object that is white is reflecting photons of all wavelengths within the visible wavelength spectrum, whereas a black object is absorbing photons of all visible wavelengths.

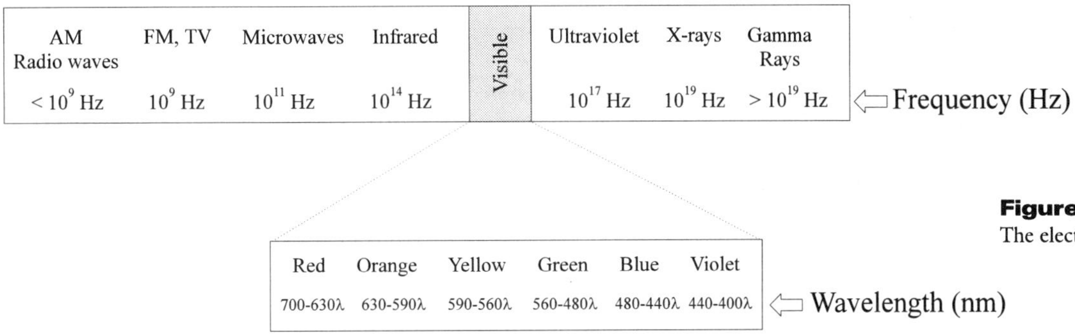

Figure 2-14.
The electromagnetic spectrum.

17 NUCLEAR PHYSICS

a. Atomic number

is the number of protons in the nucleus of an atom, which equals the number of electrons in a neutral element (Table 2-3).

TABLE 2-3. Subatomic particles

Particle	Alternate Name	Symbol	Mass Number	Atomic Number
Alpha	Helium nucleus	α	4	2
Beta	Electron	β	0	−1
Gamma		γ	0	0
Neutron		n	1	0
Positron		β^+	0	1

b. Mass number

is the total number of protons and neutrons in the nucleus of an atom.

c. Isotopes

are two atoms with the same atomic number but different mass numbers; they differ in the number of neutrons in the nucleus.

d. Atomic Mass

A "weighted average" of the mass numbers for the different isotopes of a particular element is the average mass of an atom of a particular element and is equal to the number of grams in a mole of that element.

QUESTION

^{235}U (atomic number 92) undergoes spontaneous radioactive decay after colliding with a neutron. It emits four alpha particles, two beta particles, and three gamma particles. What atom is formed?

ANSWER

You know that mass is conserved in all reactions, so all you have to do is write out the reaction, as follows:

$$^{235}_{92}U + {}^{1}_{0}n \rightarrow {}^{16}_{8}\alpha_4 + {}^{0}_{-2}\beta_2 + {}^{0}_{0}\gamma_3 + {}^{a}_{b}X$$

Adding up the top and bottom numbers results in two simple equations:

$$236 = 16 + \text{mass number (a)}$$

$$92 = 6 + \text{atomic number (b)}$$

Mass number = 220
Atomic number = 86

By looking at the periodic table, you see that radon (Rn) has an atomic number of 86. (The periodic table is included in the MCAT question booklet.) Therefore, the answer is ^{220}Rn.

18 RADIOACTIVE DECAY AND HALF-LIFE

Half-life is the time required for half the particles of a given substance to decay radioactively. For radioactive decay, the fraction of particles left (A/A_0) at time (t) is:

$$\frac{A}{A_0} = \left(\frac{1}{2}\right)^{t/t_{1/2}}$$

A = number of particles
A_0 = initial number of particles
$t_{1/2}$ = half-life
t = time

When time (t) equals the half-life ($t_{1/2}$), $A/A_0 = 1/2$.

QUESTION

If radioactive substance X has a half-life of 3 hours, approximately how long will it take for 94% of its present radioactivity to decay?

ANSWER

The half-life of X is 3 hours.

Time (Hours)	% of Original Radioactivity
0	100
3	50
6	25
9	12.5
12	6.25

Therefore, after 12 hours, only 6.25% of the original radioactivity remains and approximately 94% has decayed.

STRATEGY

On some MCAT problems dealing with half-life, it may be easier to work backward from the choices. Otherwise, working backward can serve as a method to double-check your answers.

19 ESSENTIAL PHYSICS FORMULAS

$$x = x_0 + v_0t + \frac{1}{2}at^2$$
$$v = v_0 + at$$
$$v^2 = v_0^2 + 2as$$

a = acceleration (m/s^2)
s = distance traveled (m)
x = current position (m)
t = time (sec)
v = current velocity (m/s)
x_0 = initial position (m)
v_0 = initial velocity (m/s)

$$slope = \frac{\Delta v}{\Delta t} = a$$

$$v_x = v_0 \cos(\theta)$$
$$v_y = v_0 \sin(\theta)$$

v_x = velocity in the horizontal direction (m/s)
v_y = velocity in the vertical direction (m/s)
v_0 = initial speed of the object (m/s)
θ = angle between the vector v_0 and the horizontal plane

$$F = ma$$

F = force (newtons, N, or kg·m/s^2)
m = mass (kg)
a = acceleration (m/s^2)

and

$$a_c = \frac{v^2}{r}$$
$$F_c = m \times \frac{v^2}{r}$$

a_c = centripetal acceleration (m/s^2)
F_c = centripetal force (N)
m = mass of object (kg)
r = radius of the circular path (m)
v = velocity of object (m/s)

$$F_g = G\frac{m_1 m_2}{r^2}$$

F_g = gravitational force (N)
m_1, m_2 = mass of each object (kg)
r = distance between the 2 objects (m)
G = universal gravitational constant (7×10^{-11} N·m^2/kg^2)

$$F = mg\sin(\theta) = ma$$
$$a = g\sin(\theta)$$

F = force on the object sliding down ramp (N)
g = gravitational constant (9.8 m/s^2)
a = acceleration (m/s^2)
m = mass of the object (kg)
θ = angle between the inclined plane and the horizontal axis

$$f = \mu mg\cos(\theta) = \mu F_N$$

f = frictional force (N)
m = mass of object (kg)
θ = angle between the inclined plane and the horizontal axis
μ = coefficient of friction
g = gravitational constant (9.8 m/s^2)
F_N = normal force acting on the object (N)

$$F = -kx$$

F = force (N)
k = spring constant (N/m)
x = displacement (m)

$$E = \frac{k}{2}x^2$$

E = total energy (N·m)
k = spring constant (N/m)
x = displacement (m)

$$T = 2\pi\sqrt{\frac{l}{g}}$$

T = period of motion (s)
l = length of pendulum (m)
g = gravitational constant (9.8 m/s^2)

$$T = 2\pi\sqrt{\frac{m}{k}}$$

T = period of motion (s)
m = mass at the end of the spring (kg)
k = spring constant (N/m)

$$y_{max} = y_0 + \left|\frac{(v_{0y})^2}{2g}\right|$$

y_{max} = maximum vertical height of projectile (m)
y_0 = initial height from which the projectile was launched (m)
v_{0y} = vertical component of the initial velocity of the projectile (m/s)
g = gravitational constant (9.8 m/s^2)

$$W = F \times d$$

W = work (J)
F = force (N)
d = distance (m)

$$KE = \frac{1}{2} mv^2$$

KE = kinetic energy (J)
m = mass (kg)
v = velocity (m/s)

$$PE = mgh$$

PE = potential energy (J)
g = gravitational constant (9.8 m/s^2)
m = mass (kg)
h = height (m)

$$PE + KE = \text{constant}$$

$$P = \frac{W}{t} = F \times v$$

P = power (watts)
t = time (s)
v = velocity (m/s)
W = work (J)
F = force (N)

$$KE_{bottom} = PE_{top}$$
$$\frac{1}{2} mv^2 = mgh$$
$$v = \sqrt{2gh}$$

$$p = mv$$

p = momentum (kg·m/s)
m = mass (kg)
v = velocity (m/s)

$$i = F\Delta t = \Delta p$$

i = impulse (kg·m/s)
Δp = change in momentum (kg·m/s)
F = force (N)
Δt = duration (s)

$$\tau = F \times r$$

τ = torque (N·m)
F = force (N)
r = radius (m)

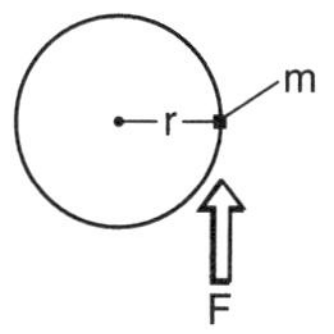

Figure 2-15.
Torque. F = applied force; m = mass; r = the moment arm. (Reprinted with permission from Roth, D: *MCAT Essentials*, Baltimore, Williams & Wilkins, 1998, p 145.)

$$v = f \cdot \lambda$$

v = velocity (m/s)
f = frequency (Hz)
λ = wavelength (m)

$$V = 10 \log \left(\frac{I}{I_0} \right) \qquad \Delta V = 10 \log \frac{I_{new}}{I_{old}}$$

V = volume of sound (dB)
I = intensity of the sound at a given point (W/m^2)
I_0 = threshold of hearing (10^{-12} W/m^2)

I_{new} = new sound intensity (W/m^2)
I_{old} = original sound intensity (W/m^2)

$$\theta_{incident} = \theta_{reflected}$$

$$n_r \sin(\theta_r) = n_i \sin(\theta_i)$$

n_r, n_i = indices of refraction of the refractive and incident media
θ_r, θ_i = angle of the refracted and incident rays with respect to a plane perpendicular to the reflecting surface

$$\sin(\theta_{critical}) = \frac{n_r}{n_i}$$

$\theta_{critical}$ = critical angle
n_r, n_i = indices of refraction of the refractive and incident media

$$\frac{1}{f} = \frac{1}{d_o} + \frac{1}{d_i} = \frac{2}{r}$$

f = focal length of lens (m)
d_i = distance of the image from the lens (m)
d_o = distance of the object from the lens (m)
r = radius of curvature of the lens (m)

$$M = \frac{-d_i}{d_o} = \frac{h_i}{h_o}$$

M = magnification ratio
d_i = distance of image (m)
d_o = distance of object (always positive, m)
h_i = height of image (m)
h_o = height of object (m)

$$D = \frac{1}{f}$$

D = diopter (m^{-1})
f = focal length (m)

$$f_{beat} = |f_1 - f_2|$$

f_{beat} = beat frequency (Hz)
f_1, f_2 = frequencies of overlapping waves (Hz)

$$f' = f\,\frac{v \pm v_d}{v \mp v_s}$$

f′ = new frequency (Hz)
f = original frequency (Hz)
v_s = velocity of sound source (m/s)
v_d = velocity of sound detector (m/s)

$$P = \frac{F}{A}$$

P = pressure (pascals [Pa = N/m^2])
F = force (newtons, N)
A = area (m^2)

$$\Delta P = \Phi \cdot R$$

ΔP = change in pressure
Φ = flow
R = resistance

$$R = \frac{8\eta L}{r^4}$$

R = resistance
L = length
η = viscosity
r = radius

$$A_1 v_1 = A_2 v_2$$

A_1, A_2 = cross-sectional area of the entering and leaving streamline bundle
v_1, v_2 = flow velocity in the entering and exiting streamline bundle

Bernoulli's Equation:

$$P + \rho g h + \tfrac{1}{2}\rho v^2 = \text{constant}$$

P = pressure
g = gravitational constant
v = flow velocity
ρ = density of the fluid
h = height of the fluid

$$F_b = V\rho g = mg$$

Fb = buoyant force
V = fluid volume displaced by object
ρ = fluid density
g = gravitational constant
m = mass of displaced fluid

$$F = qE$$

F = force (N)
q = charge (coulombs)
E = electric field strength (volts/m, V/m)

$$V = \frac{W}{q}$$

$$V = IR$$

V = voltage (volts, V)
I = current (amperes, amp = coul/sec)
R = resistance (ohms, Ω)
W = work (J)
q = charge (coulombs)

$$P = IV = I^2R = \frac{V^2}{R}$$

P = power (watts, W)
V = voltage (volts, V)
I = current (amperes, amp = coul/sec)
R = resistance (ohms, Ω)

$$R = \frac{\rho_0 L}{A}$$

R = resistance (ohms, Ω)
L = wire length (m)
ρ_0 = resistivity (property of the wire material)
A = cross-sectional area of the wire (m^2)

Resistors in series:

$$R_{eq} = R_1 + R_2 + R_3$$

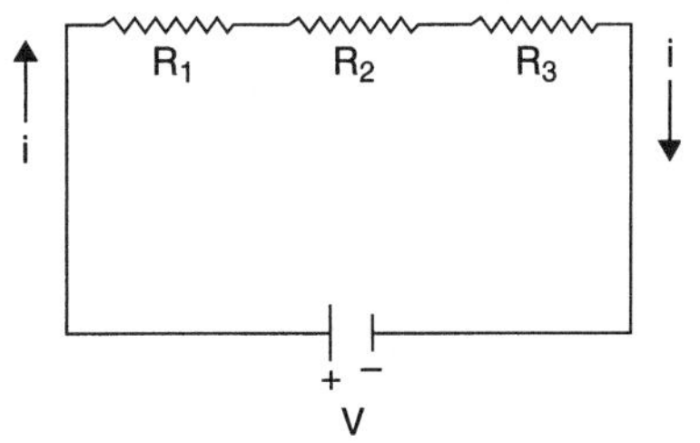

Figure 2-16. Series circuit i = current; R = net resistance; V = voltage. (Reprinted with permission from Roth, D: *MCAT Essentials*, Baltimore, Williams & Wilkins, 1998, p 132.)

Resistors in parallel:

$$\frac{1}{R_{eq}} = \frac{1}{R_1} + \frac{1}{R_2} + \frac{1}{R_3}$$

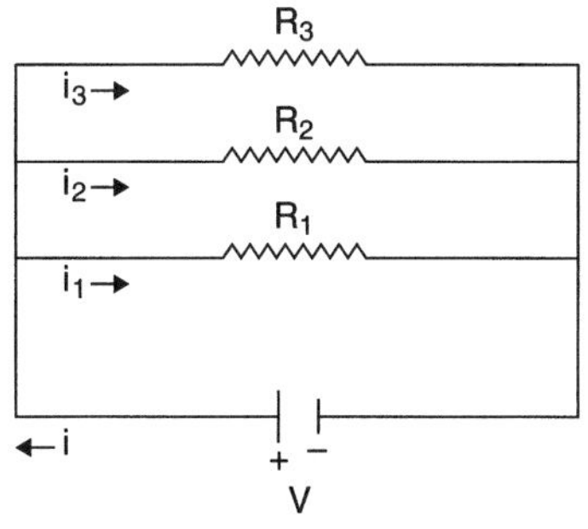

Figure 2-17. Parallel circuit. (Reprinted with permission from Roth, D: *MCAT Essentials*, Baltimore, Williams & Wilkins, 1998, p 109.)

$$C = \varepsilon_0 \frac{A}{d}$$

C = capacitance (farads, F)
A = plate area
ε_0 = dielectric constant of the medium between the two plates
d = distance separating the plates

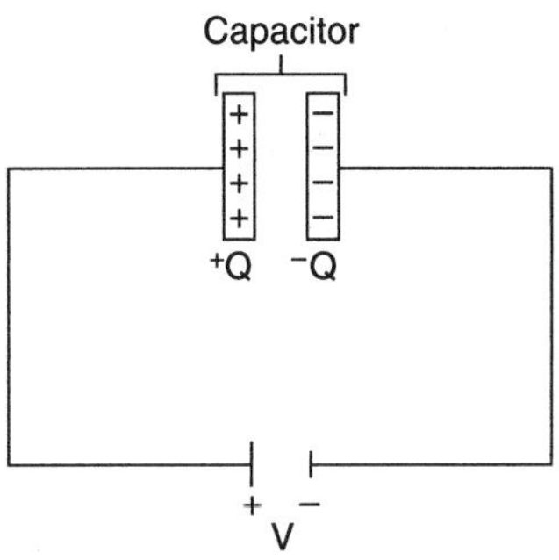

Figure 2-18. Capacitors. (Reprinted with permission from Roth, D: *MCAT Essentials*, Baltimore, Williams & Wilkins, 1998, p 28.

$$q = CV$$

$$V = Ed$$

q = charge (coulombs)
C = capacitance
V = voltage
E = electric field strength (V/m)
d = distance (m)

Capacitors in series:

$$\frac{1}{C_{eq}} = \frac{1}{C_1} + \frac{1}{C_2} + \frac{1}{C_3}$$

Capacitors in parallel:

$$C_{eq} = C_1 + C_2 + C_3$$

$$F = ILB\sin(\theta)$$

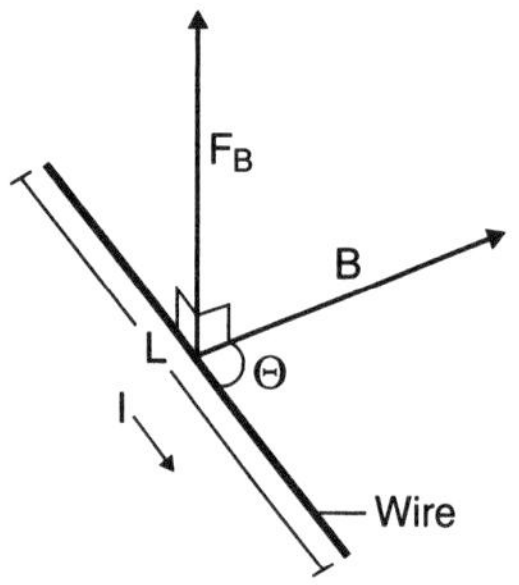

Figure 2-19. Magnetic force. (Reprinted with permission from Roth, D: *MCAT Essentials*, Baltimore, Williams & Wilkins, 1998, p 90.)

F = force (N)
L = length of wire (m)
θ = angle between vector B and wire
I = current (amp = coul/sec)
B = strength of the magnetic field (gauss)

$$E = hf = h\frac{c}{\lambda}$$

E = energy of light (J)
f = frequency (Hz)
λ = wavelength of light (m)
h = Planck's constant
c = speed of light (m/s)

$$E = mc^2$$

E = energy
m = mass
c = speed of light

$$\frac{A}{A_0} = \left(\frac{1}{2}\right)^{t/t_{1/2}}$$

A = number of particles
$t_{1/2}$ = half-life
A_0 = initial number of particles
t = time

E Inorganic Chemistry

1 PERIODIC TRENDS

a. Atomic Radius

- The **metallic atomic radius** is half the distance between the centers of neighboring atoms in a solid sample.
- The **ionic radius** is the distance between the center and the edge of an ion measured in different species.
- **Atomic radius** increases down a column and decreases across a row of the periodic table (Figure 2-20).
- Until you reach the noble gases at the end, the elements on the left are larger than the elements on the right.

b. Electronegativity

- Electronegativity is the ability of an atom to attract electrons in a chemical bond.
- Electronegativity predicts the type of bonding that occurs within a molecule (see Part II E 2).
- Electronegativity increases across a row and decreases down a column of the periodic table (Figure 2-21).
- Electronegativity increases across the periodic table, because more valence electrons are being added and the atom is approaching a stable noble gas electron configuration.
- Electronegativity is inversely related to an atom's atomic radius.

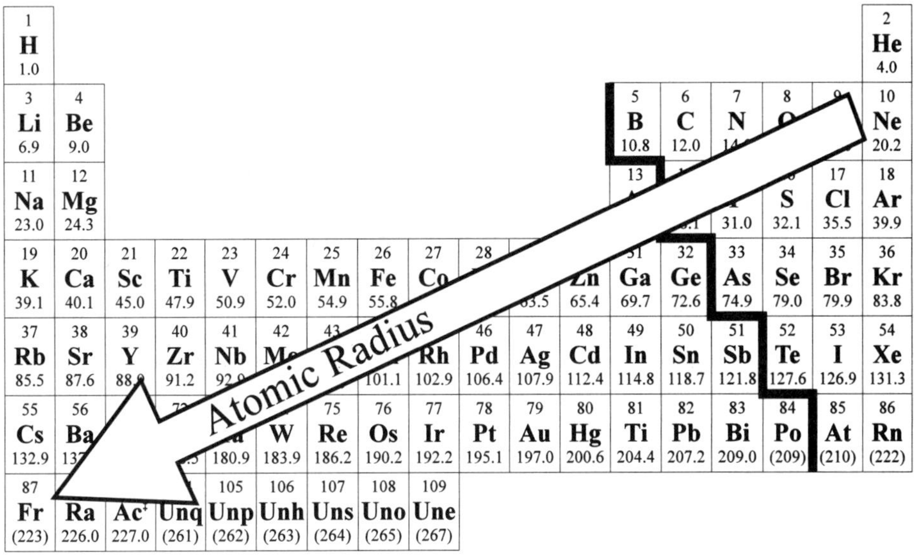

Figure 2-20. Periodic trend for atomic radius.

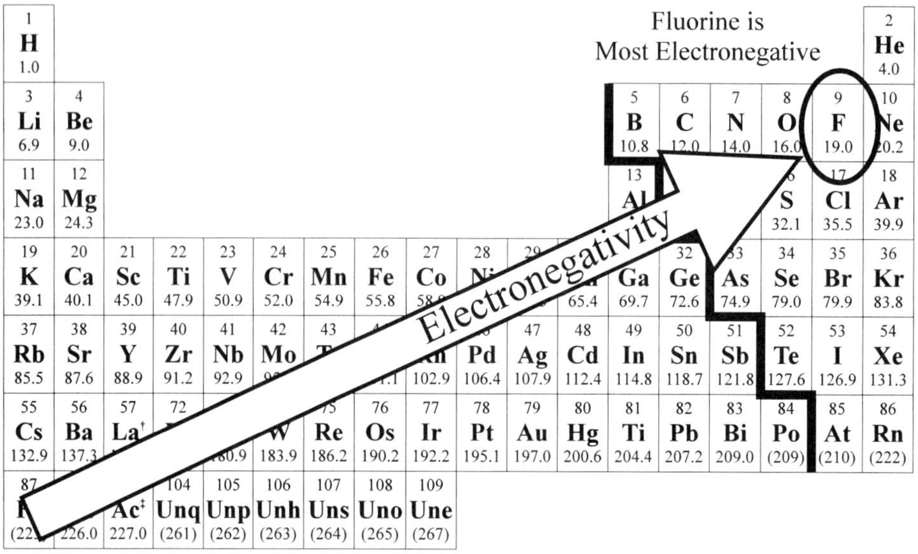

Figure 2-21. Periodic trend for electronegativity.

- Electronegativity decreases down a column of the periodic table because electrons are dispersing and the nucleus is farther away from free electrons (electric force decreases with the square of the distance).

c. Ionization Energy

- Ionization energy is the minimum energy required to remove an electron from the ground state of a gaseous atom.
- Ionization energy increases across a row and decreases down a column of the periodic table (Figure 2-22).
- The farther the electron is from the nucleus, the easier it is to remove that electron.

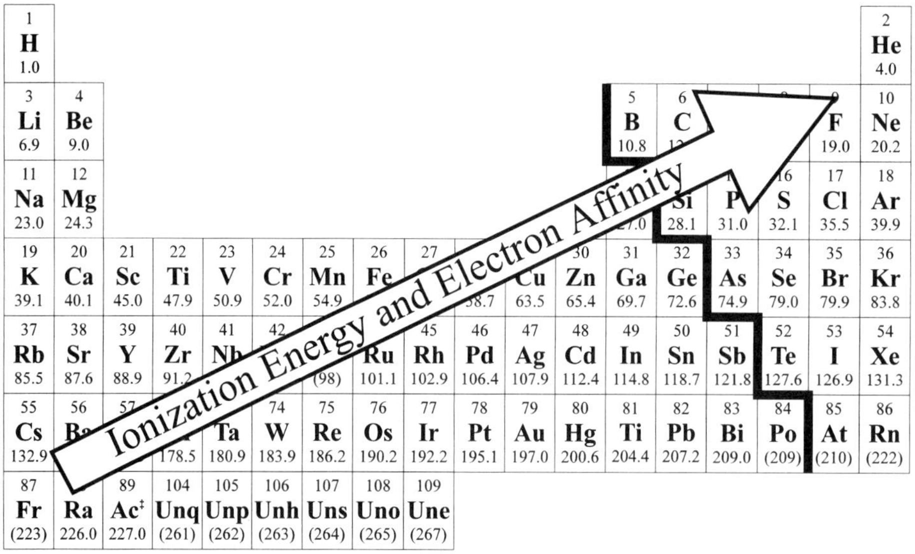

Figure 2-22. Periodic trend for ionization energy and electron affinity.

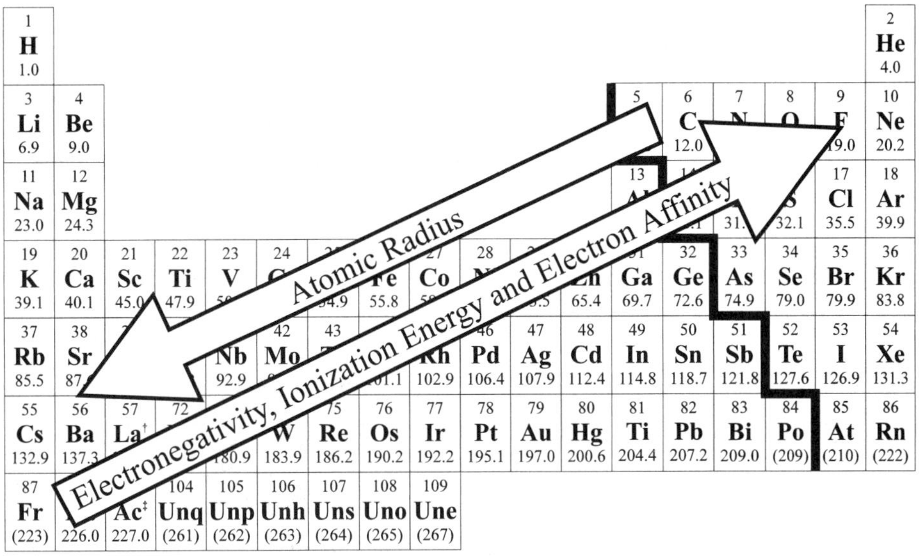

Figure 2-23.
Periodic trends: the big picture.

d. Electron Affinity

- Electron affinity is the amount of energy released when a neutral atom acquires an electron.
- Electron affinity increases across a row and decreases down a column of the periodic table (Figure 2-23).

2 BONDING: INTRAMOLECULAR VERSUS INTERMOLECULAR FORCES

a. **Intramolecular forces** (forces within a molecule) are stronger than intermolecular forces (forces between two similar molecules). The type of intramolecular bond between two atoms depends on the electronegativity difference between the two atoms.

1. **Covalent bonds** involve sharing of electrons for atoms of low electronegativity difference (approximately 0.0–1.7). Because of their lower electronegativity difference, covalent bonds are weaker than ionic bonds.
   (a) The electronegativity difference of **nonpolar covalent bonds (weak)** is less than 0.4 (e.g., O_2).
   (b) The electronegativity difference of **polar covalent bonds (stronger)** is approximately 0.4–1.7 (e.g., H_2O).

2. **Ionic bonds are the strongest chemical bonds** (e.g., $Na^{+}Cl^{-}$).

   The electronegativity difference of ionic bonds is greater than 1.7.

   Ionic bonds involve actual transfer of electrons from one atom to another when forming a chemical bond, because the electronegativity difference is high.

   In the solid state, ionic compounds form crystals; in water, they dissolve (at least slightly) to form solutions.

b. Intermolecular Forces

1. **Hydrogen bonding (Figure 2-24)**

   In compounds hydrogen bonding occurs only between hydrogen atoms and nitrogen (N), oxygen (O), or fluorine (F) atoms; the hydrogen "latches on" to the N, O, or F because all three have nonbonding electron pairs (e.g., H_2O, HF, NH_3).

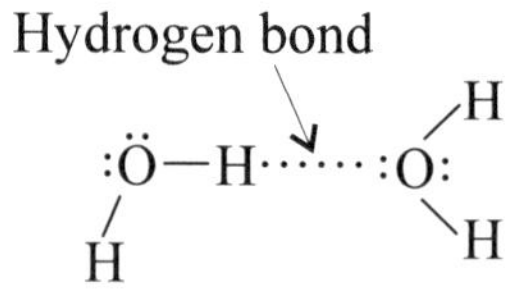

Figure 2-24.
Hydrogen bonding.

   In liquids with hydrogen bonding, the additional intermolecular attraction results in a higher boiling point than a non–hydrogen-bonded compound, such as a hydrocarbon of similar molecular weight (e.g., water and ammonia have much higher boiling points than methane).

2. **Van der Waals (dispersion) forces** are the weakest chemical forces; they are found on covalently bonded atoms that have a small (or zero) difference in electronegativity (e.g., H_2, N_2, O_2). These forces result from the constant movement of electrons, which sets up temporary differences in polarity within a nonpolar molecule. Van der Waals forces cause a temporary dipole between two nonpolar molecules. Figure 2-25 is a mnemonic about bond strength.

MNEMONIC

Ionic	Strongest	**I**onic
Polar covalent	↓	**P**illars
Covalent		**C**arefully
Hydrogen		**H**old
Dipole		**D**own
Van der Waals	Weakest	**V**eakling

Figure 2-25.
Bond strength mnemonic.

c. Formal charge

is the charge that an individual atom bears in an ion or molecule. Remember the following formula:

Formal charge = valence number of the neutral atom − (dots + bonds).

QUESTION

Determine the formal charge for the following.
(a) The aluminum atom in the compound $AlCl_3$
(b) The carbon atom in formic acid (HCOOH)
(c) The oxygen atom in the hydronium ion (H_3O^+)
(d) The nitrogen atom in glycine at a pH of 1

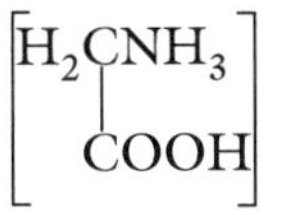
Glycine

ANSWER

To determine the formal charge of an atom, first draw the Lewis structure of the ion or molecule and then apply the formula in Part II E 2 c.

(a) 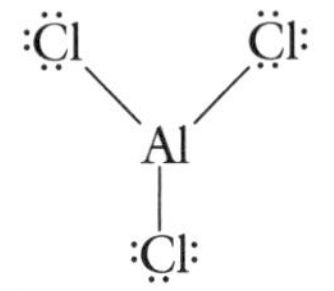
Formal charge of the aluminum atom $= 3 - (0 + 3) = \mathbf{0}$

(b) 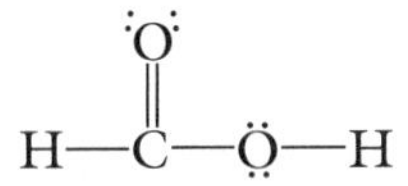
Formal charge of the carbon atom $= 4 - (0 + 4) = \mathbf{0}$

(c) 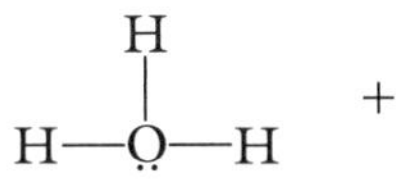
Formal charge of the oxygen atom $= 6 - (2 + 3) = \mathbf{+1}$

(d) 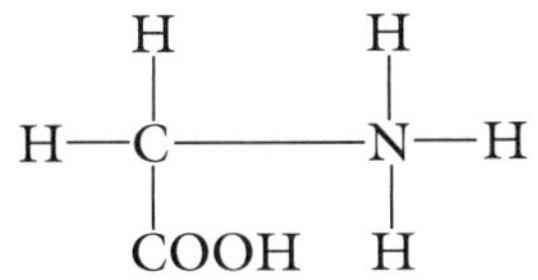
Formal charge of the nitrogen atom $= 5 - (0 + 4) = \mathbf{+1}$

3 MOLES AND STOICHIOMETRY

A **mole** is a unit of measure equal to 6.02×10^{23} atoms or molecules.

$$\text{Moles} = \frac{\text{grams of molecules}}{\text{molecular weight}}$$

Just as 1 dozen donuts always means 12 donuts, 1 mole of atoms (or molecules) is a constant 6.02×10^{23} atoms (or molecules). The concept of moles is used in calculations of the ideal gas law and solution stoichiometries.

QUESTION

Given the reaction

$$C_3H_8 + 5\ O_2 \Leftrightarrow 3\ CO_2 + 4\ H_2O$$

If 88 g of propane (C_3H_8) [MW = 44 g/mol] combust with excess oxygen, how many grams of water are produced?

ANSWER

$$\frac{88\ \text{g}}{44\ \frac{\text{g}}{\text{mole } C_3H_8}} = 2 \text{ moles of propane}$$

With excess O_2, propane (C_3H_8) is the limiting reagent. In terms of the reaction, each mole of propane combusted produces 4 moles of water. Therefore, 2 moles of propane produce 8 moles of water.

$$8 \text{ moles } H_2O \times 18\ \frac{\text{g}}{\text{mole } H_2O} = \mathbf{144\ grams\ of\ H_2O}$$

QUESTION

Calculate the mass percentage of carbon in carbon dioxide (CO_2).

ANSWER

Mass percentage is simply defined as the percentage of mass that a specific atom comprises in a given molecule. Thus, in this problem, the mass percentage of carbon in carbon dioxide can be calculated using the formula below.

$$\text{Mass percentage} = \frac{\text{molecular weight of carbon}}{\text{molecular weight of carbon dioxide}} \times 100$$

$$= \frac{12 \text{ g/mol}}{[12 + 2(16)] \text{ g/mol}} \times 100 \approx \mathbf{27\%}$$

4 QUANTUM NUMBERS

a. Definitions

- The **principal quantum number** is n.

  The number of electrons in each principal quantum level = $2n^2$.

- The **angular momentum quantum number** is *l*.

  l ranges from 0 to (n − 1).

  s: *l* = 0 (The s subshell holds 2 electrons and is spherical.)

  p: *l* = 1 (The p subshell holds 6 electrons and is dumbbell-shaped.)

d: $l = 2$ (The d subshell holds 10 electrons and includes the transition metal elements.)

f: $l = 4$ (The f subshell holds 14 electrons and includes the actinides and lanthanides.)

- The **magnetic quantum number** is m_l.

  m_l ranges from $+l$ to $-l$. Each orbital holds two electrons.

- The **spin quantum number** is m_s.

  m_s equals either $+1/2$ or $-1/2$. Paired electrons in a given orbital must have opposite spin.

b. Hund's Rule

When electrons fill orbitals of the same energy level, they fill all empty orbitals in the lowest unfilled subshell before entering a half-filled orbital. Because all electrons are negatively charged, they avoid inhabiting the same orbital as long as possible.

c. Pauli's Exclusion Principle

No 2 electrons can share the same set of 4 quantum numbers, and no 2 electrons of identical spin can share the same orbital. The order of filling the orbitals follows the diagonal rule—1s, 2s, 2p, 3s, 3p, 4s, 3d, 4p, 5s, 4d, 5p, 6s, and so forth (Figure 2-26).

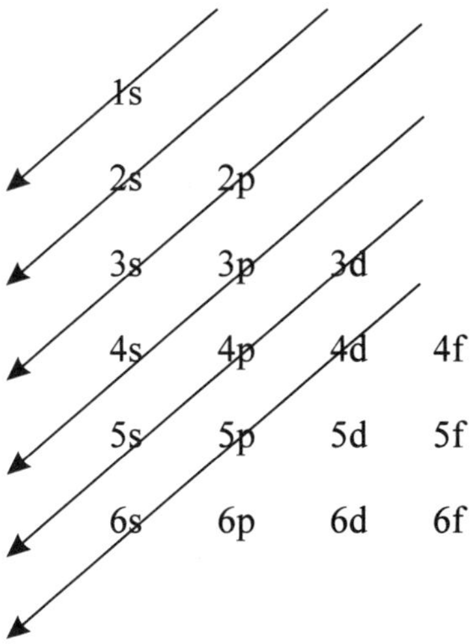

Figure 2-26. Diagonal rule.

STRATEGY

The periodic table (Figure 2-27) organizes the elements according to their respective quantum numbers. For example, the horizontal rows of the periodic table correspond to the principal quantum number. Therefore, carbon and oxygen, which sit in the second row of the periodic table, share the same principal quantum number ($n = 2$). In addition, all the transition metals have occupied d subshells.

s Orbital p Orbital

Periodic Table of the Elements

d Orbital

1 H 1.0																	2 He 4.0
3 Li 6.9	4 Be 9.0											5 B 10.8	6 C 12.0	7 N 14.0	8 O 16.0	9 F 19.0	10 Ne 20.2
11 Na 23.0	12 Mg 24.3											13 Al 27.0	14 Si 28.1	15 P 31.0	16 S 32.1	17 Cl 35.5	18 Ar 39.9
19 K 39.1	20 Ca 40.1	21 Sc 45.0	22 Ti 47.9	23 V 50.9	24 Cr 52.0	25 Mn 54.9	26 Fe 55.8	27 Co 58.9	28 Ni 58.7	29 Cu 63.5	30 Zn 65.4	31 Ga 69.7	32 Ge 72.6	33 As 74.9	34 Se 79.0	35 Br 79.9	36 Kr 83.8
37 Rb 85.5	38 Sr 87.6	39 Y 88.9	40 Zr 91.2	41 Nb 92.9	42 Mo 95.9	43 Tc (98)	44 Ru 101.1	45 Rh 102.9	46 Pd 106.4	47 Ag 107.9	48 Cd 112.4	49 In 114.8	50 Sn 118.7	51 Sb 121.8	52 Te 127.6	53 I 126.9	54 Xe 131.3
55 Cs 132.9	56 Ba 137.3	57 La† 138.9	72 Hf 178.5	73 Ta 180.9	74 W 183.9	75 Re 186.2	76 Os 190.2	77 Ir 192.2	78 Pt 195.1	79 Au 197.0	80 Hg 200.6	81 Ti 204.4	82 Pb 207.2	83 Bi 209.0	84 Po (209)	85 At (210)	86 Rn (222)
87 Fr (223)	88 Ra 226.0	89 Ac‡ 227.0	104 Unq (261)	105 Unp (262)	106 Unh (263)	107 Uns (264)	108 Uno (265)	109 Une (267)									

Metals Nonmetals

Lanthanides	58 Ce 140.1	59 Pr 140.9	60 Nd 144.2	61 Pm (145)	62 Sm 150.4	63 Eu 152.0	64 Gd 157.3	65 Tb 158.9	66 Dy 162.5	67 Ho 164.9	68 Er 167.3	69 Tm 168.9	70 Yb 173.0	71 Lu 175.0
Actinides	90 Th 232.0	91 Pa (231)	92 U 238.0	93 Np (237)	94 Pu (244)	95 Am (243)	96 Cm (247)	97 Bk (247)	98 Cf (251)	99 Es (252)	100 Fm (257)	101 Md (258)	102 No (259)	103 Lr (260)

f Orbital

Figure 2-27. Quantum number arrangement in the periodic table.

QUESTION

1. Which of the following sets of quantum numbers could represent the *first* electron ionized from a calcium atom in its ground state?

	n	l	m_l	m_s
(a)	3	2	2	$-\frac{1}{2}$
(b)	3	3	1	$-\frac{1}{2}$
(c)	4	0	0	$+\frac{1}{2}$
(d)	4	1	1	$+\frac{1}{2}$

2. Write the correct electron configuration for Cu^+ in its ground state.
3. Which ion contains three electrons in its d orbital?

   (a) N^{3-}
   (b) Mn^{2+}
   (c) Ni^+
   (d) Cu^+

ANSWER

1. The answer is (c). In any given atom, the first electron to be ionized is the one in the outermost shell. Because calcium has an atomic number of 20, its electron configuration in its ground state is $1s^2\ 2s^2\ 2p^6\ 3s^2\ 3p^6\ 4s^2$. Thus, the electrons in its outermost shell are in the $4s^2$ orbital, where $n = 4$, $l = 0$, $m_l = 0$, and $m_s = \pm\frac{1}{2}$.
2. Because Cu^+ has +1 charge, the atom has lost one electron, leaving it with a positive charge. Thus, if the atomic number of copper is 29, Cu^+ has 28 electrons. The two electrons in the 4s orbital move to fill the last vacant 3d orbital, resulting in increased stability. Therefore, the electron configuration of Cu^+ in the ground state is $1s^2\ 2s^2 2p^6 3s^2 3p^6 4s^0 3d^{10}$. This exception in the order of electron filling occurs with Cr, Cu, and Ag atoms because a half-filled (d=5) or completely filled (d=10) d subshell provides added stability.
3. The answer is (b). Looking at the periodic table, you can see the transitional metals represent atoms with electrons in their d orbital. Therefore, atoms or ions with three electrons in their d orbitals have atomic numbers of 23, 41, 73, and 105. Thus, the best way to solve this problem is to figure out the number of electrons of the ions listed.
   Remember: Number of electrons = atomic number − (charge of ion).

   N^{3-} Number of electrons $= 7 - (-3) = 10$ electrons

   Mn^{2+} Number of electrons $= 25 - (+2) = 23$ electrons

   Ni^{+} Number of electrons $= 28 - (+1) = 27$ electrons

   Cu^{2+} Number of electrons $= 29 - (+2) = 27$ electrons

   Thus, Mn^{2+} has 3 electrons in its d orbitals.

QUESTION

Why are aqueous ionic solutions of transition metals (e.g., Fe^{3+}, Cu^{2+}) colored?

ANSWER

Aqueous ionic solutions of transition metals often have 1 or more electrons in the ground state of an unfilled high-energy d orbital; therefore, these transition metal electrons can absorb light energy and enter into an excited state. For example, an electron in the 4s subshell of Fe^{3+} (ground state: $1s^2 2s^2 2p^6 3s^2 3p^6 4s^2 3d^3$) can absorb a photon of appropriate energy to enter into a higher energy orbital in the 3d subshell (excited state: $1s^2 2s^2 2p^6 3s^2 3p^6 4s^1 3d^4$). When this electron returns to its ground state (goes back to its lower energy 4s subshell), it emits this lost energy in the form of light of a higher wavelength and lower energy than that originally absorbed by the electron. This emission of energy appears as a colored solution.

5 IDEAL GAS LAW

The ideal gas law is a combination of three basic laws for ideal gases.

a. Boyle's Law

At constant temperature, the pressure of a gas is inversely proportional to the volume.

$$P_1 V_1 = P_2 V_2 \text{ at constant temperature}$$

b. Charles' Law

At constant pressure, the volume of a gas is directly proportional to the temperature.

$$\frac{V_1}{T_1} = \frac{V_2}{T_2} \text{ at constant pressure}$$

c. Avogadro's Law

At constant pressure and temperature, the volume of a gas is directly proportional to the number of moles of gas.

$$PV = nRT$$

$$PV = \frac{gRT}{MW}$$

$$P = \frac{\rho RT}{MW}$$

$$\frac{P_1 V_1}{T_1} = \frac{P_2 V_2}{T_2}$$

P = pressure (atm)
n = moles of gas
T = absolute temperature (K)
MW = molecular weight (g/mol)
V = volume (L)
R = gas constant (0.0821 L·atm/mol·K)
ρ = density (g/L)
g = grams of gas (g)

STRATEGY

Estimate before you calculate.

(1) **PV = nRT** is the key form of the ideal gas law to remember because from this equation, you can derive all its variations through the relationships among temperature, pressure, volume, and number of moles (e.g., moles = mass/molecular weight; density = grams/volume).

When doing calculations based on the ideal gas law, **round R to 0.1 L atm/mol K** to save time. Then, **estimate before you calculate.**

BEWARE

(2) **Standard temperature and pressure** (STP) is defined as 1 atm of pressure at 273 K. At STP, 1 mole of gas occupies 22.4 L. This volume (1 mole gas = 22.4 L) is true **if and only if** the gas is at STP.

The greatest deviation from the ideal gas law occurs when molecules have very low energy (low temperatures) or are very close together (high pressures), because intermolecular (e.g., Van der Waals) forces start affecting these variables.

QUESTION

Thirty grams of nitrogen gas (N_2) is placed in a 2-L container at room temperature (25°C).

(a) What is the pressure in atmospheres of the nitrogen gas?
(b) If the temperature has changed to 0°C and the pressure was held constant at 1 atmosphere, what volume would the nitrogen gas occupy?
(c) At *extremely* high pressures and *extremely* low temperatures (e.g., absolute zero), how would nitrogen gas differ in pressure and volume from an ideal gas?

ANSWER

ESTIMATE

use 0.1 for R

(a) $$PV = \frac{gRT}{MW}$$

$$P = \frac{gRT}{(V)(MW)} = \frac{(30)(0.0821)(298)}{(2)(28)} \approx \frac{(\cancel{30})(0.1)(300)}{(2)(\cancel{30})}$$

$$= 15 \text{ atm}$$

(b) You could use the formula: $P_1V_1/T_1 = P_2V_2/T_2$ to figure out the volume. Nevertheless, a key shortcut is available; the conditions being described in this part of the question are those of standard temperature and pressure (STP) and 1 mol of an ideal gas occupies 22.4 L if and only if it is at STP.

$$\text{moles} = \frac{\text{grams}}{MW}$$

$$= \frac{30}{28} \approx 1 \text{ mol } N_2 \qquad \frac{22.4 \text{ L}}{1 \text{ mol gas}} \times 1 \text{ mol } N_2 = 22.4 \text{ L}$$

(c) Because Van der Waals forces would cause a repulsive force between molecules of N_2 at small intermolecular distances, the volume would be higher and the pressure would be lower than those of an ideal gas.

6 DALTON'S LAW OF PARTIAL PRESSURES

Dalton's law. For a mixture of gases, the total pressure is the sum of the partial pressures of each of the individual gases in the mixture.

$$P_{total} = P_A + P_B + P_C$$

$$X_A = \frac{\text{moles of A}}{\text{total number of moles}}$$

P_{total} = total pressure
$P_{A,B,C}$ = partial pressures of various components
X_A = mole fraction

Dalton's law of partial pressure expressed in terms of mole fraction is:

$$P_A = P_{total}X_A$$

(Raoult's law; see Part II E 8)

7 MOLARITY, MOLALITY, AND NORMALITY

a. Molarity

The concentration of a specific molecule in a solution can be expressed as a ratio of moles of solute to liters of solution.

$$\text{Molarity (M)} = \frac{\text{moles of solute}}{\text{liters of solution}}$$

b. Molality

The concentration of a specific molecule in a solution can be expressed as a ratio of moles of solute to kilograms of solvent.

$$\text{Molality (m)} = \frac{\text{moles of solute}}{\text{kilograms of solvent}}$$

Molarity and molality of dilute aqueous solutions are roughly equivalent if water is the solvent. Remember that the density of water is 1 g/ml; therefore, 1 L of water weighs 1 kg.

c. Normality

The concentration of a specific molecule in a solution can be expressed as a ratio of solute equivalents (e.g., oxidizing/reducing equivalents, acid/base equivalents) to liters of solution.

Normality (N) = molarity × number of equivalents

For example, a 1-molar solution of H_2SO_4, which can donate 2 protons, is a 2-N solution.

d. Dilution Equation

$$M_1 V_1 = M_2 V_2$$

When you dilute an aqueous solution, the number of moles of solute stays constant.

8 COLLIGATIVE PROPERTIES

a. Definition

Physical properties of a solution that depend on the number of particles in the solution are called colligative properties. The four types are:

- Boiling-point elevation: $\Delta T_b = K_b m i$
- Freezing-point depression: $\Delta T_f = K_f m i$
- Osmotic pressure: $P = MRTi$
- Raoult's law: $P_A = P_{total} X_A$

ΔT_b = change in boiling point
K_b = molal boiling-point elevation constant
m = molality
M = molarity
T = temperature (kelvins, K)
P_A = partial pressure of gas A
P_{total} = total pressure of gaseous mixture
ΔT_f = change in freezing point
K_f = molal freezing-point depression constant
i = number of particles per molecule
R = ideal gas law constant (0.08 L/mol K—round to 0.1)
X_A = mole fraction of gas A

b. For Raoult's law,

whenever you put a solid in a liquid, the vapor pressure of the solvent decreases.

BEWARE

- Remember that the m stands for molality, not molarity.
- Remember to take into account the number of particles in the solution (i).
- The formulas for boiling-point elevation and freezing-point depression give you the **change** in the boiling point and freezing point, respectively. To derive the new freezing point (or the boiling point) of the solution, subtract this number from the freezing point or add this number to the boiling point of the solvent.

$$T_b^{new} = T_b^{pure} + K_b mi$$

$$T_f^{new} = T_f^{pure} - K_f mi$$

QUESTION

Which aqueous solution has the highest boiling point?
(a) 1 molal NaCl
(b) 2 molal $MgCl_2$
(c) 4 molal glucose
(d) 2 molal KCl

ANSWER

The equation to use is:

$$\Delta T_b = K_b m i$$

Because i = 3 for $MgCl_2$ (i.e., $MgCl_2$ splits into 1 Mg^{2+} ion and 2 Cl^- ions) and it is a 2-molal solution, it has the highest boiling-point elevation. Therefore, the correct answer is (b).

9 EQUILIBRIUM: GENERAL CONCEPTS

Equilibrium is the situation or stage when the rate of the forward reaction is equal to the rate of the reverse reaction; at that point, the concentrations of the reactants and products no longer change with time. At equilibrium, $\Delta G = 0$.

In the reaction:

$$aA(aq) + bB(g) + cC(s) \Leftrightarrow dD(aq) + eE(l) + fF(g)$$

$$K_{eq} = \frac{D^d F^f}{A^a B^b}$$

Remember that K_{eq} is the ratio of products over reactants, with the mole coefficient as the exponent. In addition, only gases and aqueous solutions figure into the K_{eq} (not solids or liquids). From the K_{eq}, you can calculate the **Gibbs free energy** (ΔG), using the following relationship:

$$\Delta G = -RT\ln(K_{eq})$$

R = gas constant
T = temperature (K)

10 LE CHATELIER'S PRINCIPLE

If the environment changes, the reaction always shifts to a new equilibrium to reduce the stress on the system.

For example, if the temperature of a system increases, the reaction shifts to absorb heat (or vice versa if the temperature decreases). If pressure increases, the reaction shifts to the side that has fewer moles of gas (and the compounds take up less space). If you add more of a reactant or product, the reaction shifts to consume some (but not all) of the added reactant or product.

QUESTION

In the exothermic reaction

$$C_3H_8(g) + 5\ O_2(g) \Leftrightarrow 3\ CO_2(g) + 4H_2O(g)$$

which way does the reaction shift if
(a) the temperature is increased?
(b) the pressure is increased?
(c) a dehydrating agent is added to the reaction vessel?

ANSWER

(a) The reaction is exothermic; therefore, heat is a product of the reaction.

$$C_3H_8 + 5\ O_2 \Leftrightarrow 3\ CO_2 + 4\ H_2O + \text{heat}$$

If the temperature is increased (i.e., more heat is added), the reaction shifts to the **left.**

(b) If the pressure is increased, the effective volume decreases, and the reaction shifts to the side that has the lower number of moles of gas. In this case, the reaction shifts to the **left.**

(c) If a dehydrating agent is added to the reaction vessel, this agent absorbs all the water. Because you are removing one of the products of the reaction (i.e., water), the reaction shifts to the **right.**

11 PHASE EQUILIBRIA

Phase diagram. Plotting the pressure of a compound versus the temperature for its three basic states (solid, liquid, or gas) lets you predict the conditions for equilibrium among the states of the compound (Figure 2-28).

Water is most dense at 4°C; therefore, an increase in pressure at the triple point favors the liquid phase. This situation explains why segment BC has a negative slope. Carbon dioxide is most dense when it is solid; therefore, segment BC in this diagram has a positive slope. **An increase in pressure at the triple point favors the most dense phase.**

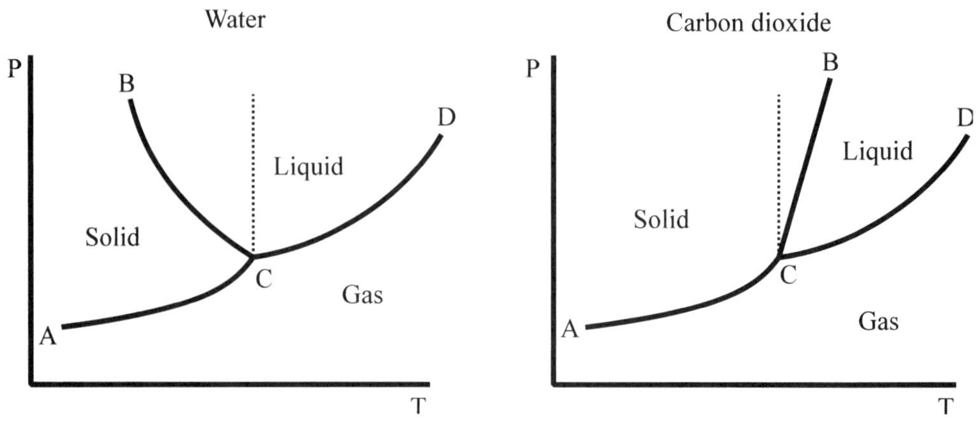

Figure 2-28. Pressure–temperature phase diagrams for water and carbon dioxide. *AC* = sublimation: a phase change from solid to gas that bypasses the liquid phase; *CD* = boiling/condensation; *D* = critical point: the temperature at which a pressure increase can no longer cause condensation; *BC* = freezing/melting; *C* = triple point (solid, liquid, and gas phases coexist in equilibrium): when an increase in pressure favors the densest phase.

12 SOLUBILITY EQUILIBRIA, PRECIPITATION, AND THE COMMON ION EFFECT

a. Solubility equilibria

is the state of equilibrium between the solid form of a compound (precipitate) and its aqueous form in a specific solvent.

$$BaSO_4(s) \Leftrightarrow Ba^{2+}(aq) + SO_4(aq)$$

$$K_{sp} = [Ba^{2+}][SO_4^{2-}]$$

K_{sp} = solubility product constant

The solubility constant (K_{sp}) is a measure of the amount of solid that is able to be dissolved in a saturated aqueous solution. Therefore, the lower the K_{sp}, the more insoluble the compound. In nonequilibrium conditions:

$$Q = [Ba^{2+}][SO_4^{2-}]$$

Q = nonequilibrium ion product

Equilibrium is reached when $Q = K_{sp}$.

b. Precipitation

is the formation of an insoluble, solid compound from its ions in solution.

- If $Q > K_{sp}$, the solution precipitates (the gunk settles at the bottom of the beaker).
- If $Q < K_{sp}$, the solution does not precipitate (all of the compound dissolves in solution).

c. Common Ion Effect

A compound is less soluble in a solution that contains an ion identical to one of its dissociation products. Le Chatelier's principle fully explains the common ion effect.

For example, $BaSO_4$ is more soluble in a 1-M NaCl solution than in a 1-M solution of $BaCl_2$ because the Ba^{2+} is an ion present in both the compound and the solvent. The Ba^{2+} in the solvent shifts the reaction to the left, favoring formation of the $BaSO_4$ precipitate.

QUESTION

One liter of a 0.05 M Fe^{3+} solution is prepared at a pH of 7. [K_{sp} of $Fe(OH)_3 = 6.3 \times 10^{-38}$]

(a) Will a precipitate form?
(b) At what pH will a precipitate start to form?
(c) Will the addition of HCl increase or decrease the solubility of $Fe(OH)_3$?

ANSWER

(a) For a precipitate to form, Q must be greater than K_{sp}. Thus, to solve this problem, we need to calculate the value of Q:

$$Q = [Fe^{3+}][OH^-]^3$$

$$pOH = 14 - pH = -\log[OH^-]$$

$$pOH = 14 - 7 = -\log[OH^-]$$

$$\text{Concentration of } (OH^-) = 1 \times 10^{-7}$$

$$Q = (5 \times 10^{-2})(1 \times 10^{-7})^3 = 5 \times 10^{-23};$$
which is greater than K_{sp} of 6.3×10^{-38}

Because Q is greater than K_{sp}, a precipitate will form.

(b) A precipitate will start to form as Q becomes greater than K_{sp}. Thus,

$$K_{sp} = 6.3 \times 10^{-38} = [Fe^{3+}][OH^-]^3$$

$$6.3 \times 10^{-38} = [5 \times 10^{-2}][OH^-]^3$$

$$\text{Concentration of } OH^- \text{ when precipitate begins to form} = \sqrt[3]{\frac{6.3 \times 10^{-38}}{5 \times 10^{-2}}} \approx 1 \times 10^{-12}$$

$$pOH = -\log(1 \times 10^{-12}) = 12$$

$$pH = 14 - pOH = 14 - 12 = 2$$

Therefore, a precipitate begins to form when the pH rises above 2.

(c) Look at the solubility reaction:

$$Fe(OH)_3(s) \rightarrow Fe^{3+}(aq) + 3OH^-(aq)$$

Adding HCl will neutralize and decrease the concentration of OH^-. Based on Le Chatelier's principle, decreasing the concentration of OH^- will shift the reaction to the right, thus decreasing the amount of precipitate that is formed.

13 CALORIMETRY AND HEAT TRANSFER

a. Calorimetry

is a technique that permits the measurement of heat absorbed or released from a physical process such as a chemical reaction. A change in phase or temperature can be tracked as a transfer of heat in potential energy.

For simple heating of a compound without a change in phase, use the following equation:

$$q = mc\Delta T$$

c = specific heat: the number of joules or calories it takes to heat 1 gram of a particular compound 1 Kelvin

q = heat added (calories or joules)
m = mass
ΔT = change in temperature

b. Heat Transfer

For the amount of heat added or released from a change in phase of a compound at a specific temperature:

$$q = mL$$

q = heat added (calories or joules)
m = mass
L = latent heat (heat of fusion or vaporization): the number of joules or calories it takes to melt/freeze (equal but opposite in sign) or vaporize/condense (equal but opposite in sign)

A phase change can also happen at constant temperature (see Figure 2–28). Heat is still transferred.

$$c_{water} = 1\ \frac{\text{cal}}{\text{g}\cdot{}^\circ\text{C}} = 4.18\ \frac{\text{J}}{\text{g}\cdot{}^\circ\text{C}}$$

c = specific heat of water

MNEMONIC

Heat (q) = MCAT (mcΔT). "The heat is on" when you are taking the MCAT.

QUESTION

How much heat does it take to bring 5 g of ice at −10°C to 5 g of steam at 120°C? It is given that the specific heat of water, steam, and ice is 1 kcal/g °C; the heat of fusion of water is 20 kcal/g; and the heat of vaporization of water is 40 kcal/g.

ANSWER

This problem consists of the following steps:

1. Heat ice at −10°C to ice at 0°C

$$q_1 = mc\Delta T = 5{\cdot}1{\cdot}10 = 50 \text{ kcal}$$

2. Heat ice at 0°C to water at 0°C (melting)

$$q_2 = mL = 5{\cdot}20 = 100 \text{ kcal}$$

3. Heat water at 0°C to water at 100°C

$$q_3 = mc\Delta T = 5{\cdot}1{\cdot}100 = 500 \text{ kcal}$$

4. Heat water at 100°C to steam at 100°C (boiling)

$$q_4 = mL = 5{\cdot}40 = 200 \text{ kcal}$$

5. Heat steam at 100°C to steam at 120°C

$$q_5 = mc\Delta T = 5{\cdot}1{\cdot}20 = 100 \text{ kcal}$$

$$q_{total} = q_1 + q_2 + q_3 + q_4 + q_5 = 950 \text{ kcal}$$

14 THERMODYNAMICS

a. Enthalpy (ΔH)

is the change in heat during a reaction that occurs at constant pressure. If a negative ΔH means that the reaction gives off heat (exothermic), a positive ΔH means that the reaction absorbs heat (endothermic).

TABLE 2-4. Free energy of a reaction

If ΔG is	The reaction is
Negative	Spontaneous
Zero	At equilibrium
Positive	Nonspontaneous

b. Entropy (ΔS)

is the amount of unusable energy (disorder) in a reaction. ΔS corresponds to the change in the randomness or disorder during a reaction. If ΔS is positive, the reaction gets more random and disordered (e.g., the transition from solid to liquid). If it is negative, the reaction gets more ordered.

As a general rule, the **entropy of gases > liquids > solids.**

c. Free energy of a reaction (ΔG)

This quantity tells us whether the reaction is spontaneous (Table 2-4).

d. Gibbs-Helmholtz equation (Table 2-5)

$$\Delta G = \Delta H - T\Delta S$$

ΔG = Gibbs' free energy (J) ΔH = enthalpy (J)
T = temperature (K) ΔS = entropy (J/K)

e. Laws of Thermodynamics

1. **First law of thermodynamics** states that the internal energy of an isolated system (E) is constant. To change the internal energy (E) of a system, you

TABLE 2-5. Dependence of ΔG on the sign and magnitude of ΔH and ΔS

If ΔH is	And ΔS is	ΔG is
Positive	**Negative**	Always positive A nonspontaneous reaction at all temperatures
Negative	**Positive**	Always negative A spontaneous reaction at all temperatures
Positive	**Positive**	Positive at low temperatures Negative at high temperatures
Negative	**Negative**	Negative at low temperatures Positive at high temperatures

must either do work (w) or add or remove heat (q); and, as a result, the system is no longer isolated.

$$E = q + w$$

2. **Second law of thermodynamics.** In a spontaneous reaction, entropy always increases—as long as you take into account not just the system but the entire environment.

3. **Third law of thermodynamics.** The entropy of a perfect crystal at absolute zero is 0; in other words, a perfect crystal is in perfect order at absolute zero. However, this state can never be attained (i.e., some entropy always exists).

f. Thermodynamics and the Facts of Life

MNEMONIC

The laws of thermodynamics are like the facts of life.

1. **First law of thermodynamics.** A no-win situation. You can never win (get more energy than you put in); you can only break even ($\Delta E = q + w$).
2. **Second law of thermodynamics.** Murphy's law. You will not be lucky enough to break even—you will always lose. (A spontaneous reaction always involves a loss of energy because of an increase in entropy.)
3. **Third law of thermodynamics.** Nobody's perfect. Some entropy is always present (unless you have a perfect crystal at absolute zero).

15 ENTHALPY: HEAT OF FORMATION, BOND ENERGY, AND HESS'S LAW

a. Heat of Formation

The heat of formation (ΔH_f) is the heat of the reaction that produces a compound in its standard state from its elements. The heat of a reaction (ΔH_{rxn}) equals the difference between the product's and the reactant's heat of formation (ΔH_f).

$$\Delta H_{rxn} = \Sigma H_f(\text{products}) - \Sigma H_f(\text{reactants})$$

ΔH (also known as the enthalpy change) signifies the change in enthalpy caused by the reaction. For example, a reaction that gives off 40 kcal per mole of reactant (i.e., raises the temperature of 1 kg of water by 40 degrees) has a ΔH of -40 kcal/mol. For the reaction

$$2A + B \rightarrow A_2B$$

$\Delta H_f A = 20$ kcal/mol
$\Delta H_f B = -10$ kcal/mol
$\Delta H_f A_2B = 40$ kcal/mol

To get ΔH for this reaction, subtract the reactants' heats of formation from the products' heats of formation. Be careful to take into account the number of moles of each product and reactant. ΔH for this reaction would be calculated as follows:

$$\Delta H = \left(40\ \frac{\text{kcal}}{\text{mole}}\right)(1\ \text{mole}) - \left[\left(-10\ \frac{\text{kcal}}{\text{mole}}\right)(1\ \text{mole}) + \left(20\ \frac{\text{kcal}}{\text{mole}}\right)(2\ \text{mole})\right] = 10\ \frac{\text{kcal}}{\text{mole}}$$

b. Hess's law

states that ΔHs are additive; therefore:

$$X \xrightarrow{\Delta H = a} Y$$

$$Y \xrightarrow{\Delta H = b} Z$$

$$X \xrightarrow{\Delta H = a+b} Z$$

c. Calculating ΔH from Bond Energies

Breaking bonds is an endothermic process ($\Delta H > 0$) requiring an input of energy. Forming bonds is an exothermic process ($\Delta H < 0$) involving the release of heat. You can use bond enthalpies or energies (the two terms are used interchangeably) to calculate the enthalpy of a reaction. Look at the following reaction:

$$CH_3OH(g) + \tfrac{3}{2}\,O_2(g) \rightarrow CO_2(g) + 2H_2O$$

The heat required to break the bonds of the reactants:

$$\Delta H = 3{\cdot}(C{-}H) + (C{-}O) + \tfrac{3}{2}{\cdot}(O{=}O) + (O{-}H)$$

$$\Delta H = 3{\cdot}(412\ \text{kJ}) + 360\ \text{kJ} + \tfrac{3}{2}{\cdot}(498\ \text{kJ}) + 463\ \text{kJ} = 2806\ \text{kJ}$$

The heat released when the new bonds form to make the products:

$$\Delta H = 2{\cdot}(C{=}O) + 4{\cdot}(O{-}H)$$

$$\Delta H = 2{\cdot}(803\ \text{kJ}) + 4{\cdot}(463\ \text{kJ}) = 3458\ \text{kJ}$$

$$\Delta H = (\text{Heat needed to break bonds}) - (\text{Heat released when making bonds})$$

$$\Delta H = 2806\ \text{kJ} - 3458\ \text{kJ} = -652\ \frac{\text{kJ}}{\text{mole}}\ CH_3OH$$

16 CHEMICAL KINETICS

Activation energy. The minimum kinetic energy needed for a reaction to proceed (Figure 2-29). The activation energy allows reactants to progress to the transition state (D) of a reaction before yielding products.

As Figure 2-29 shows, enzymes (biological catalysts) and other catalysts increase the rate of the reaction by lowering the activation energy of **both** the forward and reverse

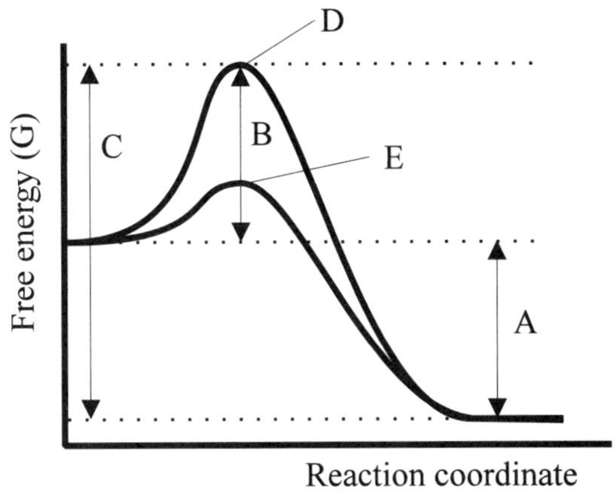

Figure 2-29. Activation energy diagram. *A* = ΔG of the reaction; here, ΔG is negative, so the reaction is spontaneous; a reaction with a positive ΔG is nonspontaneous. *B* = activation energy of the forward reaction. *C* = activation energy of the reverse reaction. *D* = transition state (activated complex); it is the most unstable arrangement of atoms/molecules in the reaction. *E* = path of the catalyzed or enzymatic reaction.

reactions, but they do **not** change *ΔG*.

A rise in temperature, which means an increased number of molecular collisions (increased kinetic energy), results in an increased rate of reaction.

A reaction proceeds along a reaction coordinate from reactants to products.

QUESTION

For the reaction

$$A + B \rightarrow C$$

the following data were obtained:

Experiment No.	[A]	[B]	Rate
1	0.35	0.20	3.0
2	0.70	0.20	12.0
3	0.35	0.40	6.0
4	0.70	0.40	24.0

What is the rate law for this reaction?

ANSWER

Comparing reactions 1 and 2 shows that as the concentration of A doubles, (whereas the concentration of B remained constant), the rate of reaction increases fourfold. The rate order with respect to reactant A is calculated by solving for n in the equation $2^n = 4$. Here, the rate order (n) is 2. In comparing reactions 1 and 3, as the concentration of B doubles (whereas the concentration of A remains constant), the rate of reaction increases twofold. Therefore, the rate order with respect to reactant B is 1 ($2^n = 2$). **Therefore, the rate = $k[A]^2[B]$, and the overall order for the reaction is 3.**

17 REDOX REACTIONS AND VOLTAIC/ELECTROLYTIC CELLS

a. Redox reactions

involve the oxidation and reduction (transfer of electrons) of reactants in the formation of products.

MNEMONIC

"**Leo** says **Ger**."

Loss of **e**lectrons is **o**xidation; **g**ain in **e**lectrons is **r**eduction.

b. Voltaic Cell

In a voltaic cell, anion flow goes from anode to cathode.

MNEMONIC

"**An Ox** and **red cat**."

Oxidation occurs at the **an**ode (−); **red**uction occurs at the **cat**hode (+).

c. Electrolytic Cell

In an electrolytic cell, anions migrate to the anode and cations migrate to the cathode (i.e., electron flow is opposite that of a voltaic cell) [Figure 2-30].

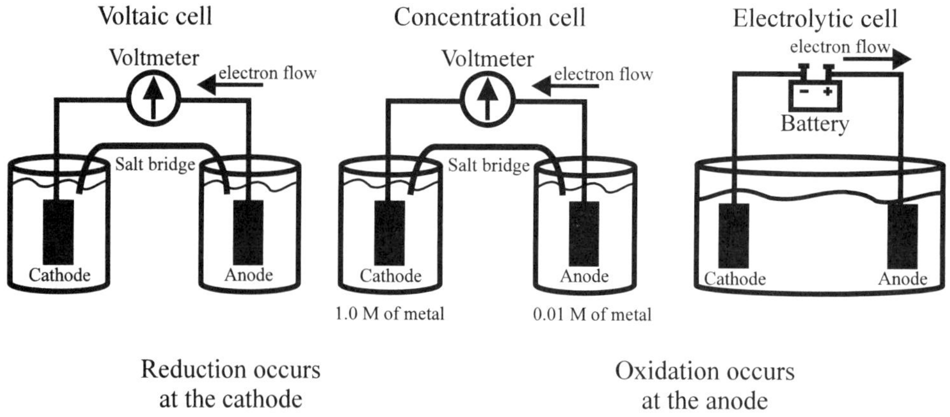

Figure 2-30.
Voltaic versus electrolytic cell.

18 REDOX, NERNST EQUATION, AND FREE ENERGY

The **Nernst equation** relates the voltage E derived from a voltaic cell to the free energy ΔG and equilibrium constant K_{eq} of the chemical reaction driving the battery.

$$E_{cell} = E^0 - \frac{0.06}{n} \log(Q)$$

E_{cell} = voltage derived from a chemical battery
n = number of electrons transferred in the redox reaction
Q = nonequilibrium ion product (mass action expression for the chemical battery reaction)
E^0 = standard reduction potential for the voltaic cell (all reactants and products at 1 M)

$$\Delta G = -nFE$$
$$= -RT\ln(K_{eq})$$

n = charge of the ionic species in solution
F = Faraday's constant, 96,500 coul/mol of electrons
T = temperature (Kelvin)
R = 8.31 J/K
K_{eq} = equilibrium constant of the reaction

QUESTION

A 10-amp battery is used to drive the following half-reaction:

$$Au^{2+}(aq) + 2e \rightarrow Au(s)$$

The battery is connected to this circuit, which runs for 30 minutes. How much solid gold is formed?

ANSWER

To answer this question, you must know the definition of a coulomb (coul).

1 coulomb = a unit of charge = (1 amp)(sec)

Therefore, in this reaction:

charge = (10 amp)(30 min)(60 sec/min) = 18,000 coul

Now, use Faraday's law to determine the moles of electrons produced:

[(18,000 coul)/(96,500 coul/mol electron)] = ~0.2 mol electrons

Then use stoichiometry to derive the moles of gold formed:

0.2 mol electrons × (1 mol Au/2 mol e^-) = 0.1 mol Au (s)

To find the mass (grams) of gold formed, multiply the moles of gold by its molecular weight:

0.1 mol Au × 197 g/mol = **~20 g of solid gold formed**

19 ACID-BASE DEFINITIONS (TABLE 2-6)

TABLE 2-6. Definition of acid and base

Chemical Type	Arrhenius Definition	Bronsted-Lowry Definition	Lewis Definition
Acid	Produces H^+ or H_3O^+ upon dissociation in water	H^+ (proton) donor	Electron (e^-) acceptor
Base	Produces OH^- upon dissociation in water	H^+ (proton) acceptor	Electron (e^-) donor

STRATEGY

If a question asks how a certain molecule (e.g., coordination complex, reactant) functions in a given reaction, the answer may use these terms.

20 ACID-BASE CHEMISTRY

TEST CORRELATION

On the physical sciences section of the MCAT, you may get a passage about physiological buffers in your body. The major physiological buffer of blood is bicarbonate (HCO_3^-), which maintains blood pH at its normal level of 7.4. You must know how buffers act, how to interpret a titration curve involving a buffer, and how to use the Henderson-Hasselbalch equation.

a. Henderson-Hasselbalch equation

$$pH = pK_a + \log\left(\frac{[A^-]}{[HA]}\right)$$

$$pOH = pK_b + \log\left(\frac{[BH^+]}{[B]}\right)$$

$pK_a = -\log(K_a)$
$pH = -\log([H^+])$
K_a = equilibrium constant of acid dissociation

$[HA]$ = concentration of weak acid (M)
$[A^-]$ = concentration of conjugate base (M)
$[B]$ = concentration of weak base (M)
$[BH^+]$ = concentration of conjugate acid (M)

These equations show that the greater the K_a, the lower the pK_a, and the stronger the acid (the lower the pH).

pH works on a logarithmic scale. For example, there is a 100-fold difference in hydrogen ions between a solution with a pH of 2 and a solution with a pH of 4.

When thinking about K_b and pOH, remember that

$$K_w = K_a \times K_b = 1 \times 10^{-14}$$

and that

$$pOH = 14 - pH$$

b. Strong Acid/Strong Base

A strong acid or base dissociates **completely** in water (i.e., moles of strong acid = moles of H^+).

- The six strong acids are HCl, HBr, HI, H_2SO_4, HNO_3, and $HClO_4$. A strong acid has a large K_a. K_a is not useful for strong acids and bases; theoretically, it would be infinite.
- The strong bases are the metal hydroxides from rows 1 and 2 of the periodic table (alkali and alkali earth metals), including NaOH, KOH, and $Ca(OH)_2$, with the exception of Mg $(OH)_2$, which is a weak base.

c. Titration curves

show the pH as a function of the amount of acid [H^+] or base [OH^-] added.

d. Equivalence point

occurs in a titration when the moles of acid equal the moles of base (i.e., equal numbers of equivalents of the acid/base and the titrant have been combined) [Table 2-7].

In the titration of a weak acid with a strong base, the equivalence point is reached when the moles of weak acid equal the moles of strong base (Figure 2-31). Note that this does not mean that concentrations of H^+ equal moles of OH^- (since you usually titrate a weak acid/base with a strong base/acid—otherwise the equivalence point would always be at a pH of 7).

Take, for example, the addition of NaOH to acetic acid CH_3COOH. At low pH, before the NaOH is added, the majority of the acetic acid is protonated. However, as the NaOH concentration increases, an increasing fraction of acetate

TABLE 2-7. When pH = pK_a or pH = equivalence point

When pH = Equivalence Point	When pH = pK_a
Steepest part of the titration curve	Flattest part of the titration curve
At this point, there is 100% of one species (either A^- or HA)	At this point, there is 50% A^-, 50% HA
Least buffering capacity at this point of the curve	Greatest buffering capacity at this point of the curve
At this point, moles of acid = moles of base	At this point, ($[A^-]/[HA]$) = 1

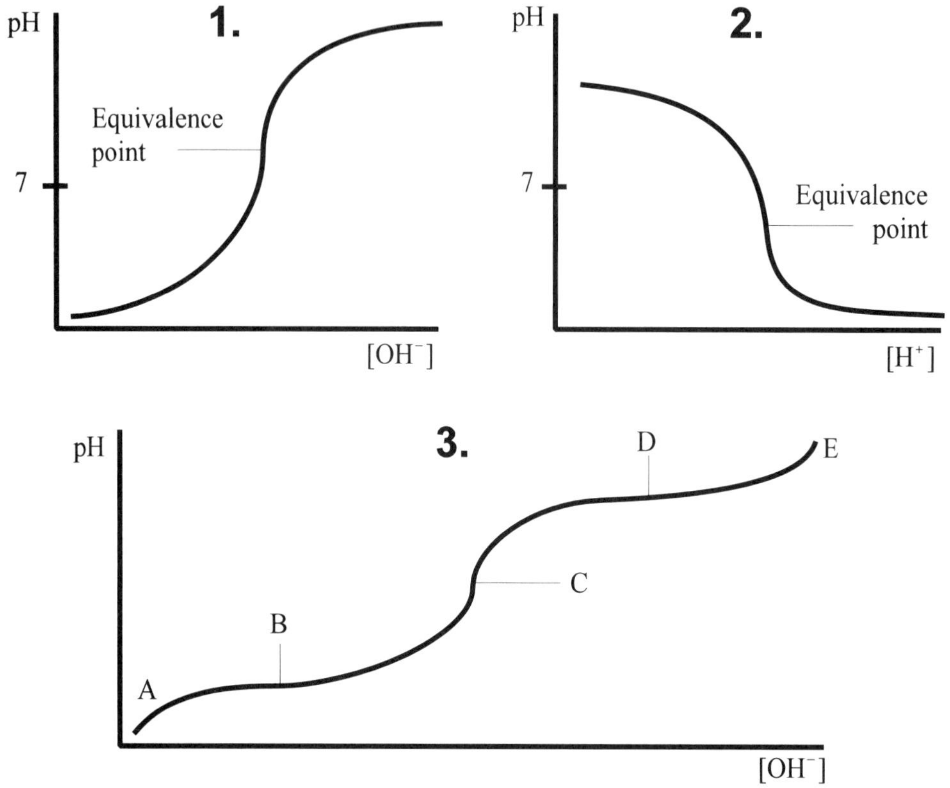

Figure 2-31. Titration of *(1)* a weak acid with a strong base; *(2)* a weak base with a strong acid; and *(3)* a weak diprotic acid with a strong base. *A* = 100% H_2CO_3 (equivalence point #1); *B* = 50% H_2CO_3, 50% HCO_3^- (pH = pK_{a1}); *C* = 100% HCO_3^- (equivalence point #2); *D* = 50% HCO_3^-, 50% CO_3^{2-} (pH = pK_{a2}); *E* = 100% CO_3^{2-} (equivalence point #3).

CH_3COO^- is produced. At the pK_a, the concentration of CH_3COOH is equal to the concentration of CH_3COO^-. For concentrations of OH^- greater than needed to get to the equivalence point, the concentration of CH_3COO^- is greater than the concentration of CH_3COOH.

For a weak acid added to a strong base, the equivalence point is above the neutral pH of 7. For a weak base added to a strong acid, the equivalence point is below the neutral pH of 7. At points B and D, when pH = pK_a, the compound shows the greatest buffering capacity to resist changes in pH (i.e., the flat parts of the titration curve).

F Introduction to the Biological Sciences

Do not get bogged down on any one question or passage.

The last thing you want to see after 3 hours on the verbal reasoning, physical sciences, and essay sections is another section. Then, just when you have had enough, the AAMC hits you with the biological sciences section. Like the physical sciences section, this section has 77 questions to be completed in 100 minutes. Once again, you want to spend 1.25 minutes per question (which leaves you a little extra time for answering hard questions and for checking your answers). Do not get bogged down on any one question or passage; if a particular passage gives you a lot of trouble, skip it and return to it at the end. You can use "batch fill-in" on the answer sheets, but never go to the next passage without filling in the answers from the previous one. The MCAT does not have a penalty for guessing, so answer all questions.

The biggest non–content-related problem that students have with the biological sciences section is fatigue. You begin taking the biological sciences section after hours of previous testing. Most college students have experience with 3- or 4-hour tests, but few have experienced an all-day affair like the MCAT.

- During the break between the essay and the biological sciences section, take a walk outside and load up on sugar (e.g., a candy bar, an endurance bar [Power Bar], a Coke, or even one of the carbo-loading sports drinks).
- Be aware that most people catch their "second wind" and experience increased alertness in the middle of the biological sciences section (the "late afternoon recovery"). Once you finish this section, review your work for careless mistakes.

According to the AAMC, 65% of the biological sciences section tests concepts from biology and only 35% asks about organic chemistry topics. However, students say that the mix has been about 50–50 on recent exams. Given that the majority of premedical students have strong biology backgrounds and that the AAMC grades the MCAT on a curve, you better know your stuff! Most students have taken more than enough biology courses and tests before they take the MCAT. However, your success on this section does not depend on knowledge of advanced biology. Whereas courses in upper-division biology help you in medical school, much of the advanced biology does not help on the biological sciences section of the MCAT (with the exception of physiology and biochemistry). Instead, you should master the basic biological concepts and processes. Do **not** get lost relearning all the details from all your biology classes. For example, you should master the reactants, products, location, and purpose of glycolysis and the Krebs cycle, but you do not need to memorize all of the intermediate steps.

When studying biology, stress the high-yield concepts associated with the endocrine system, physiology, neurobiology, biochemistry, and cell biology.

Organic chemistry is often the premedical student's worst nightmare. It is curious that medical school requires two semesters of organic chemistry. Is it inertia from some 50 years ago, when the biochemical pathways were first discovered? More cynically, is it because admissions committees want to see how you fare under the pressure of blind memorization for no apparent purpose? **The MCAT, however, has been revamped, and the organic chemistry tested on the MCAT is mostly passage-based and all multiple choice. You do not need to memorize every reaction, reagent, and mechanism all over again.** Instead, focus your preparation on reviewing the important concepts of organic chemistry, such as S_N1/E_1 S_N2/E_2 reactions, Markovnikov/anti-Markovnikov addition, and the structures and physical/chemical properties of the different functional groups. Often, the important reactions surface in the passage. In addition, review the different organic chemistry laboratory procedures, such as separation, recrystallization, nuclear magnetic resonance (NMR), infrared (IR) spectroscopy, and chromatography.

Although the test writers state that organic chemistry makes up only 35% of the biological sciences section of the MCAT, many students who have recently taken the exam agree that the split between organic chemistry and biology in the biological sciences section is 50–50.

Know important concepts such as S_N1/S_N2 substitution and Grignard reactions; if you **understand** these reactions, you will be able to deduce the answers to more difficult reaction-based questions presented on the actual exam. Most important, **don't sweat it.** Everyone hates this section, and you need not know most of the brutal details of organic chemistry to do well on the MCAT.

G Organic Chemistry

1 IUPAC NOMENCLATURE AND FUNCTIONAL GROUPS

a. International Union of Pure and Applied Chemistry (IUPAC) Nomenclature

The rules of naming molecules follow this international convention system (Table 2-8). You probably already know that organic chemistry has its own numbering system.

TABLE 2-8. Organic nomenclature for number

Number	Prefix	Number	Prefix
1	meth- (form-)	**6**	hex-
2	eth- (acet-)	**7**	hept-
3	prop-	**8**	oct-
4	but-	**9**	non-
5	pent-	**10**	dec-

b. Functional Groups

In addition, you need to know the **functional groups** in order to name the organic molecules. Functional groups make a molecule distinctive by changing its properties and reactivity. Table 2-9 shows the most important groups to know.

STRATEGY

Use the process of elimination to determine the name of a compound.

Check the multiple-choice answers if you are confused. Start by eliminating answers with the wrong prefix or suffix; then choose from what remains.

- When a molecule has more than one chain or functional group, always name the longest chain first. In addition, assign side chains by the lowest number possible. Often two answers to a question will make sense, but only one follows this IUPAC convention.
- Many common molecules have other common non-IUPAC names, such as acetone (IUPAC name is propanone) or formic acid (methanoic acid). For purposes of the MCAT, know the IUPAC nomenclature system, not these common names; they may appear in a passage, but in most cases the test gives the modern name for the molecule.

TABLE 2-9. Common functional groups

Name	Group	Suffix	Properties	Example
Alkanes	R-CH_2-R	"ane"	1. Formula of C_nH_{2n+2} 2. Nonpolar 3. Boiling and melting points rise with number of carbons, but they decrease with branching 4. All alkanes > 3 carbons have more than one isomer	CH_4 methane
Alkenes	R-CH=CH-R	"ene"	Similar to alkanes—formula of C_nH_{2n}	C_3H_6 propene
Alkynes	R-C≡C-R	"yne"	Similar to alkanes and alkenes—formula of C_nH_{2n-2}. The C≡C bond is shorter and stronger than C–C or C=C.	C_4H_6 butyne
Aromatic Rings	Ph-R	"benzene" "phenyl-"	1. Very stable (Kekulé's ring) 2. Bonds intermediate in length and strength between single and double bonds (hybrid bonds due to resonance)	C_6H_6 benzene C_7H_8 methyl benzene, or toluene
Alcohols	R-OH	"ol"	1. High boiling points due to hydrogen bonding 2. Excellent solutes; dissolve readily in water (polar) 3. Excellent protic solvents due to hydrogen bonding	C_2H_5OH ethanol
Carboxylic Acids	R-COOH	"oic acid"	1. Not as strong as inorganic acids (e.g., HCl); soluble in aqueous base 2. Polar: can form hydrogen bonds 3. Acids with four or fewer carbons are soluble in water; the rest are insoluble 4. Very high boiling points; higher than corresponding alcohols	CH_3-COOH ethanoic acid
Esters	R-COOR	"ate"	1. Polar: can form hydrogen bonds 2. Characteristic odors (like flowers) 3. Larger esters are insoluble in water but soluble in nonpolar organic solvents	C_2H_5-COO-CH_3 methyl propanoate
Ethers	R-O-R	"ether"	1. Very weak polarity 2. Relatively insoluble in water 3. Excellent organic solvents	C_2H_5-O-C_2H_5 diethyl ether
Aldehydes	R-CHO	"aldehyde"	1. Polar compounds 2. High boiling points (lower than alcohols) 3. Capable of hydrogen bonding (acceptor) 4. Only smaller aldehydes are soluble in water	CH_2O formaldehyde
Ketones	R-CO-R	"one"	Similar to aldehydes	CH_3-CO-CH_3 propanone (acetone)
Amines	R-NH_2 R-NH-R′ R-N-R′R″	"amine"	1. Polar—form hydrogen bonds 2. Soluble in water or organic solvents 3. Soluble in dilute acid	CH_3-NH-CH_3 dimethyl amine

Using the numeric prefixes and functional group suffixes, you should be able to name any compound given on the examination.

QUESTION

Give the proper IUPAC nomenclature for the following compounds:

(1)
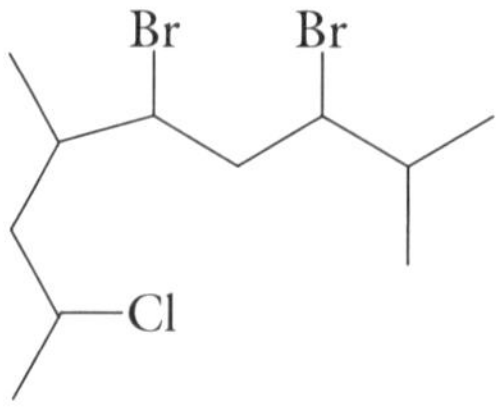

(2)
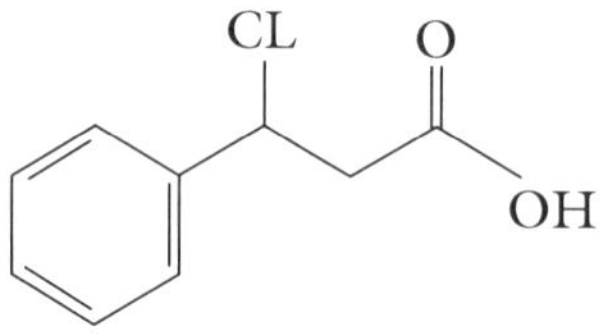

(3)
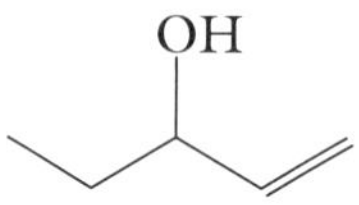

(4)
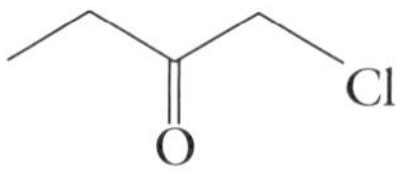

(5)
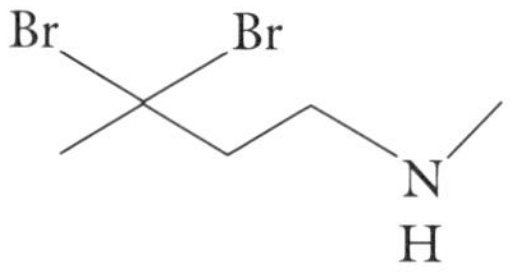

ANSWER

(1) 3,5-dibromo-8-chloro-2,6-dimethylnonane

(2) 3-chloro-3-phenylpropanoic acid (Remember: The carboxyl group carbon is the lowest numbered carbon)

(3) 1-penten-3-ol

(4) 1-chloro-2-butanone

(5) N-methyl-3,3-dibromo-1-butanamine

Use molecular models to review stereochemistry.

2 STEREOCHEMISTRY

a. Definition

Isomers are different compounds with the same molecular formulas. These compounds often have different physical properties and react differently with the same reagents.

b. Types

The several types of isomers are described next.

1. **Structural isomers** have the same molecular formula but differ in the connectivity of their atoms. The classic examples of structural isomers, the basic type of isomer, are ethyl alcohol (CH_3CH_2OH) and dimethyl ether (CH_3OCH_3). Both have the molecular formula C_2H_6O, but each has different physical and chemical properties (e.g., melting points, boiling points, solubility) and different chemical reactivity because of their different functional groups. The first three alkanes (methane, ethane, and propane) have no structural isomers. Butane has two such isomers:

$CH_3-CH_2-CH_2-CH_3$

Butane (C_4H_{10})

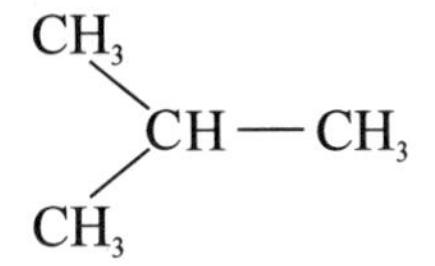

Isobutane (C_4H_{10})

All alkanes with more than three carbons have at least two structural isomers, and the number of isomers increases with more carbons (e.g., decane has 75 structural isomeric forms). Don't worry about memorizing isomers; just know what a structural isomer is and how to identify two isomers versus two identical structures written differently.

2. **Stereoisomers** do not differ in the connectivity of their atoms but have a different arrangement of atoms in space, for example:

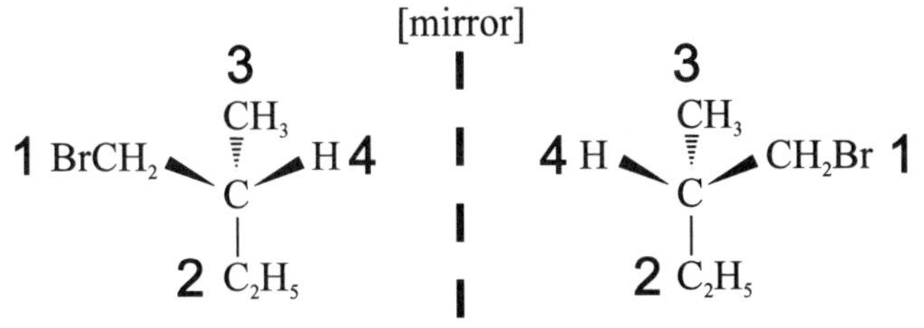

[R]-1-bromo-2-methylbutane [S]-1-bromo-2-methylbutane

3. **Geometric isomers (*cis/trans*, or Z/E, isomers)** differ in the spatial arrangement of atoms around a double bond. When these isomers have two similar chemical groups connected to the central atoms, they can be named via the *cis* (same side) or *trans* (opposite side) nomenclature.

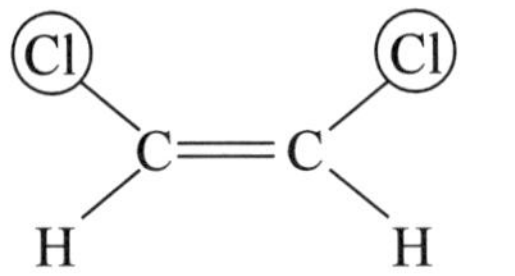

cis-1,2 dichloroethene

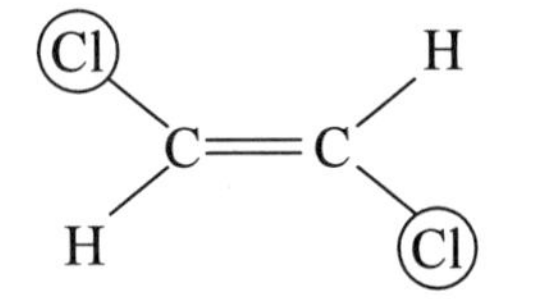

trans-1,2 dichloroethene

When all of the chemical groups connected at the central atoms are different, however, the Z/E nomenclature system must be used. The Z/E nomenclature uses the priority system to classify the attached groups. Generally, the attached atom with the higher atomic weight is assigned the higher priority (e.g., Br has a higher priority than Cl, which in turn has a higher priority than the carbon atom in CH_3). If the two highest priority groups are on the same side of the double bond, a Z isomer is present. In an E isomer, molecules with the two highest priority groups are on different sides of the double bond.

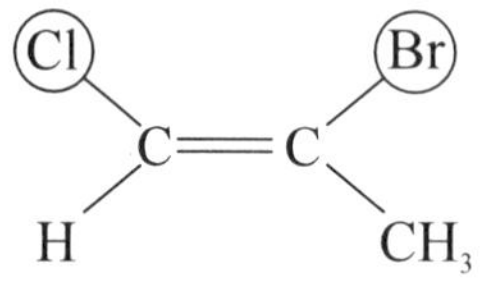

(Z)-1-chloro-2-bromopropene
two high-priority groups (Cl, Br) on **same** side of the double bond

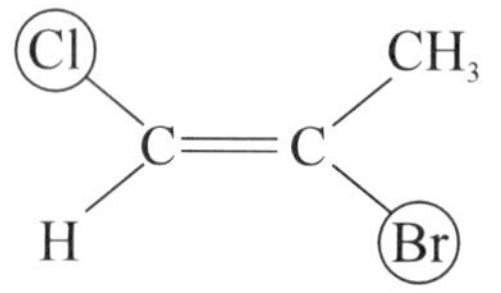

(E)-1-chloro-2-bromopropene
two high-priority groups (Cl, Br) on **different** sides of the double bond

4. **Optical isomers** have chiral centers, which means that the central atom has four different groups attached to it (i.e., it lacks a plane of symmetry). The three types of optical isomers are **enantiomers, diastereomers, and meso compounds.**

   (a) **Enantiomers (R/S isomers)** are **nonsuperimposable mirror images** of one another. Compounds must have at least one asymmetric or **chiral** carbon to have a pair of enantiomers. Such a carbon must lack a plane of symmetry; that is, if a carbon has two identical substituents (such as two hydrogen atoms), it is not a chiral carbon.

   Enantiomers are named using the R/S system. The groups surrounding a carbon are ranked with the largest group (oxygen, nitrogen) given the highest priority, the second largest group (nitrogen, carbon) given second priority, the next largest group given third priority, and the smallest group (hydrogen) given the lowest priority. Note that you need four different substituent groups on the same carbon to use this method (this is the definition of chirality). Position the molecule so that the lowest ranked group is in the back, and rotate your hand from the highest ranked group to the next-highest ranked group.

MNEMONIC

> If your hand moves clockwise (as if you were making a right turn with a car), you call the carbon an R carbon. If you turn your hand left, it is an S carbon (R = "right turn").

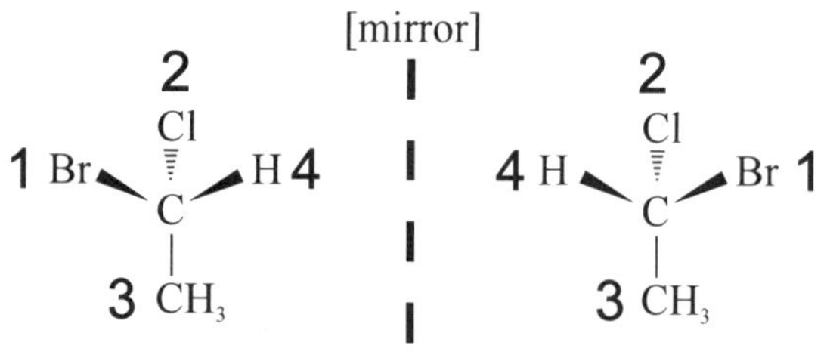

[S]-1-bromo-1-chloroethane [R]-1-bromo-1-chloroethane

Enantiomers do not differ from one another in most physical or chemical properties, but they do differ in optical activity. One enantiomer will rotate plane-polarized light clockwise (the ***d*** isomer), and the other will rotate plane-polarized light counterclockwise (***l*** isomer).

Optical activity is calculated using the following formula:

$$\alpha_{sp} = \frac{\alpha_{obs}}{cl}$$

α_{sp} = specific rotation of the compound
l = path length (dm)
c = concentration (g/ml)
α_{obs} = experimentally observed rotation

Stereochemistry and the direction of rotation have no known relationship. You cannot predict which enantiomer rotates the light to the right (**dextrorotatory, *d***) and which rotates it to the left (**levorotatory, *l***).

Enantiomeric pairs are hard to separate. A mixture of equal amounts of the two enantiomers is called a **racemic mixture.** Since a racemic mixture contains exactly 50% *d* isomers and 50% *l* isomers, the individual isomer's rotation of polarized light cancels out. Therefore, racemic mixtures do not rotate polarized light (i.e., they are optically inactive).

(b) **Diastereomers** are stereoisomers that are not enantiomers (non–mirror-image isomers). They differ in the arrangement of atoms in space but are not mirror images.

Chiral diastereomers are isomers that result from chiral carbons but are not enantiomers. They require **at least two chiral carbons.**

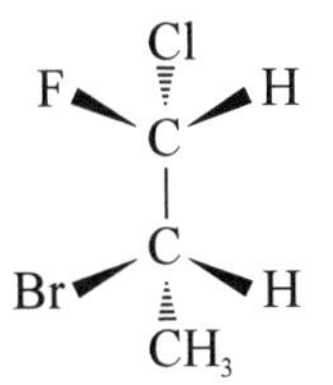

[1R,2S]-1-chloro-1-fluoro-2-bromopropane

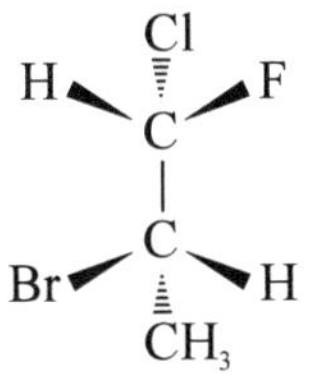

[1S,2S]-1-chloro-1-fluoro-2-bromopropane

MNEMONIC

Diastereomer: At least two chiral carbons

(c) **Meso compounds** are achiral but have asymmetric carbons. They reduce the number of stereoisomers from 2^n (where n is the number of chiral carbons). Although each carbon is asymmetric, the molecule as a whole has a plane of symmetry.

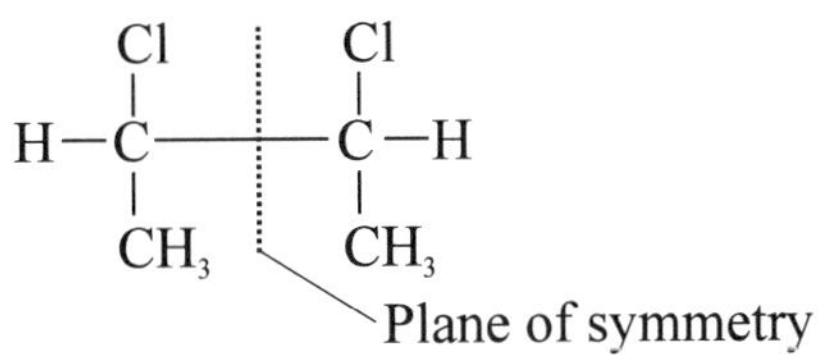

meso-2,3-dichlorobutane

8. **Conformational (rotational) isomers** differ from each other only by rotation around a carbon–carbon single bond. The molecule can rapidly switch from one rotational isomer to another and thus can usually arrive at the most stable rotational isomer (Figure 2-32). Normally the three conformations are:

- **Anti,** which is the most stable arrangement
- **Gauche,** which is less stable (an H–CH_3 gauche interaction is more stable than a CH_3–CH_3 interaction)
- **Eclipsed,** which is the least stable arrangement

Another example of a conformational isomer pair is the chair (most stable—all bonds are in the anti-conformation) versus the boat (less stable—not all bonds are in the anti-conformation) form of cyclohexane. The chair form of cyclohexane minimizes the angle strain, torsional strain, and nonbonded strain of the molecule. Remember that on the cyclohexane molecule, the most stable conformation occurs when the bulky groups occupy the equatorial positions.

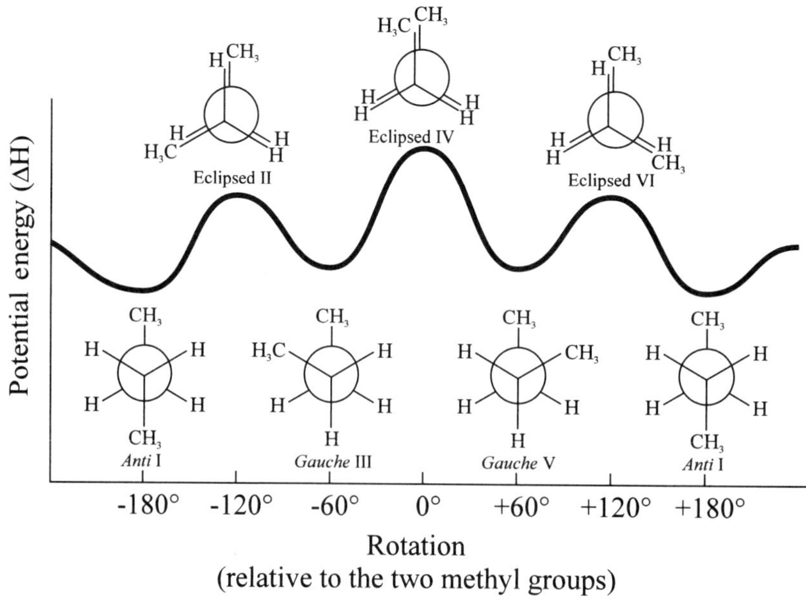

Figure 2-32.
Internal rotation of n-butane. Note the three conformations: *anti*—methyl groups are: ±180° rotation—is the most stable (the methyl groups are furthest apart); *gauche*—±60° apart rotation—is less stable than anti; *eclipsed*—0°, ±120° apart rotation—is the least stable arrangement (the most steric interaction).

QUESTION

Give the proper IUPAC nomenclature for the following compounds:

(1)

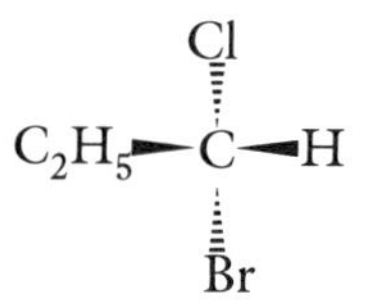

(2)

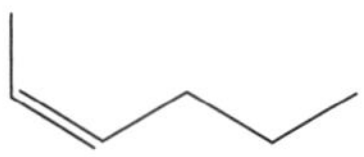

(3) 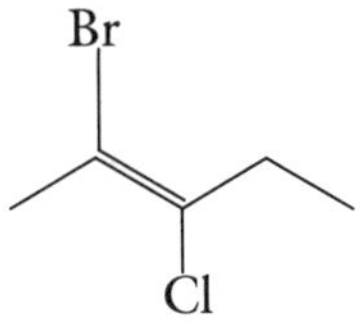

(4) 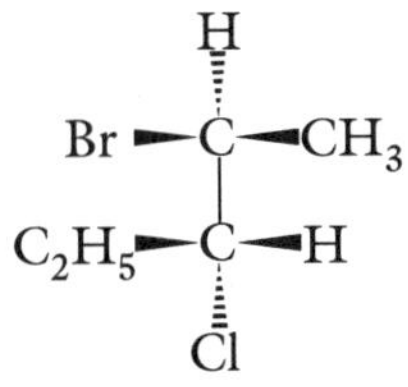

(5) 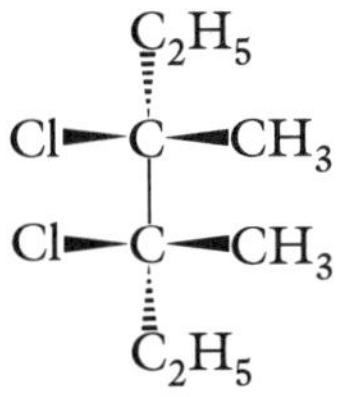

ANSWER

(1) (R)-1-bromo-1-chloropropane

(2) Cis-2-hexene

(3) (E)-2-bromo-3-chloro-2-pentene

(4) (2S,3R)-2-bromo-3-chloropentane

(5) Meso-3,4-dichloro-3,4-dimethyl hexane

3 STABILITY, PHYSICAL PROPERTIES, AND REACTIVITY

The energetic stability of molecules depends on their type of branching, their cis/trans configuration, and the presence of electron-donating or electron-withdrawing groups.

a. Branching

increases the stability of hydrocarbons and the intermolecular repulsion because of increased van der Waals forces, therefore decreasing their boiling point. For example, the branched molecule 2-methylbutene:

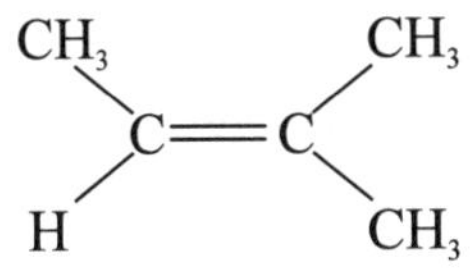

2-methylbutene

will have a lower boiling point than CH_2=CH–CH_2–CH_2–CH_3 (n-pentene), even though both have the same molecular formula (C_5H_{10}).

Increased stability of molecular compounds is associated with a reduction in the boiling point of the compound. In addition, boiling point is largely dependent on intermolecular forces (e.g., hydrogen bonding).

Cis isomers have higher boiling points than trans isomers because of a net dipole that exists in cis isomers, creating stronger intermolecular forces. Trans isomers have higher melting points because they can stack tighter in a solid matrix than their cis counterpart.

b. *Cis/trans* isomers

like *cis*-2-butene and *trans*-2-butene differ in stability:

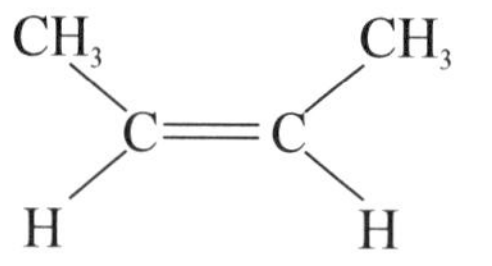

cis-2-butene

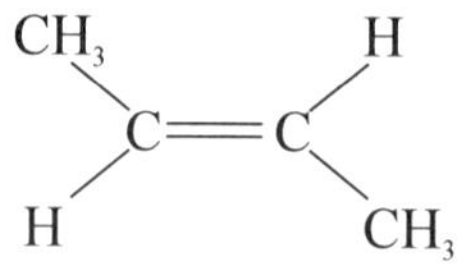

trans-2-butene

The *trans* isomer will be more stable than the *cis* isomer because the methyl groups are further apart in the *trans* conformation. This separation leads to less steric interaction and thus to a thermodynamically favored conformation.

Note that the molecule cannot rotate from one form to another because a double bond cannot rotate; therefore, this isomer relationship is different from gauche–anti stability. The *cis* form can exist and will not convert unless the double bond is broken and then reformed.

c. Electron-donating and electron-withdrawing groups

also affect the stability of organic molecules.

According to the Lewis definition, acids are compounds that accept electrons. An electron-withdrawing group makes an organic compound more suitable for accepting electrons and therefore more acidic.

- **Effects on acidic compounds and their conjugate bases**

  Electron-donating groups destabilize the conjugate bases of acidic compounds and decrease the acidity of the compound. Once the acid loses a proton, it has an excess of electrons. Examples of electron-donating groups are OH, NH_2, and OR.

  Electron-withdrawing groups stabilize conjugate bases and therefore increase the acidity of acidic compounds by helping the compounds share the excess electrons of the conjugate base. Examples of electron-withdrawing groups are CO, COOH, and NO_2.

- **Effects on aromatic stability and substitution**

  Electron-donating groups stabilize additions to a benzene ring and increase the reaction rate of electrophilic aromatic substitution. They direct additional substitution to the ortho and para sites. Note that the halogens, which decrease the reaction rate but still direct ortho and para substitution, are an exception to this rule.

BEWARE

> Electron-withdrawing groups decrease the rate of electrophilic aromatic substitution and direct the substitution to the meta site.

4 SUBSTITUTION/ELIMINATION REACTIONS

a. Substitution Reactions of Alkyl Halides

Table 2-10 describes how different types of alkyl halides (primary, secondary, and tertiary) undergo substitution/elimination reactions.

TABLE 2-10 Substitution/elimination reactions of alkyl halides

Reacting Molecule	S_N1	E_1	S_N2	E_2
Primary alkyl halide	Does not react because it cannot form a sufficiently stable carbocation	Does not react because it cannot form stable carbocation	Reacts readily and quickly, fastest in polar aprotic solvent with strong unhindered nucleophile	Reacts favorably with strong, sterically hindered base (e.g., t-butoxide)
Secondary alkyl halide	Reacts slowly if it has an excellent leaving group in a polar protic solvent (E_1 also occurs)	Reacts with good leaving group, in polar protic solvent (enhanced in basic solution)	Reacts only with strong nucleophile (which is not too bulky/branched) in a polar aprotic solvent	Reacts with strong, sterically hindered base
Tertiary alkyl halide	Reacts readily (not that quickly) in a polar (nucleophilic) protic solvent	Reacts in non-nucleophilic protic solvent and is enhanced in basic solution	Does not react (steric hindrance)	Reacts somewhat in presence of a strong base

These four reactions have two categories:

1. **Nucleophilic substitution (S_N).** In this reaction, an incoming nucleophile uses a pair of electrons to form a new carbon bond while displacing the leaving group. This reaction is also called nucleophilic displacement reaction.
2. **Elimination (E).** This reaction occurs when two elements leave a molecule to form a pi bond, thereby changing a carbon–carbon single bond into a carbon–carbon double bond.
3. S_N2 and E_2 are second-order reactions in that two different molecules are involved in their rate-limiting step. The **rate of the reaction, therefore, depends on the concentration of the nucleophile:**

$$\text{rate of } S_N2 \text{ or } E_2 = k\,(\text{electrophile})(\text{nucleophile})$$

4. On the other hand, the S_N^1 and E_1 are first-order reactions, in that the rate-limiting step involves one molecule. The **rate of these reactions is independent of the concentration of the nucleophile.**

$$\text{rate of } S_N^1 \text{ or } E_1 = k\,(\text{electrophile})$$

b. S_N2 Reaction

In this one-step reaction, a nucleophile attacks an electrophile while a leaving group simultaneously leaves. This reaction is often called **backside displacement** (Figure 2-33).

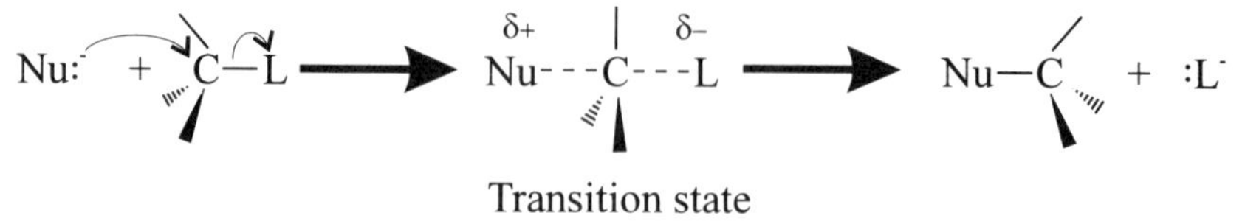

Figure 2-33.
S_N2 reaction: backside displacement.

- The reaction depends on the presence of a strong nucleophile and a good leaving group.
- The stereochemistry of the molecule **inverts** (i.e., R turns to S, and vice versa).
- This reaction is **highly dependent on steric interaction,** which means that primary alkyl halides react best, whereas tertiary alkyl halides barely react at all. Small nucleophiles (e.g., OH) work better than bulky nucleophiles.
- S_N2 works best in **polar aprotic solvents** [e.g., dimethyl sulfoxide (DMSO), N,N-dimethylformamide (DMF)].
- Poor leaving groups (such as OH^-) can be enhanced by compounds such as TsCl (the tosyl group bonds with the O to form a better leaving group).

c. E_2 Reaction

Although similar to S_N2 in that a strong nucleophile attacks an electrophile with a good leaving group, in this reaction, the nucleophile acts as a base and takes a proton from the electrophile, which leads to β **elimination** of the leaving group and the formation of a carbon–carbon double bond (Figure 2-34).

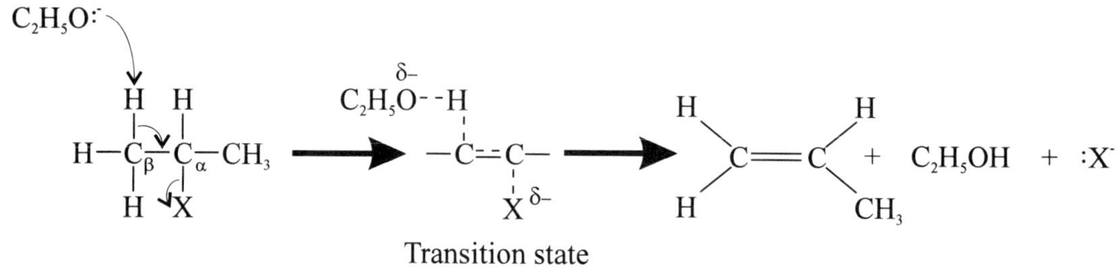

Figure 2-34.
E_2 reaction.

- This reaction is favored over S_N2 if the nucleophile or electrophile is bulky or sterically hindered. E_2 occurs most often when the nucleophile is an especially **strong, bulky base** (e.g, t-butoxide).

BEWARE

d. S_N1 reaction

is a two-step reaction (Figure 2-35). First, the leaving group is pulled away, forming a carbocation, the rate-limiting step of the reaction. Then, the carbocation is attacked by the nucleophile. Carbocation rearrangement can occur.

- **Stereochemistry is not inverted.** The formation of the carbocation leads to **racemization** because the nucleophile can attack from either side of the carbon, leading to a product that does not rotate polarized light.
- In the first step, loss of the leaving group, the solvent molecule takes part in a **solvolysis** reaction, which works best with **polar protic solvents** (such as formic acid). Polar protic solvents facilitate the solvolysis reaction, leading to the formation of a carbocation intermediate, the rate-determining step.
- This reaction is also improved with tertiary halide electrophiles, which can stabilize the formation of the carbocation.

The formation of the carbocation is the rate-limiting step.

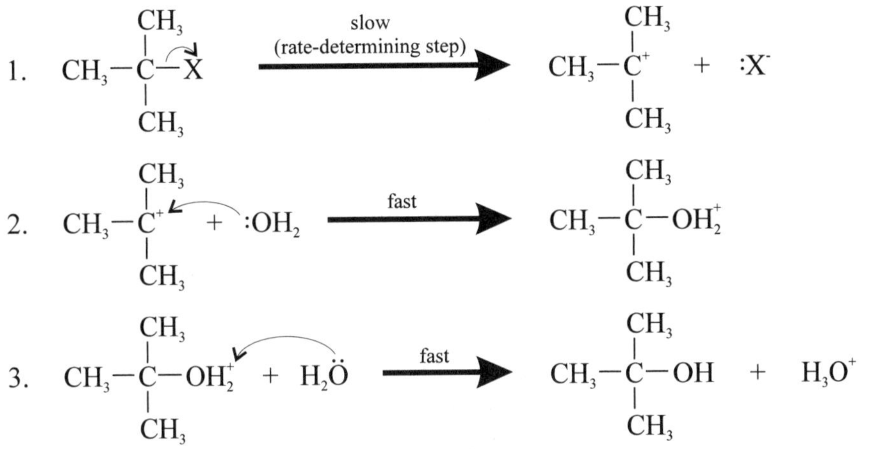

Figure 2-35.
S_N1 reaction.

e. E_1 Reaction

is a two-step alternative to S_N1 reaction (Figure 2-36). After the leaving group leaves, the nucleophile picks off a β proton and forms a carbon–carbon double bond. The reaction is favored under circumstances similar to those that favor S_N1: polar protic solvents and tertiary halides.

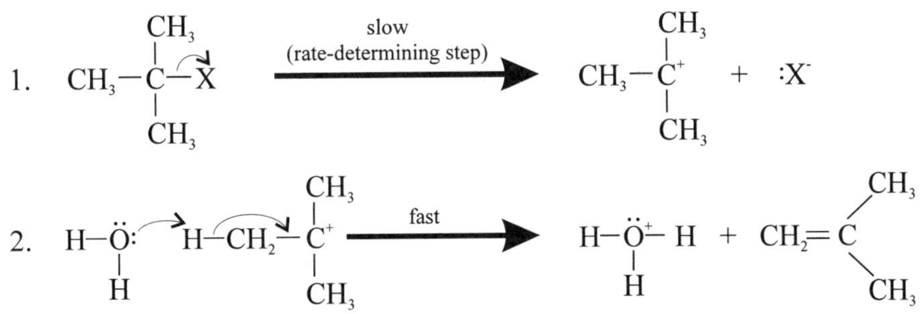

Figure 2-36.
E_1 reaction.

High temperatures favor elimination reactions. If the MCAT sketches a reaction with heat (Δ) as one reactant, but you don't know the product, the best answer choice is the one in which the molecule formed has a double bond.

STRATEGY

QUESTION

All of the following statements about organic substitution and elimination reactions are true EXCEPT:

(a) The rate of an S_N1/E_1 reaction does not depend on the concentration of the nucleophile.

(b) S_N2 reactions are favored by the use of polar aprotic solvents (e.g., DMSO, DMF).

(c) S_N2 reactions result in a product that is a racemic mixture and optically inactive.

(d) E_2 reactions are favored by high temperatures and the use of a strong, bulky base (e.g., t-butoxide).

ANSWER

The answer is **c.** Because S_N2 reactions are one-step reactions in which a nucleophile attacks an electrophile while a leaving group is simultaneously displaced, this results in a backside displacement that causes the stereochemistry of the molecule to invert. S_N1 reactions result in a product that is a racemic mixture and optically inactive through the formation of a carbocation intermediate, which is the rate-determining step of the reaction.

5 MARKOVNIKOV'S RULE AND ITS EXCEPTIONS

a. Markovnikov's rule

Whenever a molecule H–X (X is a halogen) is added to an alkene, the halogen bonds to the more substituted carbon and the hydrogen bonds to the less substituted carbon.

1. The guiding principle for this reaction is that **the more stable carbocation must be formed,** which happens when the positive charge of the carbocation is on the more substituted carbon. The halogen thus attacks the more substituted carbon, as Markovnikov's rule predicts.

2. The other important feature of the Markovnikov reaction is the chronology of the mechanism: **the carbocation forms first** as the proton bonds with the less substituted carbon; then the halogen anion bonds to the positively charged (more substituted) carbon. This chronology is important because the stability of the carbocation affects the specific formation of the product.

b. The basic concepts

behind this law affect the selectivity/regiochemistry of many other organic reactions. An example of Markovnikov addition follows:

STRATEGY

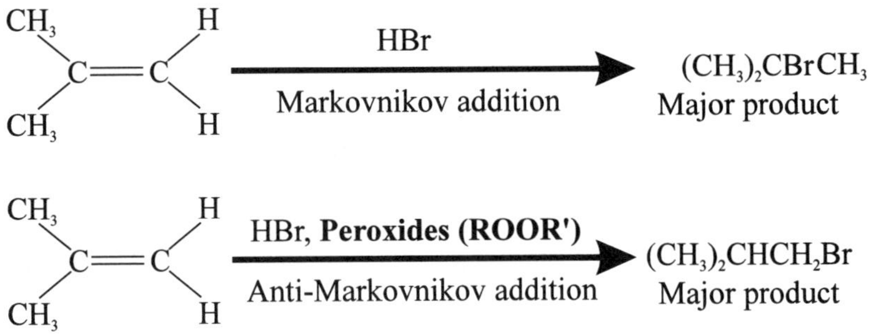

c. Exceptions

Not all H–X addition reactions happen according to Markovnikov's rule, however; this rule merely describes the thermodynamically favored reaction (i.e., the reaction that occurs in the absence of large amounts of energy or in the absence of a catalyst). Peroxides are excellent catalysts of anti-Markovnikov addition reactions.

The same principle applies to other addition reactions involving alkenes, such as the addition of H_2O to an alkene to form an alcohol. Under normal conditions (high temperatures, hydrating environment), the addition of H_2O to an alkene in the presence of an acid will form a Markovnikov alcohol so that the OH group is on the more substituted carbon. However, using a process called **hydroboration** (B_2H_6), an alcohol can be formed from an alkene so that the OH goes to the less substituted carbon (anti-Markovnikov addition).

6 GRIGNARD REACTIONS

a. Definition

A Grignard reaction yields a compound with a carbon–magnesium bond; the carbon bonded to this magnesium can then act as a nucleophile and form a carbon–carbon bond with any electrophilic carbon.

Chemical industries use **Grignard reactions to synthesize carbon–carbon bonds,** which prove to be very useful in a variety of organic reactions. In some cases, organolithium reagents can be used in place of Grignard reagents.

1. A Grignard reagent can be formed by mixing an alkyl halide with magnesium, stirring in an ether solvent (a popular lab question on the MCAT).

$$CH_3{-}CH_2{-}CH_2{-}Br + Mg \xrightarrow{(C_2H_5)_2O} CH_3{-}CH_2{-}CH_2{-}Mg{-}Br$$

(propylmagnesium bromide)

Because of its carbon–metal bond, a Grignard reagent is an organometallic compound.

2. The most common Grignard reaction is the synthesis of alcohols from aldehydes and ketones.

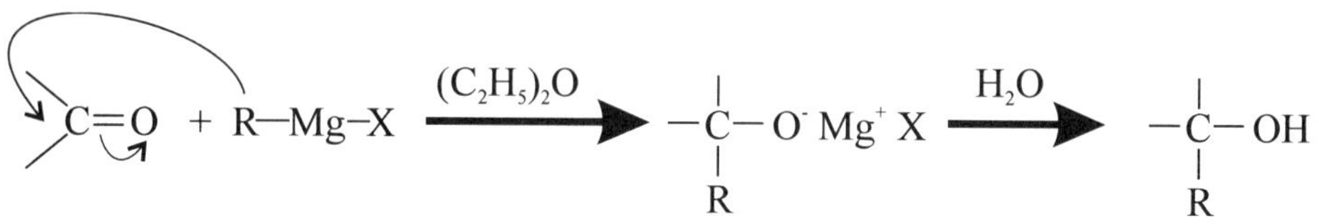

This reaction is simple. The R group acts as a nucleophile and attacks the carbon, which causes the oxygen to form a bond with the MgX portion of the Grignard reaction. The final step is an "H_2O wash," which cleaves the O–MgX bond and leaves the hydrocarbon in its alcohol form.

3. The other Grignard reactions roughly follow the model of the preparation of alcohols. For the MCAT, just remember and understand the preceding reaction and apply it to questions about other Grignard reactions.

STRATEGY

b. One other Grignard reaction

that is worth committing to memory is the formation of carboxylic acids by bubbling gaseous CO_2 into an ether solution of the Grignard reagent or by pouring the Grignard reagent over dry ice.

QUESTION

Provide the structure as well as the IUPAC name of the missing products/intermediates in the following multi-step reactions.

(a) 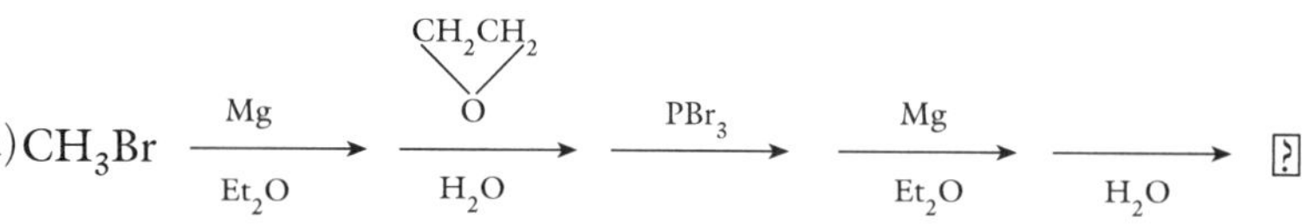

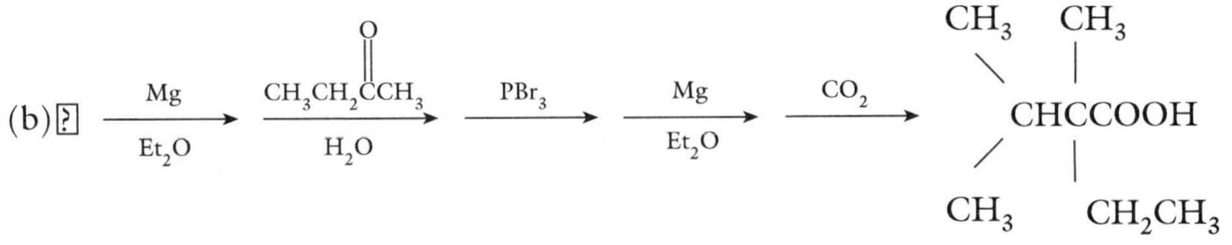

$$\text{(c) } CH_3CH_2Br \xrightarrow[Et_2O]{Mg} CH_3CH_2MgBr \xrightarrow[H_2O]{H_2C{=}O} \boxed{?} \xrightarrow{KMnO_4} CH_3CH_2COOH$$

ANSWER

$$\text{(a) } CH_3Br \xrightarrow[Et_2O]{Mg} CH_3MgBr \xrightarrow{\text{CH}_2\text{CH}_2\text{O (ethylene oxide)}} CH_3CH_2CH_2OH$$

$$\xrightarrow{PBr_3} CH_3CH_2CH_2Br \xrightarrow[Et_2O]{Mg} CH_3CH_2CH_2MgBr$$

$$\xrightarrow[H_2O]{} CH_3CH_2CH_3 \text{ (n-propane)}$$

(b) **Working backwards**:

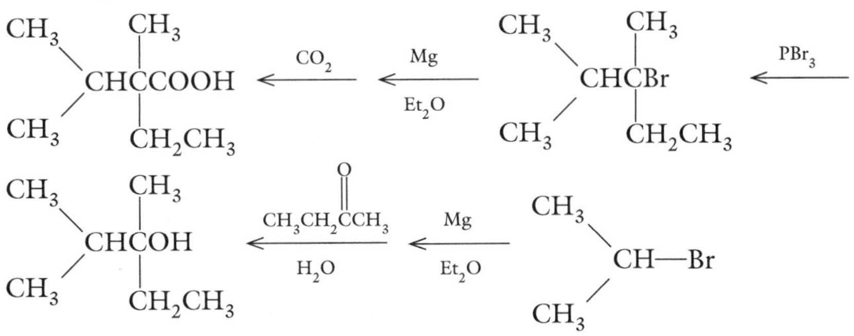

(2-bromopropane)

$$\text{(c) } CH_3CH_2Br \xrightarrow[Et_2O]{Mg} CH_3CH_2MgBr \xrightarrow[H_2O]{H_2C{=}O} CH_3CH_2CH_2OH \text{ (1-propanol)}$$

$$\xrightarrow{KMnO_4} CH_3CH_2COOH$$

7 OXIDIZING AND REDUCING AGENTS

a. An oxidizing agent

is a chemical compound or mixture of compounds in solution that brings about the oxidation of another compound (i.e., a loss of electrons); the oxidizing agent is in turn reduced (because for each oxidation reaction there must be a reduction reaction). Oxidizing agents increase the number of carbon/oxygen bonds and reduce the number of carbon/hydrogen and hydrogen/oxygen bonds (e.g., the transformation of an alcohol to an aldehyde).

b. A reducing agent

is a chemical compound or mixture of compounds in solution that brings about the reduction of another compound (i.e., a gain of electrons); the reducing agent is in turn oxidized. Reducing agents decrease the number of carbon/oxygen bonds and increase the number of carbon/hydrogen and hydrogen/oxygen bonds (e.g., the transformation of a ketone/aldehyde to an alcohol).

c. Oxidation and reduction reactions

are considered fundamental concepts within organic chemistry (Table 2-11). Many different oxidizing and reducing agents may prove useful for converting one organic compound to another, for example:

$$CH_3CH_2OH + KMnO_4 \rightarrow CH_3COOH \quad \text{(oxidation of an alcohol to a carboxylic acid)}$$

TEST CORRELATION

Oxidation and reduction reactions are very popular reactions on the MCAT; they test your knowledge of the interconversion of various organic chemical functional groups. In addition, the concept of redox appears again and again on the general chemistry section. Therefore, you must be able to identify oxidizing and reducing agents, know how they function in the reaction, and know what products they yield.

TABLE 2-11. Major oxidizing and reducing agents and the reactions/conversions they can direct

Oxidizing Agents	Reactions/Conversions
$KMnO_4$	Primary alcohols → carboxylic acids
Cr_2O_7	Primary alcohols → aldehydes → carboxylic acids
CrO_4	Secondary alcohols → ketones Tertiary alcohols (do not react)
OsO_4	Alkenes → diols
O_3	Alkenes → ketones (ozonolysis)
Reducing Agents	
$LiAlH_4$	Aldehydes → alcohols Ketones → alcohols Carboxylic acids → alcohols
$NaBH_4$	Aldehydes → alcohols Ketones → alcohols (less reactive than $LiAlH_4$)

QUESTION

Provide the structure and IUPAC name of the missing products in the following reactions:

(a) $CH_3CH_2OH \xrightarrow{KMnO_4} \boxed{?}$

(b) $(CH_3)_2C{=}CH_2 \xrightarrow[ROOR']{HBr} \xrightarrow[(C_2H_5)_2O]{Mg} \xrightarrow[H_2O]{CO_2} \xrightarrow{LiAlH_4} \boxed{?}$

(c) $(CH_3)_3COH \xrightarrow{CrO_3} \boxed{?}$

ANSWER

(a) Because $KMnO_4$ is a strong oxidizing agent, it will oxidize a primary alcohol into a carboxylic acid:

$$CH_3CH_2OH \xrightarrow{KMnO_4} CH_3COOH$$

(ethanol) ethanoic acid (acetic acid)

(b) Expect to see a few multi-step reactions on the MCAT. The best way to attack this problem is one step at a time:

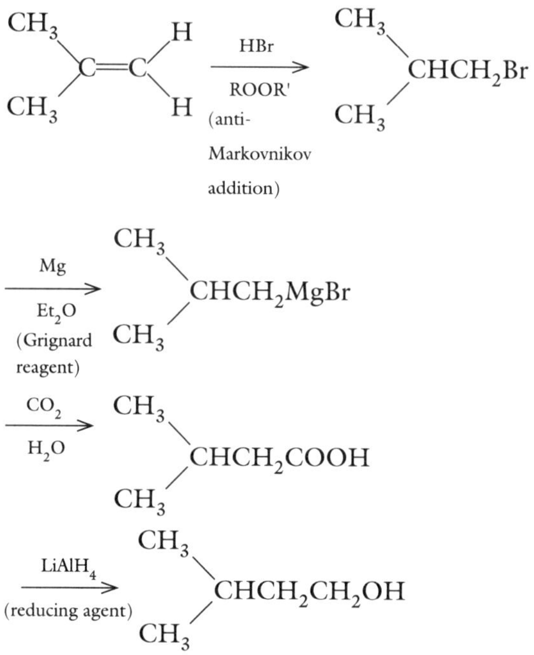

(3-methyl-1-butanol or 3-methylbutanol; isopentanol is the common name, not the IUPAC nomenclature)

(c) Tertiary alcohols cannot be oxidized. Thus, *no reaction* occurs and the product remains 2-methyl-2-propanol (tert-butyl alcohol is the common name, not the IUPAC nomenclature).

8 OTHER ORGANIC REACTIONS

Most other organic reactions are not worth memorizing. Nevertheless, you should review these reactions so you can understand them if they are on the MCAT examination.

- Hydrogenation of alkenes (with Pt as the catalyst)
- Diels-Alder reaction (dienes to cyclic alkenes—just look at it; it's pretty complex)
- Ester synthesis (usually in the presence of a dehydrating agent)
- Friedel–Crafts alkylation/acylation ($AlCl_3$ serves as a Lewis acid to destabilize the aromatic ring)
- Williamson ether synthesis (S_N2 reaction of alkyl halide with alkoxide)

- Ozonolysis
- Three ways of synthesizing a carboxylic acid: Grignard addition of carbon dioxide, oxidation of aldehydes and primary alcohols, and hydrolysis of nitriles (examples of each are found in Part II G 10)
- Diazonium salts: Interconversion of functional groups on aromatic rings
- Reactions involving Schiff bases

9 CHEMICAL PURIFICATION

a. Extraction

is the separation of a compound from a solid material by precipitating it out of solution or the separation of components from a liquid mixture using a separatory funnel (when the compound you want does not mix with the solvent of choice).

b. Centrifugation

is separating materials by using a machine that applies a centrifugal force to induce sedimentation.

c. Filtration

is the separation of a solid from a liquid or gas via a membrane that allows the liquid or gas to pass through without the solid.

d. Distillation

is the separation of multiple liquids by boiling off the liquid that has the lower boiling point and then collecting it in a condensation tube.

e. Fractional distillation

is most effective for separating two liquids that have similar boiling points (that differ by a few degrees).

f. Recrystallization

is precipitating a crystal by repeatedly manipulating the temperature of the solution, which removes impurities and purifies the crystal.

g. Sublimation

is the purification of a solid by vaporizing it directly to the gaseous phase. Condense the vapor using a cold finger, which is a piece of glassware with cold water running through it.

h. Electrophoresis

is the separation of proteins or nucleic acids (DNA/RNA) in a gel based on size, net charge, or both (Figure 2-37). Sodium dodecyl sulfate (SDS) electrophoresis separates proteins on the basis of size only. It is useful only for determining the molecular weights of single-subunit proteins, because SDS denatures proteins into single subunits. Migration of denatured compounds on SDS electrophoresis is inversely proportional to the molecular weight of the denatured compound. If the molecular weight of a multiple-subunit protein needs to be determined, then gel filtration can be used.

i. Gel filtration

is the separation of proteins or nucleic acids (DNA/RNA) based on molecular weight. In gel filtration, a glass column is filled with Sephadex beads that contain micropores of a specific diameter. The liquid containing the protein or nucleic acid is run through the column. Water is then used as an eluent. Large molecules exit

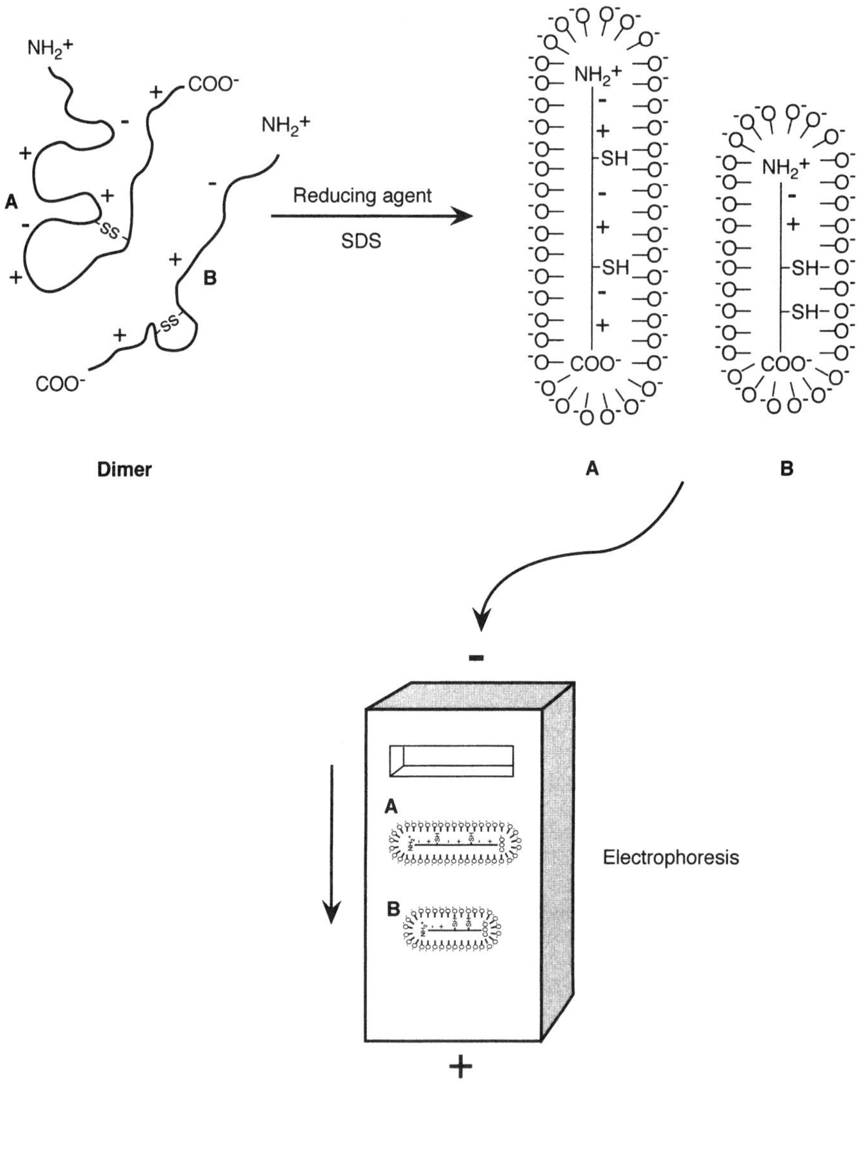

Figure 2-37. Proteins can be separated on the basis of their size by sodium dodecyl sulfate (SDS) polyacrylamide gel electrophoresis. Proteins are heated with SDS and a reducing agent, which breaks the disulfide bonds. The SDS forms negatively charged micelles around the protein. When these proteins are run through a cross-linked polyacrylamide gel in an electric field, all micelle-proteins move toward the positive pole. The small molecules *(B)* migrate through the gel faster than the large molecules *(A)*. (Reprinted with permission from Davidson VL, Sittman DB: *NMS Biochemistry,* 3rd ed. Baltimore, Williams & Wilkins, 1994, p 40.)

the column first; smaller molecules get stuck in the micropores of the beads, taking more time to elute down the column. Unlike SDS electrophoresis, denaturing agents are not used; therefore, the molecular weights of multiple-subunit proteins can be determined. Gel filtration also can be used to purify proteins (e.g., enzymes, snake venom).

j. Chromatography

is the separation of components based on the strength of their affinity for an adsorbent.

1. **Phases.** Chromatography systems consist of two phases:
   (a) **Stationary phase (adsorbent)** is the foundation onto which the mixture of compounds is loaded. This phase usually consists of a specific type of medium that has specific affinities for various chemical compounds.
   (b) **Mobile phase (eluent)** is usually an organic solvent that moves through the adsorbent at specific rates, depending on the relative polarities of the compound, adsorbent, and eluent.
2. **Types** of chromatography include:
   (a) **Thin-layer chromatography.** The adsorbent is silica gel or aluminum oxide (polar). The eluent is a nonpolar organic solvent (e.g., hexane, benzene). The driving force is capillary action.

$$\text{Ratio of fronts } (R_f) \text{ value} = \frac{\text{Distance the compound migrated}}{\text{Distance the eluent migrated}}$$

   The R_f value is inversely proportional to the polarity of the compound. Assuming that a relatively nonpolar eluent is used, the higher the compound's R_f value for a specific eluent, the more nonpolar the compound will be. The more nonpolar the eluent is, the lower the R_f value for a specific compound will be, because the more nonpolar eluent is less likely to carry along the polar adsorbent.

   (b) **Column chromatography.** The adsorbent is silica gel or aluminum oxide (polar). The eluent is a nonpolar organic solvent (e.g., hexane, benzene). The driving force is gravity. Similar to thin-layer chromatography, the more nonpolar a compound is, the more rapidly the compound will elute.
   (c) **Gas chromatography.** The adsorbent is a polar-coiled column. The eluent is a nonpolar, chemically inert gas (e.g., hydrogen, nitrogen, or helium). The driving force is vapor pressure. The retention time, which is the time it takes for the specific compound to elute through the column, is measured. The more polar the compound is, the longer retention time it will have.
   (d) **High-performance liquid chromatography.** The adsorbent is a polar-coiled column. The eluent is a nonpolar, organic liquid (e.g., hexane, benzene). The driving force is pressure. Conceptually, high-performance liquid chromatography is similar to gas chromatography.

10 HIGH-YIELD ORGANIC CHEMISTRY REACTIONS

a. Alkanes

1. Preparation

(a) Hydrogenation of Alkenes

$$CH_2{=}CH_2 \xrightarrow[\text{Pt, Pd, or Ni}]{H_2} CH_3CH_3$$

(b) Hydrolysis of a Grignard Reagent

$$CH_3CH_2Br \xrightarrow[Et_2O]{Mg} CH_3CH_2MgBr \xrightarrow{H_2O} CH_3CH_3$$

(c) Reduction of an Alkyl Halide

$$CH_3CH_2CH_2Br \xrightarrow[Zn]{H_2} CH_3CH_2CH_3$$

2. Reactions

Free Radical Halogenation

$$Br_2 \xrightarrow{\text{heat or light}} 2\ Br\cdot \quad \text{[Chain Initiating Step]}$$

$$\left.\begin{array}{l} Br\cdot + CH_3CH_3 \longrightarrow HBr + CH_3CH_2\cdot \\ CH_3CH_2\cdot + Br_2 \longrightarrow CH_3CH_2Br + Br\cdot \end{array}\right] \text{[Chain Propagating Steps]}$$

$$\left.\begin{array}{l} Br\cdot + Br\cdot \longrightarrow Br_2 \\ CH_3CH_2\cdot + CH_3CH_2\cdot \longrightarrow CH_3CH_2CH_2CH_3 \\ CH_3CH_2\cdot + Br\cdot \longrightarrow CH_3CH_2Br \end{array}\right] \text{[Chain Terminating Steps]}$$

b. Alkyl Halides

1. Preparation

(a) Halogenation of Alcohols

$$CH_3CH_2OH \xrightarrow[\text{or HBr}]{PBr_3} CH_3CH_2Br$$

(b) Free Radical Halogenation of Alkanes

$$CH_3CH_3 \xrightarrow[\text{Heat or light}]{Br_2} CH_3CH_2Br + HBr$$

(c) Hydrohalogenation of Alkenes—Markovnikov Addition

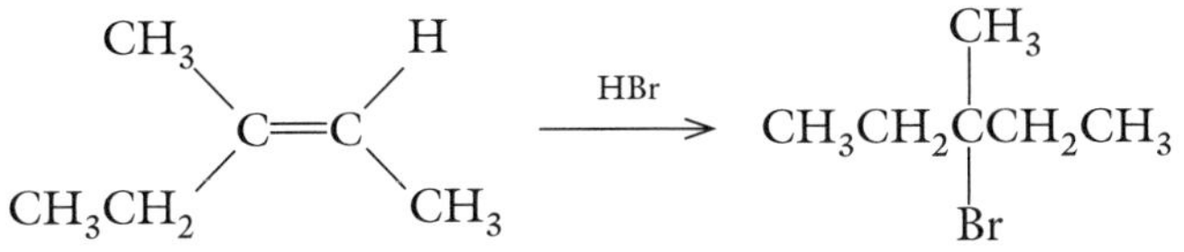

(d) Addition of Halogens to Alkenes and Alkynes

$$CH_2{=}CH_2 \xrightarrow{Br_2} BrCH_2CH_2Br \text{ (anti-addition)}$$

$$HC{\equiv}CH \xrightarrow{2Br_2} Br_2CHCHBr_2$$

2. Reactions

(a) Substitution Reactions

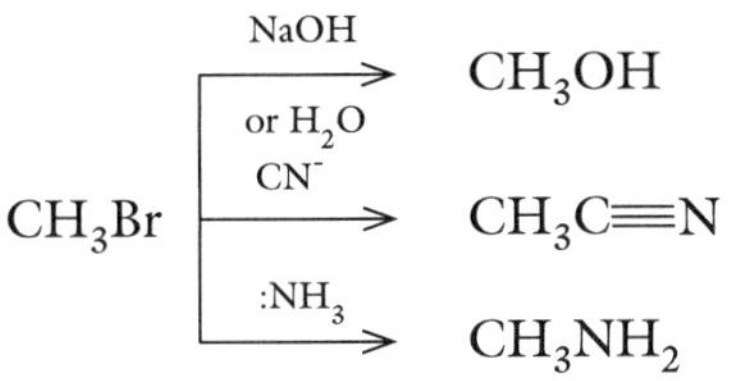

(b) Williamson Synthesis of Ethers

$$CH_3Br + {}^{-}OCH_2CH_3 \longrightarrow CH_3OCH_2CH_3$$

(c) Friedel–Crafts Reaction

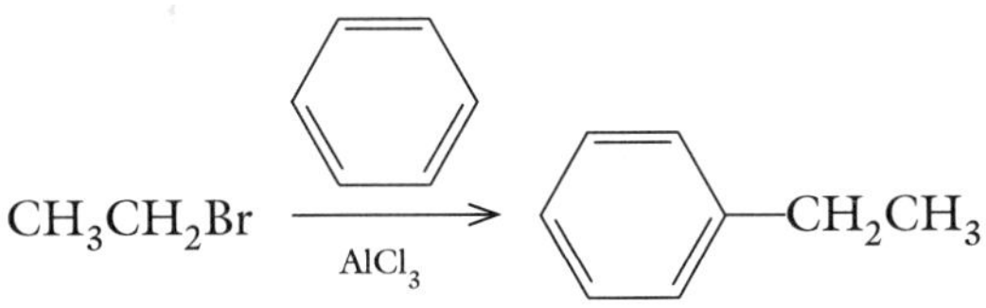

(d) Dehydrohalogenation of Alkenes (E_2 Reaction) with a Strong, Bulky Base

$$CH_3CH_2Br \xrightarrow[E_2]{NaOC(CH_3)_3} CH_2{=}CH_2$$

(e) Grignard Reactions

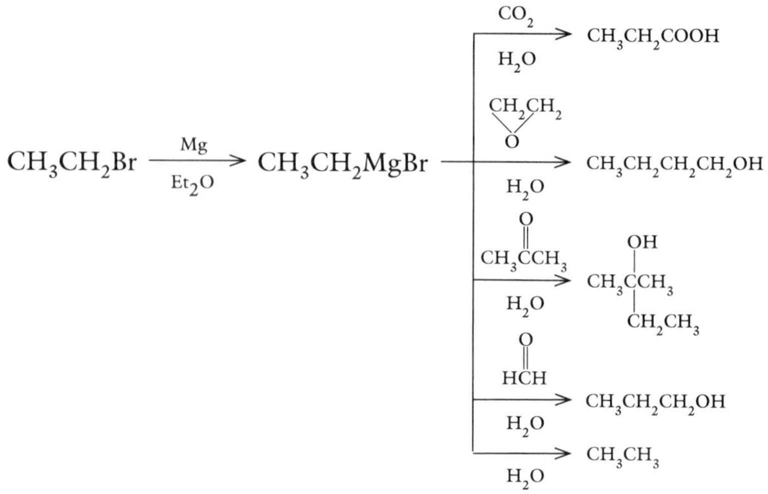

(f) Reduction to an Alkane

$$CH_3CH_2Br \xrightarrow[Zn]{H_2} CH_3CH_3$$

c. Alkenes

1. Preparation

(a) Dehydrohalogenation of Alkyl Halides (E_2 Reaction) with a Strong, Bulky Base

$$CH_3CH_2Br \xrightarrow[E_2]{NaOC(CH_3)_3} CH_2{=}CH_2$$

(b) Dehydration of Alcohols

$$CH_3CH_2CH_2OH \xrightarrow{H^+} CH_3CH{=}CH_2$$

(c) Reduction of Alkynes

$$HC{\equiv}CH \xrightarrow[\text{Lindlar Catalyst}]{H_2} CH_2{=}CH_2 \quad \text{(syn addition)}$$

2. Reactions

(a) Reduction to Alkanes

$$CH_2{=}CH_2 \xrightarrow[\text{Pt, Pd, or Ni}]{H_2} CH_3CH_3 \quad \text{(syn addition)}$$

(b) Addition of Halogens

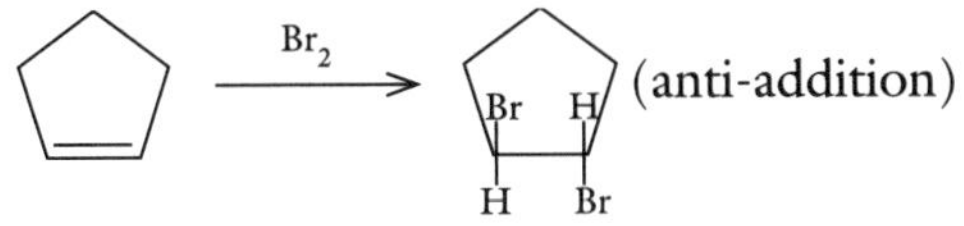

(c) Hydrohalogenation of Alkenes

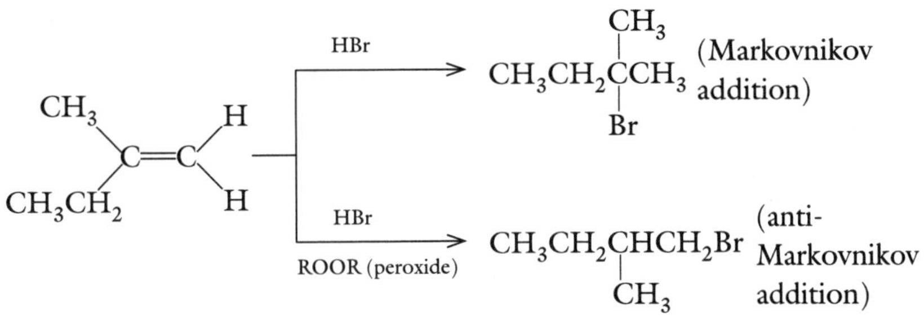

(d) Hydration of Alkenes

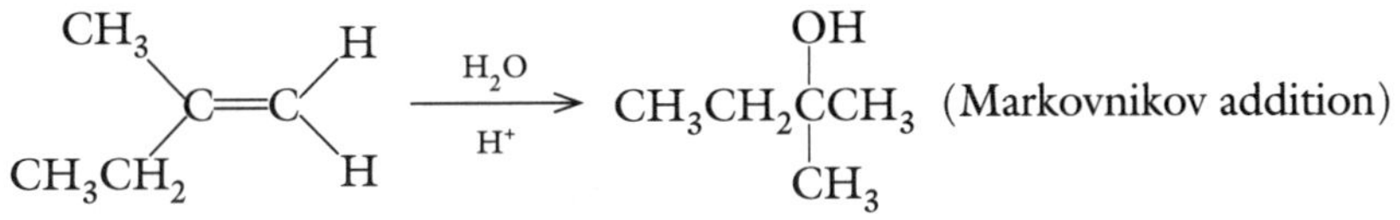

(e) Halohydrin Formation of Alkenes

-OH Group Adds by Markovnikov Addition

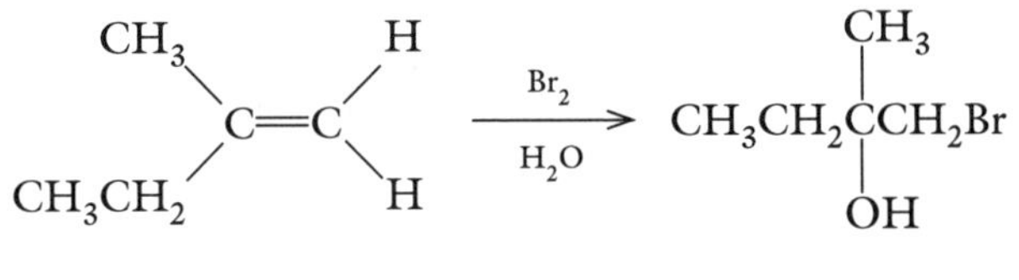

(f) Oxymercuration–Demercuration

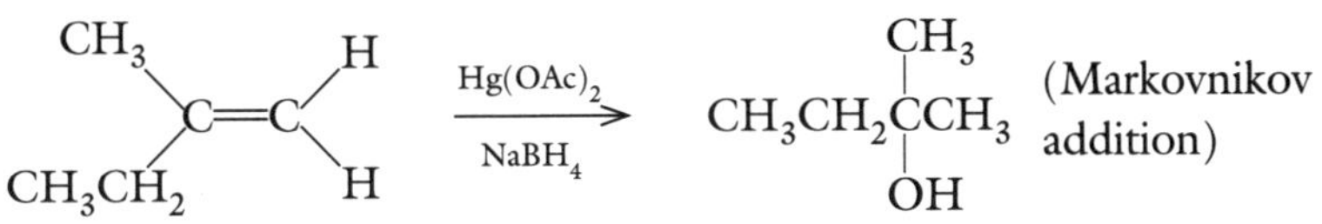

(g) Hydroboration–Oxidation

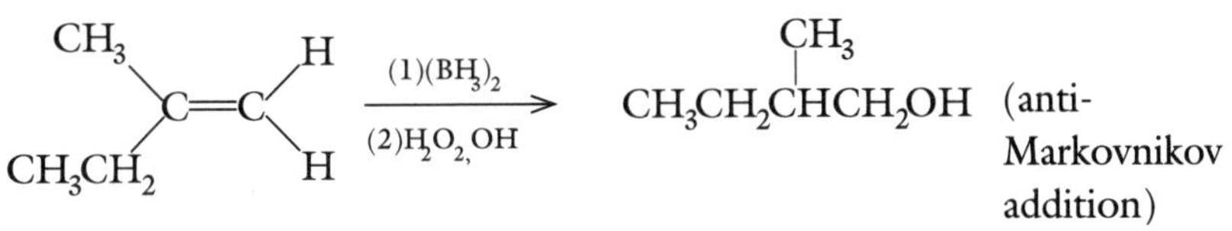

(h) Ozonolysis Cleavage of Alkanes

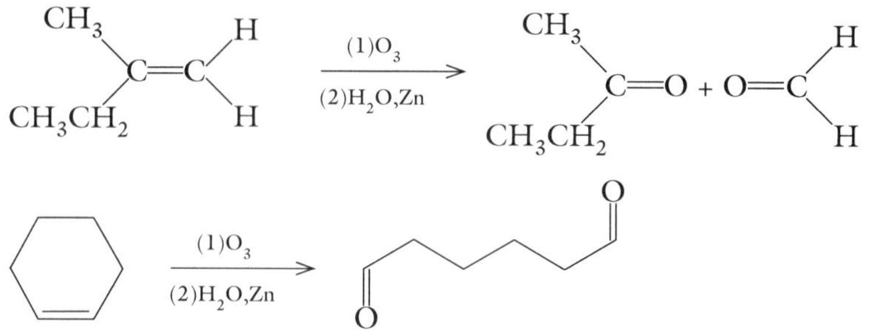

d. Alcohols

1. Preparation

(a) Preparation from Alkenes

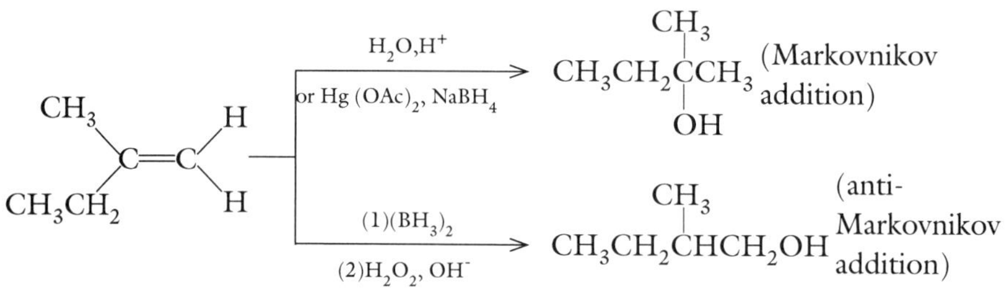

(b) Grignard Synthesis from Alkyl Halides

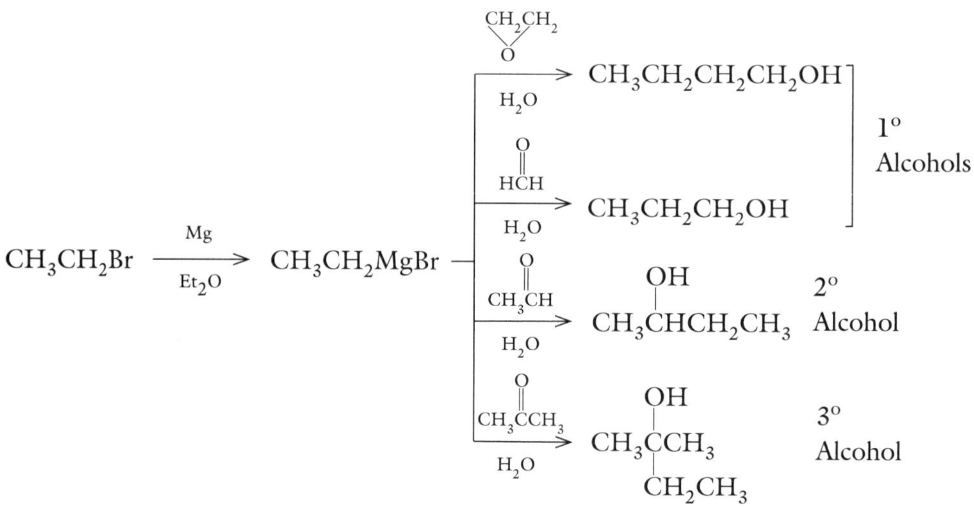

(c) Hydrolysis of Alkyl Halides

$$CH_3CH_2Br \xrightarrow[S_n2]{NaOH} CH_3CH_2OH$$

(d) Reduction of Carboxylic Acids

$$CH_3CH_2COOH \xrightarrow{LiAlH_4} CH_3CH_2CH_2OH$$

2. Reactions

(a) Conversion to Alkyl Halides

$$CH_3CH_2OH \xrightarrow[\text{or conc. HBr}]{PBr_3} CH_3CH_2Br \xrightarrow{CH_3ONa} CH_3CH_2OCH_3$$

(b) Dehydration of Alcohols to Alkenes

$$CH_3CH_2CH_2OH \xrightarrow{H^+} CH_3CH{=}CH_2 + H_2O$$

(c) Esterification (Alcohol + Carboxylic Acid = Ester)

$$CH_3CH_2OH + (CH_3)_2CHCOOH \xrightarrow{H^+} (CH_3)_2CHCOOCH_2CH_3$$

(d) Oxidation

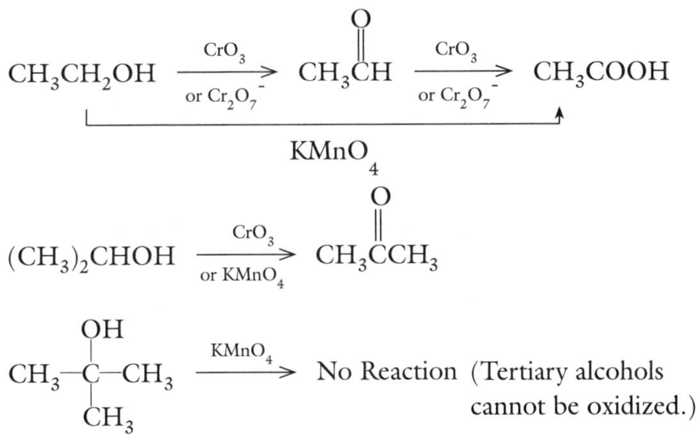

(e) Addition of Tosyl Chloride

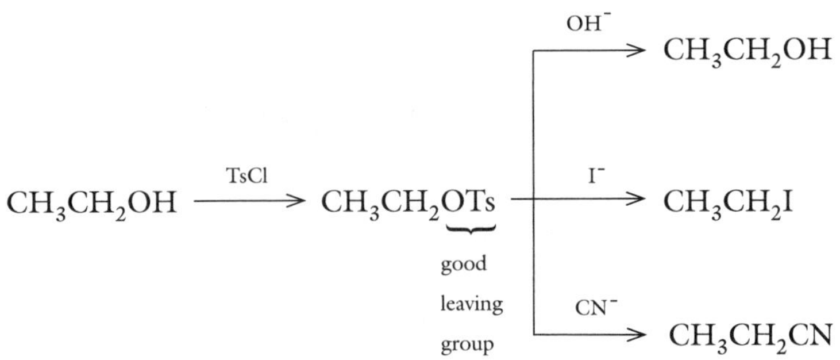

e. Ethers

1. Preparation

(a) Williamson Synthesis of Ethers

$$CH_3CH_2OH \xrightarrow{Na} CH_3CH_2O^- \xrightarrow{CH_3Br} CH_3CH_2OCH_3$$

(b) Alkoxymercuration–Demercuration

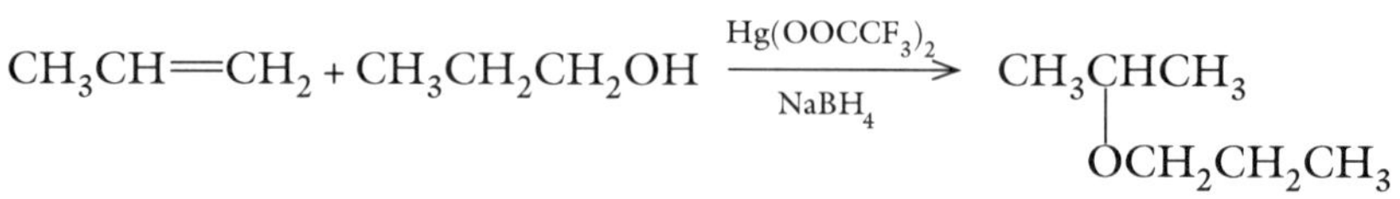

(Markovnikov addition)

2. Reactions

Cleavage by Acids

$$CH_3CH_2OCH_3 \xrightarrow{HBr} CH_3CH_2Br + CH_3OH$$

f. Aldehydes and Ketones

1. Preparation

(a) Oxidation of Alcohols

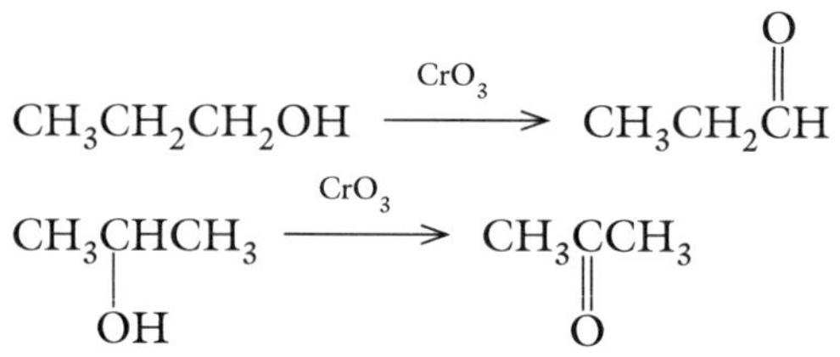

(b) Friedel–Crafts Acylation

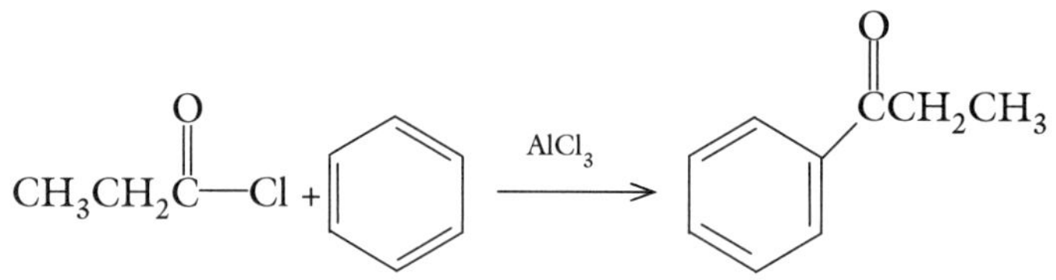

(c) Reaction of Acyl Chlorides with Organolithium Reagents

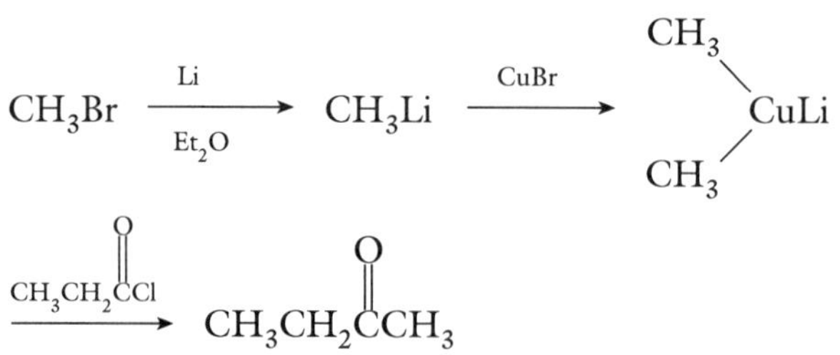

2. Reactions

(a) Oxidation and Reduction

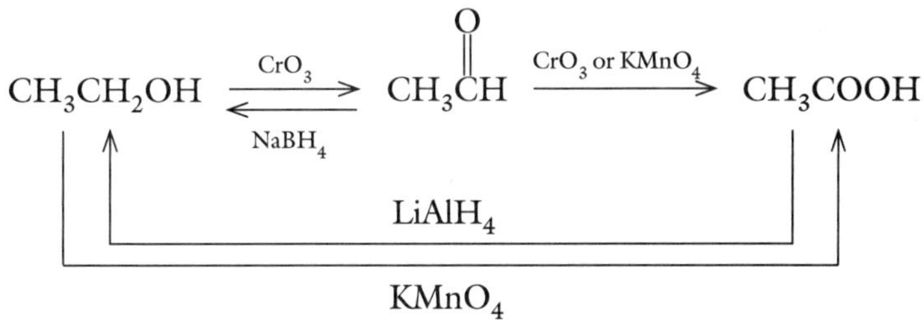

(b) Reduction to Hydrocarbons (Wolff–Kishner reduction)

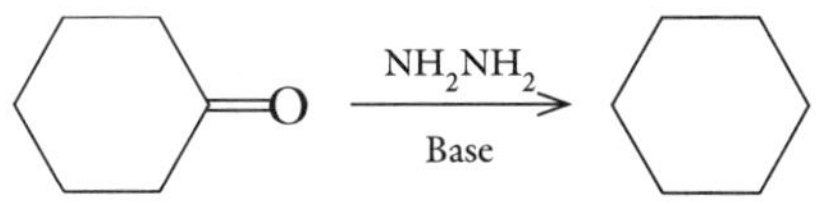

(c) Grignard Reactions

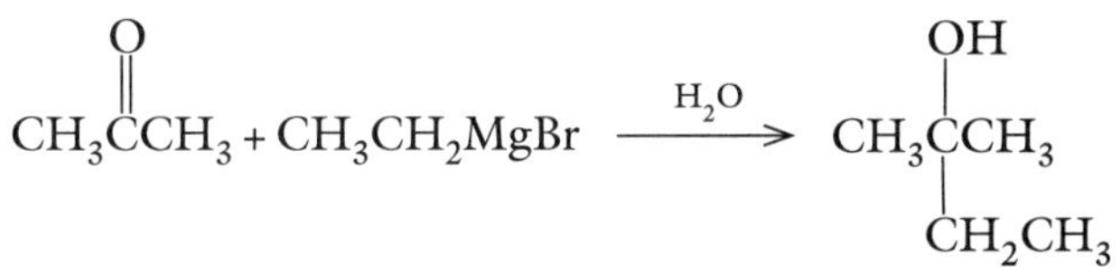

(d) Cyanohydrin Formation

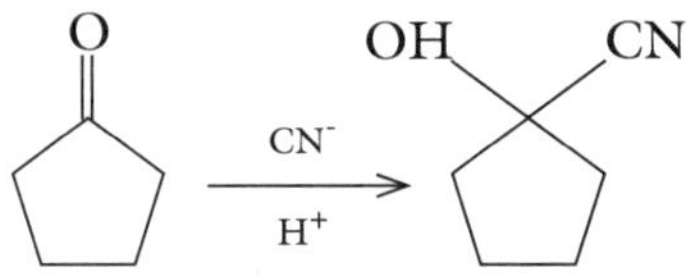

g. Carboxylic Acids

1. Preparation

(a) Oxidation of Primary Alcohols and Aldehydes

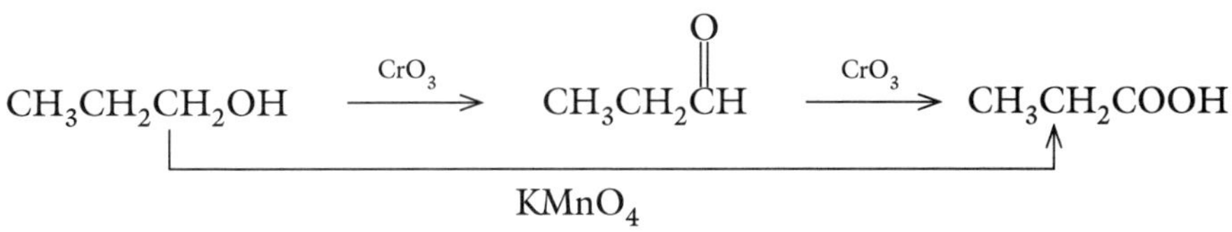

(b) Carbonation of Grignard Reagents

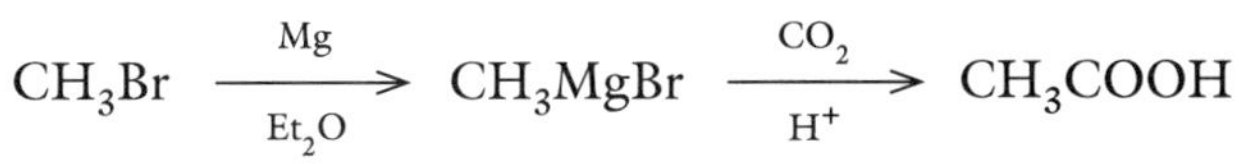

(c) Hydrolysis of Nitriles

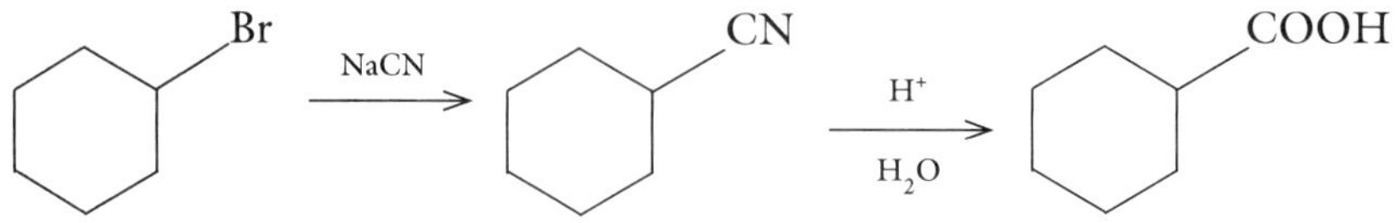

2. Reactions

(a) Conversion to Functional Derivatives

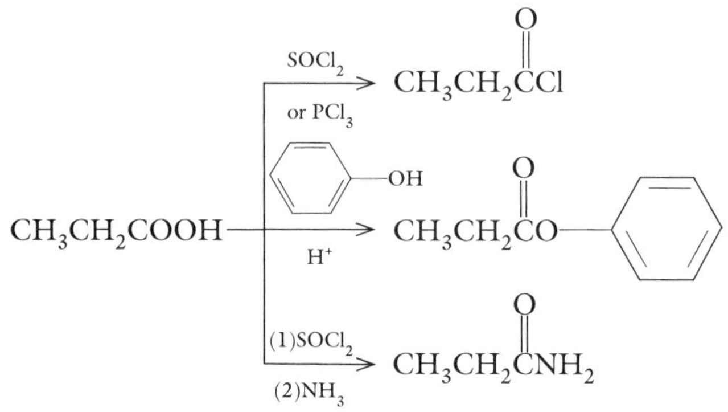

(b) Reduction

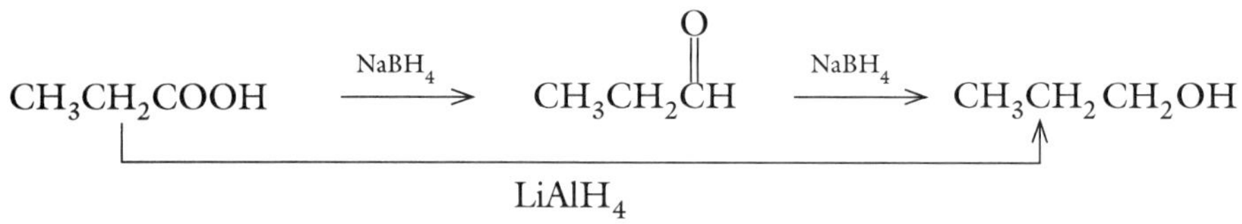

h. Acyl Halides

1. Preparation

From Carboxylic Acids

$$CH_3CH_2COOH \xrightarrow{SOCl_2} CH_3CH_2\overset{O}{\overset{\|}{C}}Cl$$

2. Reactions

(a) Conversion to Carboxylic Acids and Carboxylic Acid Derivatives

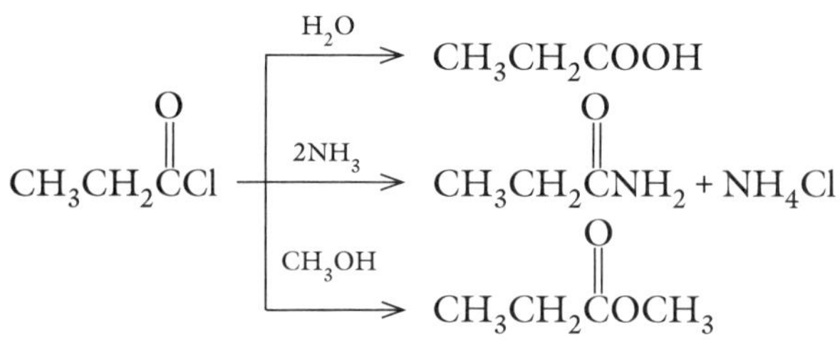

(b) Friedel–Crafts Acylation

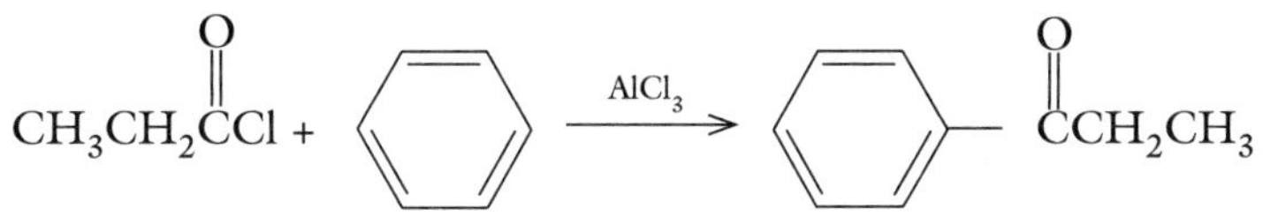

(c) Reaction with Organolithium Compounds

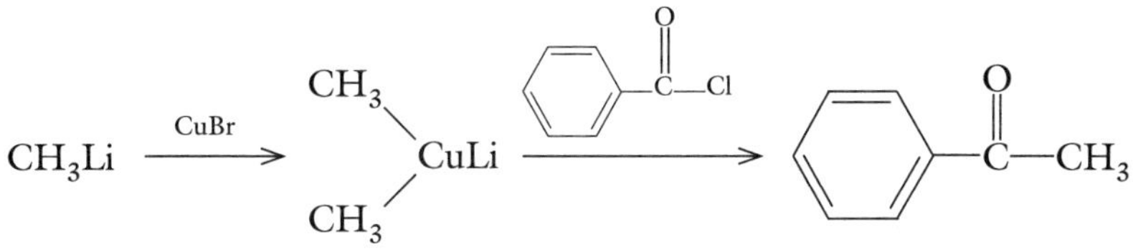

i. Esters

1. Preparation

(a) From Alcohols and Carboxylic Acids

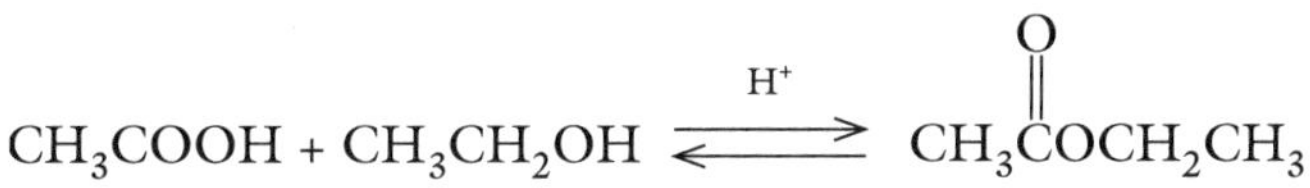

(b) From Acyl Halides

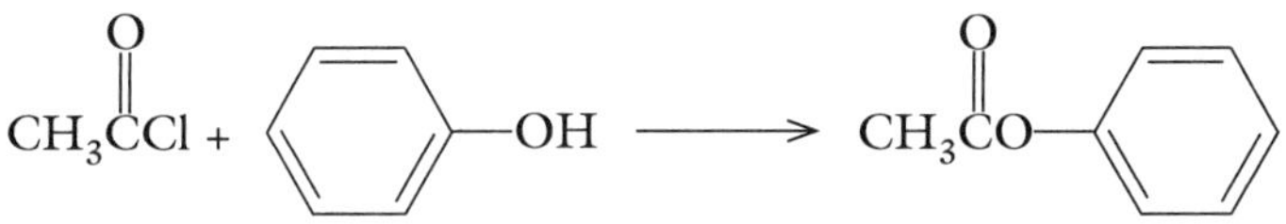

2. Reactions

(a) Conversion to Carboxylic Acids (Hydrolysis), Amides (Ammonolysis), and Other Esters (Transesterification)

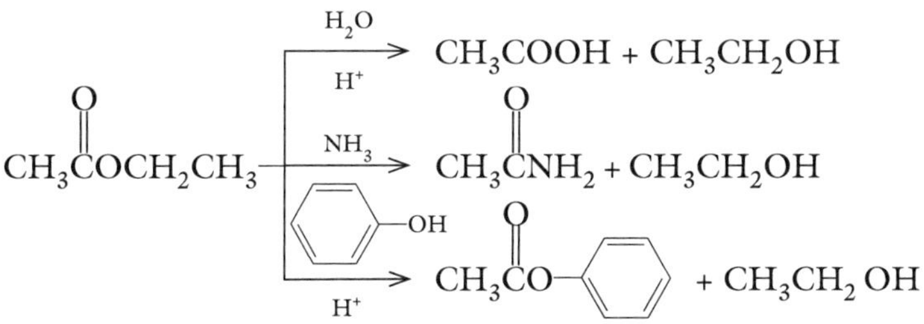

(b) Reactions with Grignard Reagents

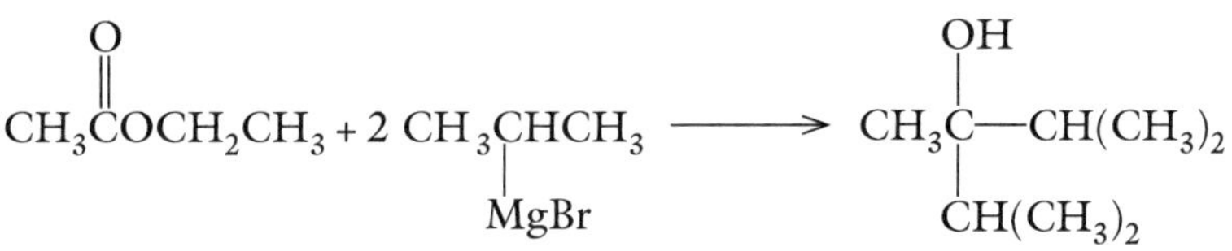

(c) Reduction

$$CH_3\overset{O}{\overset{\|}{C}}OCH_2CH_3 \xrightarrow[\text{or LiAlH}_4\text{, Et}_2\text{O, H}_2\text{O}]{\text{Ni, H}_2} 2\ CH_3CH_2OH$$

$$CH_3\overset{O}{\overset{\|}{C}}OCH_3 \xrightarrow[\text{or LiAlH}_4\text{, Et}_2\text{O, H}_2\text{O}]{\text{Ni, H}_2} CH_3CH_2OH + CH_3OH$$

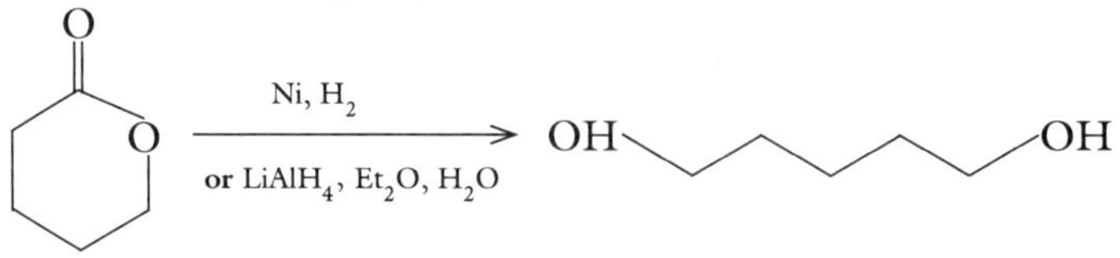

j. Aromatic Compounds

Reactions

1. Electrophilic Aromatic Substitution

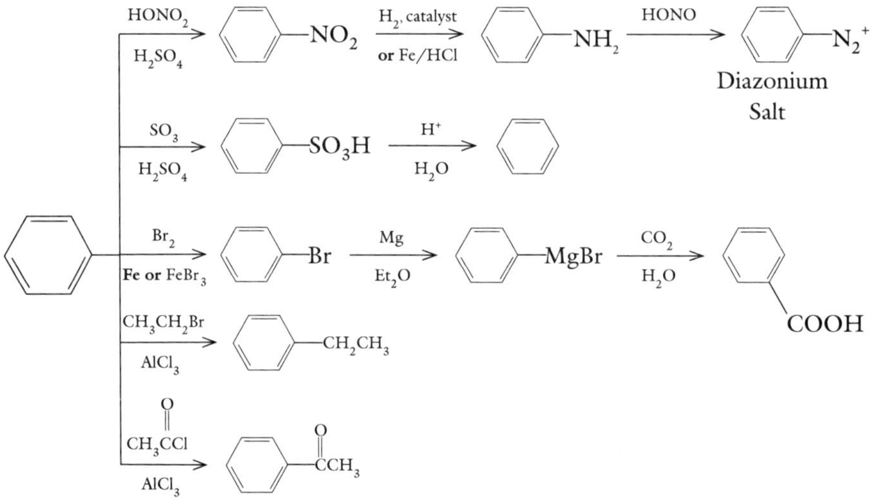

2. Reactions Involving Diazonium Salts

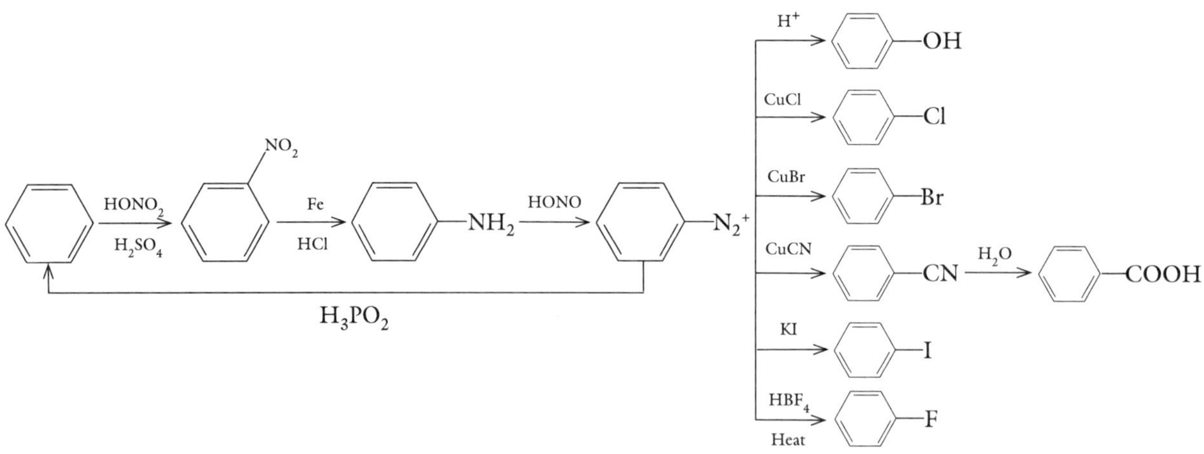

H Biology

1 DIFFERENCES BETWEEN PROKARYOTES AND EUKARYOTES

a. Characteristics of Prokaryotes

The differences between prokaryotes and eukaryotes enable specially designed antibiotics to selectively kill prokaryotic cells (i.e., bacteria) by inhibiting prokaryotic cell membrane synthesis, protein synthesis, transcription, and DNA replication.

- Prokaryotes have no membrane-bound organelles (i.e., no nuclear membrane, no mitochondria, no lysosomes, no endoplasmic reticulum).
- Transcription and translation can occur at the same time (because no nuclear membrane or nucleus is present to separate the two processes).
- Ribosomes are 70S (composed of 30S and 50S ribosomal subunits).
- Prokaryotes have peptidoglycan cell walls (consisting of amino acids and polysaccharides), which is the site of action of many antibacterial drugs (e.g., penicillins, cephalosporins).
- Most adenosine triphosphate (ATP) synthesis occurs at the cell membrane (because prokaryotes lack mitochondria), with enzymes found free in the cytoplasm.
- Prokaryotes have no true nucleus or nucleoid region where DNA is located (i.e., no nuclear membrane).
- Mechanisms of gene transfer in prokaryotes are transduction, transformation, and conjugation.
- Antibiotic resistance is transferred by conjugation via plasmids.
- Prokaryotes contain a single, circular strand of DNA.
- Cells divide by binary fission.

b. Characteristics of Eukaryotes

- Eukaryotes have membrane-bound organelles (i.e., nuclear membrane, mitochondria, lysosomes, and endoplasmic reticulum).
- Transcription and translation must occur independently (transcription takes place in the nucleus and translation takes place in the ribosomes).
- Ribosomes are 80S (composed of 40S and 60S ribosomal subunits) bound to rough endoplasmic reticulum (can also be found free in cytoplasm), except mitochondrial ribosomes, which are 70S.
- Eukaryotes may or may not have a cellulose cell wall.
- Most ATP synthesis occurs in the mitochondria.
- Nuclear material found as linear, double-stranded DNA wrapped around histone proteins (chromosomes).
- Cells divide by mitosis, with gametogenesis by meiosis.

c. Comparison of Prokaryotes and Eukaryotes (Table 2–12).

TABLE 2-12. Comparison of prokaryotes and eukaryotes

Feature	Prokaryotes	Eukaryotes
Organelles	Absent	Present
Nucleus	Absent	Present
Nucleolus	Absent	Present
Genetic information	Single chromosomes‡	Multiple chromosomes
DNA	Naked	Packaged with proteins
Cell division	Cleavage/binary fission	Mitosis and meiosis
Protein synthesis	Coupled to transcription in the same compartment	RNA made in the nucleus; translated in the cytoplasm
Metabolism (primary)	Anaerobic and aerobic	Aerobic
Respiratory enzymes	Plasma membrane	Mitochondria
Cell wall	Present	Extracellular matrix
Cytoskeleton	Absent	Present
Endocytosis* or exocytosis†	Absent	Present

*Endocytosis is the process by which cells acquire extracellular materials by an invagination of the plasma membrane.
†Exocytosis is the process by which cells discard intracellular materials, and it occurs via fusion of intracellular vesicles with the plasma membrane.
‡A chromosome refers to a single molecule of DNA, and its associated proteins, that contains many genes.
Reprinted with permission from Davidson VL, Sittman DB: *NMS Biochemistry*, 3rd ed. Baltimore, Williams & Wilkins, 1994, p 92.

2 VIRUSES

a. Definition

Viruses are obligate intracellular parasites; that is, they cannot live outside a host. A virus uses the metabolic machinery of its host to replicate. Viruses have no organelles. Viruses that inhabit animals are called animal viruses, viruses that infect plants are called plant viruses, and viruses that infect bacteria are called bacteriophages (or phages for short).

Viruses consist of nucleic acid and enzymes encased in a protein coat.

Viruses consist of:

- Protein coat (both an inner and outer protein coat or only an inner coat)
- Nucleic acid (either DNA or RNA, but not both)
- Envelope (lipoprotein membrane that surrounds the protein coat) can be found on some viruses.

Retroviruses (e.g., HIV) can make DNA from RNA (reverse transcription) and contain the enzyme reverse transcriptase.

b. Life Cycle

1. **Sequences.** A virus can follow one of three sequences in its life cycle.

   (a) **Lytic cycle.** A virus undergoing a lytic cycle attaches to the plasma membrane of the cell it is infecting, releases its nucleic acid material into the cell, replicates, and transcribes its nucleic acid material. Some RNA viruses can transcribe mRNA from their RNA directly, whereas others (retroviruses) reverse-transcribe the RNA to DNA right after it enters the cell. In either case, the virus makes many copies of its genome (DNA or RNA) and translates many copies of the viral proteins necessary for the protein coat(s). The cellular machinery is then used to assemble hundreds to thousands of viruses. Once a sufficient number of viruses have been constructed, the cell lyses and the viruses are released into the environment (i.e., the bloodstream) to infect other cells. This cycle always ends in cell death.

(b) **Lysogenic cycle.** In this cycle, the virus, after attaching to the plasma membrane and injecting its genetic material into the cell, integrates its genetic material into the host cell's genome or, alternatively, can persist in the cell as an extrachromosomal plasmid. The virus can thus lie dormant for many rounds of cell division, replicating its genetic material when the host cell replicates and never producing any new viruses or killing the host cell. In some instances, the virus can even give the host cell a survival advantage by passing on resistance to antibiotics or heavy metals (very useful in bacterial molecular biology).

Many viruses that enter the lysogenic cycle switch to the lytic cycle in a process known as **lytic induction;** this switch to an active phase is often in response to extracellular stress or DNA damage. In this situation, the virus makes new viruses and lyses the host cell as would any normal lytic virus.

(c) **Chronic infection.** In these cases (e.g., HIV or bacteriophage M13), the virus can enter a mixed stage called chronic or persistent infection. The virus does not kill the cell, but viruses are made and released at the plasma membrane surface through a budding process, the least common of the three types of viral life cycles.

2. **Switching Between Cycles.** A few viruses, such as bacteriophage lambda or hepatitis, can switch between the lytic and lysogenic (or even chronic infection) cycle (Figure 2-38); those viruses with more flexibility in their life cycle

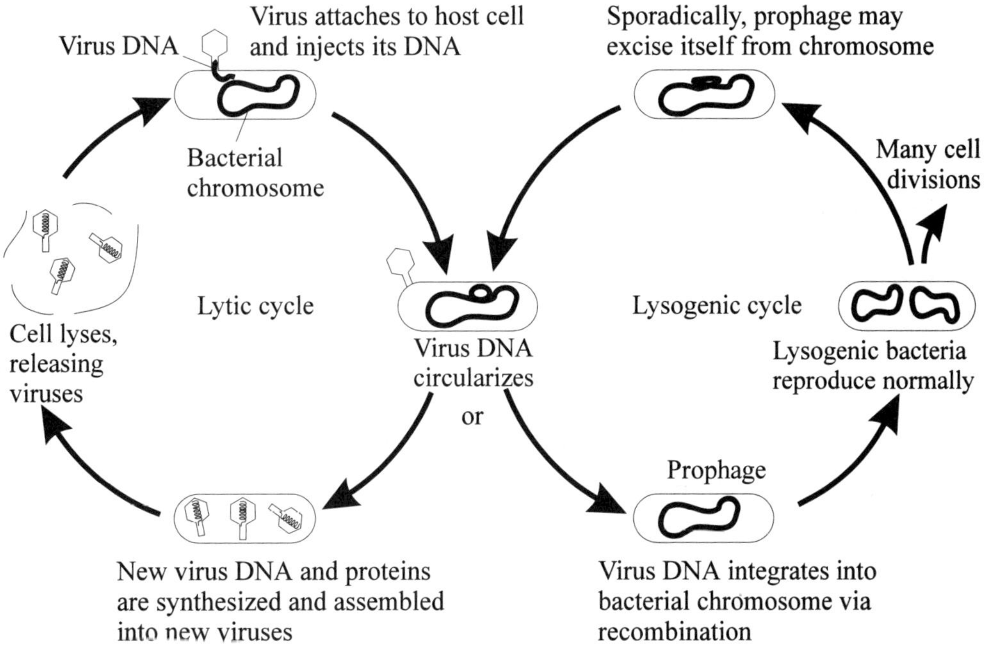

Figure 2-38.
The lytic and lysogenic cycles of bacteriophage lambda.

have a definite survival advantage. A virus that can choose between the lytic and lysogenic cycles can regulate the number of cells it kills per unit time, which allows the host organism to survive while a number of cells are lysed to release new viruses.

3 ORGANELLES AND MEMBRANE TRANSPORT (TABLE 2-13)

a. Passive Transport (Simple Diffusion) [Figures 2-39 and 2-40; Table 2-14] Molecules move down a gradient.

b. Facilitated, or carrier-mediated, transport

exhibits saturation kinetics (see Figure 2-40B).

c. Active Transport

Molecules move up a concentration gradient, using ATP.

TABLE 2-13. Organelles and their functions

Organelle	Function
Ribosome	Is the site of protein synthesis (translation)
Rough endoplasmic reticulum (RER)	Has ribosomes bound to it, therefore functioning in the synthesis, chemical modification, and ultimate secretion of proteins
Smooth endoplasmic reticulum (SER)	Is the site of steroid synthesis and detoxification of drugs and poisons
Sarcoplasmic reticulum	Has voltage-dependent calcium channels used for muscle contraction. This specialized type of smooth endoplasmic reticulum is found in all types of muscle cells that sequester calcium ions.
Golgi apparatus	Receives proteins from the endoplasmic reticulum. Site of protein modification, packaging, and secretion. Site for protein glycosylation and polysaccharide synthesis.
Lysosomes	Contain enzymes (e.g., acid hydrolases) for the digestion of endocytosed particles and old organelles
Mitochondria	Is the site of the majority of ATP synthesis. (The Krebs cycle, electron transport chain, and oxidative phosphorylation all occur in the mitochondria.)
Centrioles	Participate in cell division (mitosis and meiosis). The spindle appartus arises from the centrioles on each pole of the dividing cell and attaches to the centromere of the sister chromatids.
Nucleus	Is the site of DNA replication and gene transcription
Nucleolus	Is the site of rRNA synthesis

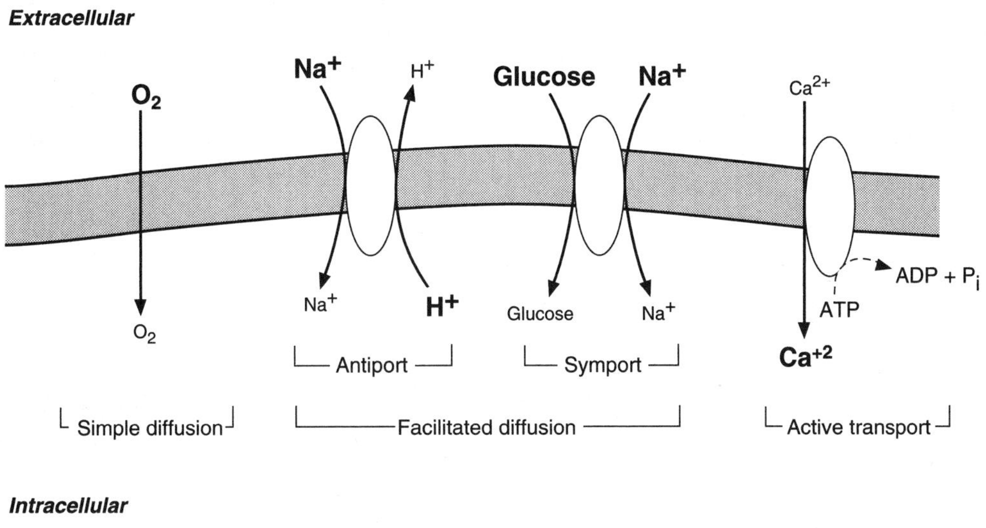

Figure 2-39. Membrane transport. In passive transport (simple diffusion), molecules move down a gradient. Facilitated, or carrier-mediated, transport exhibits saturation kinetics. Active transport moves a molecule up a concentration gradient, using ATP.

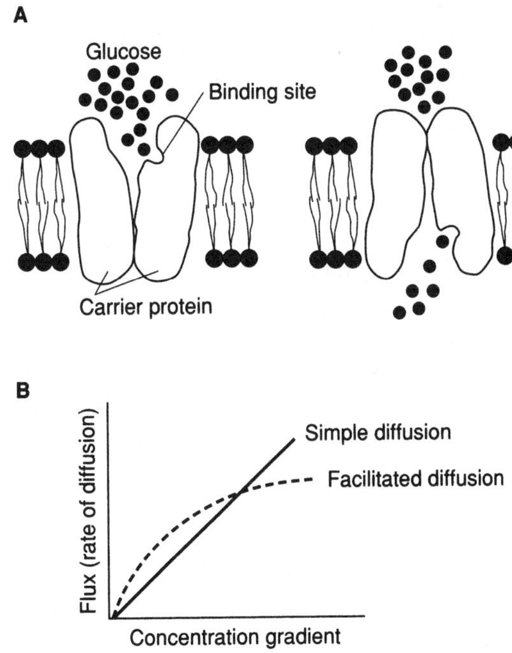

Figure 2-40. *(A)* The transmembrane carrier protein responsible for the facilitated diffusion of glucose undergoes a conformational change when glucose binds to it. The conformational change allows glucose to diffuse across the membrane down its concentration gradient. *(B)* In facilitated diffusion, the diffusion rate reaches a maximum when all the binding sites on the carrier protein are filled. Although the slope of the line may vary, the rate of membrane transport with simple diffusion is directly proportional to the concentration gradient of the molecule being transported, whereas facilitated (carrier-mediated) diffusion, like enzymes, exhibits saturation kinetics. (Reprinted with permission from Bullock J, Boyle J, Wang MB: *NMS Physiology,* 3rd ed. Baltimore, Williams & Wilkins, 1995, p 4.)

TABLE 2-14. Characteristics of different types of transport

Type	Electrochemical Gradient	Carrier-mediated	Metabolic Energy	Na^+ Gradient	Inhibition of Na^+-K^+ Pump
Simple diffusion	Downhill	No	No	No	
Facilitated diffusion	Downhill	Yes	No	No	
Primary active transport	Uphill	Yes	Yes		Inhibits (if Na^+-K^+ pump)
Cotransport	Uphill*	Yes	Indirect	Yes, same direction	Inhibits
Countertransport	Uphill*	Yes	Indirect	Yes, opposite direction	Inhibits

* One or more solutes are transported uphill; Na^+ is transported downhill.
Reprinted with permission from Bullock J, Boyle J, Wang MB: *NMS Physiology*, 3rd ed. Baltimore, Williams & Wilkins, 1995, p 4.

4 ENZYME KINETICS AND CATALYSIS

Enzymes are biologic catalysts that lower the activation energy of a reaction but are not consumed by the reaction.

a. Definitions

Enzymes are complex proteins that function as biologic catalysts, increasing the rate of both forward and reverse chemical reactions by lowering their energy of activation. Enzymes do **not** change the free energy or the equilibrium constant of the reactions they catalyze (Figure 2-41)

Zymogen is an enzyme that is secreted in an inactive form that, under proper physiological conditions, undergoes proteolytic cleavage and is activated. Many digestive enzymes are secreted as zymogens to protect the intestinal organs from autodigestion (e.g., pepsinogen is secreted by chief cells of the stomach and is activated by H^+, which is secreted by the parietal cells of the stomach).

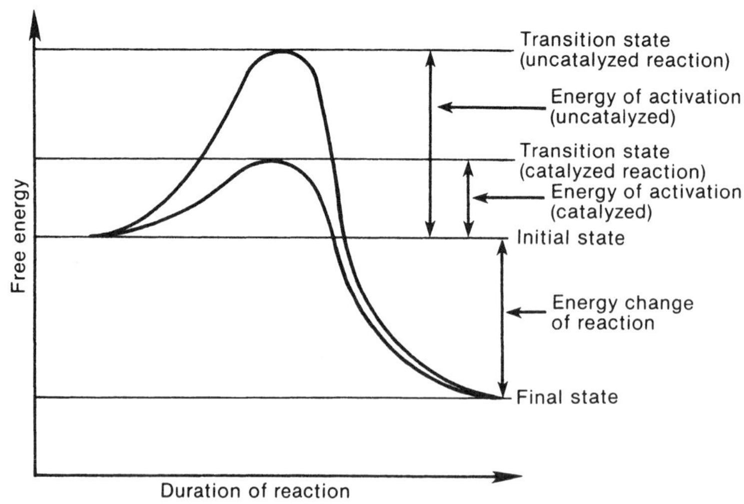

Figure 2-41. Diagrammatic representation of the free energy of activation of a chemical reaction. (Reprinted with permission from Davidson VL, Sittman DB: *NMS Biochemistry*, 3rd ed. Baltimore, Williams & Wilkins, 1994, p 87.)

b. Enzyme Kinetics

$$E + S \underset{k_2}{\overset{k_1}{\rightleftharpoons}} ES \xrightarrow{k_{cat}} E + P$$

k_1 = rate of forward reaction
k_2 = rate of reverse reaction
k_{cat} = rate of catalyzed reaction
E = enzyme
S = substrate
ES = enzyme-substrate intermediate
P = product

c. Michaelis-Menten equation

is used to describe the preceding reaction between an enzyme and a substrate. Do not memorize the derivation of this equation. Just understand why it produces the graph shown in Figure 2-42.

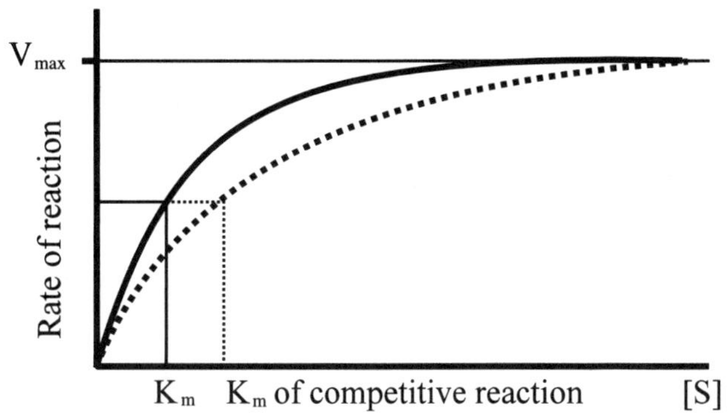

Figure 2-42. Enzyme kinetics. The *solid line* indicates an enzymatic reaction. The *dotted line* indicates an enzymatic reaction in the presence of a competitive inhibitor.

The final equation is as follows:

$$v = \frac{v_{max}[S]}{K_m + [S]}$$

v = reaction rate in forward direction
V_{max} = maximum rate of reaction (lots of substrate per molecule of enzyme)
K_m = Michaelis-Menten constant for a given enzyme-catalyzed reaction
[S] = concentration of substrate

The K_m is a very important concept; for when the concentration of substrate equals K_m, the reaction proceeds at half its maximal rate (which is a very efficient use of the enzyme). If the enzyme concentration is less than K_m, the enzyme is not used efficiently because there is too much substrate and not enough enzyme. On the other hand, if the enzyme concentration becomes larger than K_m, there will be too much free enzyme and not enough free substrate. For this reason, most enzymes in biologic systems tend to exist at concentrations close to K_m. An added benefit of having an enzyme concentration close to K_m is that small changes in the enzyme concentration have large effects on the speed of the reaction (since changes are on the steepest part of the curve), which makes it easier to regulate biologic reactions through the regulation of the enzyme concentration.

At low substrate concentrations, the rate of reaction depends primarily on the rate of formation of the enzyme–substrate complex (i.e., $k_{rxn} \approx k_1$).

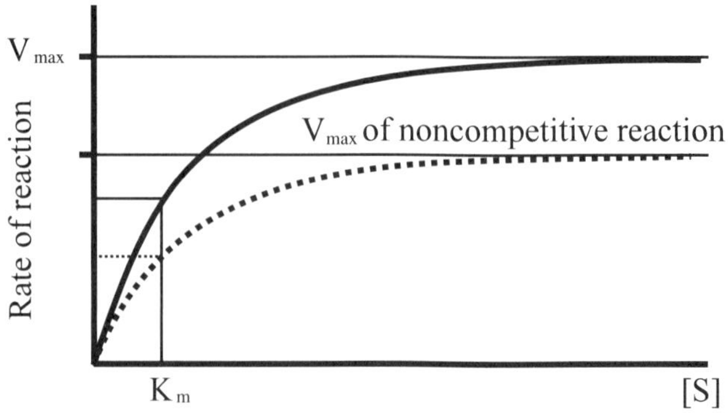

Figure 2-43. Effect of a noncompetitive inhibitor on enzyme kinetics. The *solid line* indicates an uninhibited enzymatic reaction. The *dotted line* indicates that an inhibitor accomplishes these effects by binding to the enzyme at a site other than its active site.

Competitive inhibitors are substrates that inhibit an enzyme by binding to its active site. These substrates "compete" with the substrate inhibitors for the active site. Competitive inhibitors increase K_m but do not change the V_{max}. This type of inhibition can be overcome by increasing substrate concentration [S] (see Figure 2-42).

Noncompetitive inhibitors bind to a site other than the active site of the enzyme. This type of inhibitor does not prevent binding of the substrate to the active site of the enzyme. Noncompetitive inhibitors do not change K_m but decrease V_{max} (Figure 2-43).

Enzyme denaturation occurs at high temperatures, decreasing the rate of reaction at very high temperatures owing to thermal breakdown of the enzyme. Therefore, increasing the temperature increases the rate of an enzyme-catalyzed reaction to a certain extent, until the enzyme starts to denature, resulting in a decreased rate of reaction (Figures 2-44 and 2-45).

5 METABOLISM: BASIC PRINCIPLES

Organisms must use a series of reactions to metabolize (break down) organic molecules and release energy that can be used for biologic processes. The universal energy currency of the cell is **ATP.** Cells dephosphorylate ATP to adenosine diphosphate **(ADP)** and inorganic phosphate (P_i) in a reaction that releases approximately 7 kcal of energy per mole of ATP.

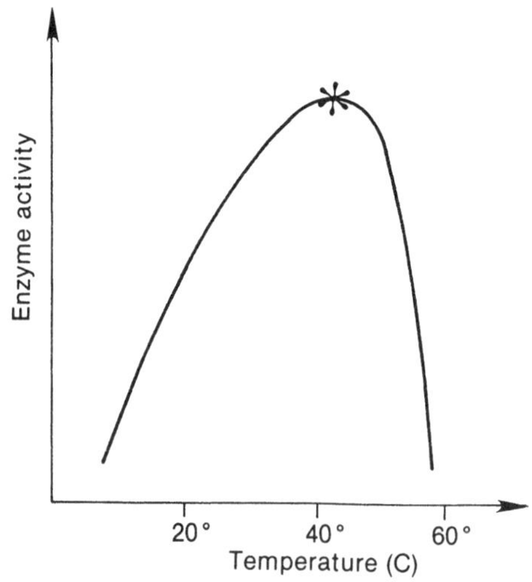

Figure 2-44. Effect of temperature on the activity of an enzyme. The apparent optimum point shown here (*) is the result of an initial increase in reaction rate due to a rise in temperature, followed by a decrease in enzymatic activity as the temperature continues upward with increasing thermal denaturation of the proteinaceous enzyme molecule. (Reprinted with permission from Davidson VL, Sittman DB: *NMS Biochemistry,* 3rd ed. Baltimore, Williams & Wilkins, 1994, p 93.)

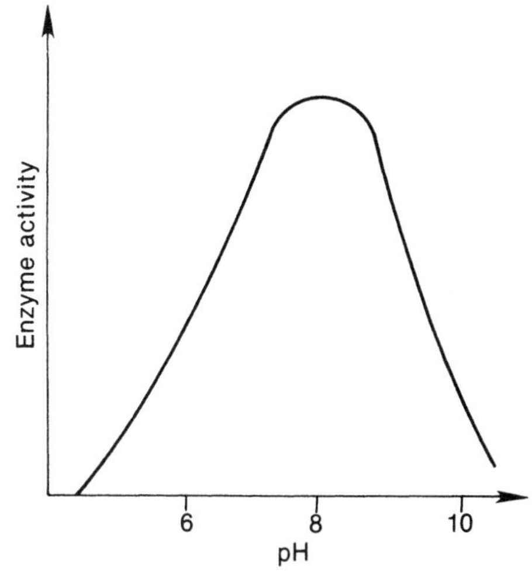

Figure 2-45.
A typical pH-activity plot of an enzyme-catalyzed reaction. (Reprinted with permission from Davidson VL, Sittman DB: *NMS Biochemistry,* 3rd ed. Baltimore, Williams & Wilkins, 1994, p 92.)

Although organisms can metabolize many different organic substrates to fulfill their energy requirements, sometimes the substrates are first converted to **glucose,** a hexose sugar that is the most common substrate catabolized by organisms. Consequently, you should focus your studies on the metabolism of glucose, although you should be aware that other reactions allow cells to metabolize substrates without conversion to glucose (such as the β-oxidation of fatty acids) [Figure 2-46].

> The metabolism of glucose in eukaryotic (and many prokaryotic) cells is a complex series of reactions, described next. The MCAT frequently describes a part or all of the metabolism of glucose (possibly including a diagram); therefore, give yourself time to analyze the Krebs cycle so you can answer passage-based and discrete questions about the different steps.

TEST CORRELATION

a. Steps in Aerobic Respiration: Catabolism of Glucose

1. **Glycolysis**, which occurs in the cytosol, converts glucose to two molecules of pyruvic acid. See Figure 2-47 for the specific steps in this pathway. During glycolysis, two molecules of ATP are produced through substrate-level phosphorylation, a process that involves the direct coupling of a step in the catabolism of a substrate to the phosphorylation of an ADP molecule. In other words, the substrate is dephosphorylated and the ADP picks up the phosphate to form ATP. This process is not the most common method of ATP synthesis; most ATP is produced by oxidative phosphorylation via chemiosmotic coupling.

2. The **Krebs cycle** occurs in the mitochondrial matrix, which is the innermost part of the mitochondria (within the cristae). This cycle is also known as the citric acid or tricarboxylic acid (TCA) cycle (know all of these names). As the pyruvate molecules enter the mitochondrial matrix, they lose a carboxyl group and are converted to a two-carbon compound called acetyl coenzyme A, or acetyl CoA. Acetyl CoA then enters a circular series of reactions. In one turn of the Krebs cycle, two molecules of carbon dioxide are produced; they are in

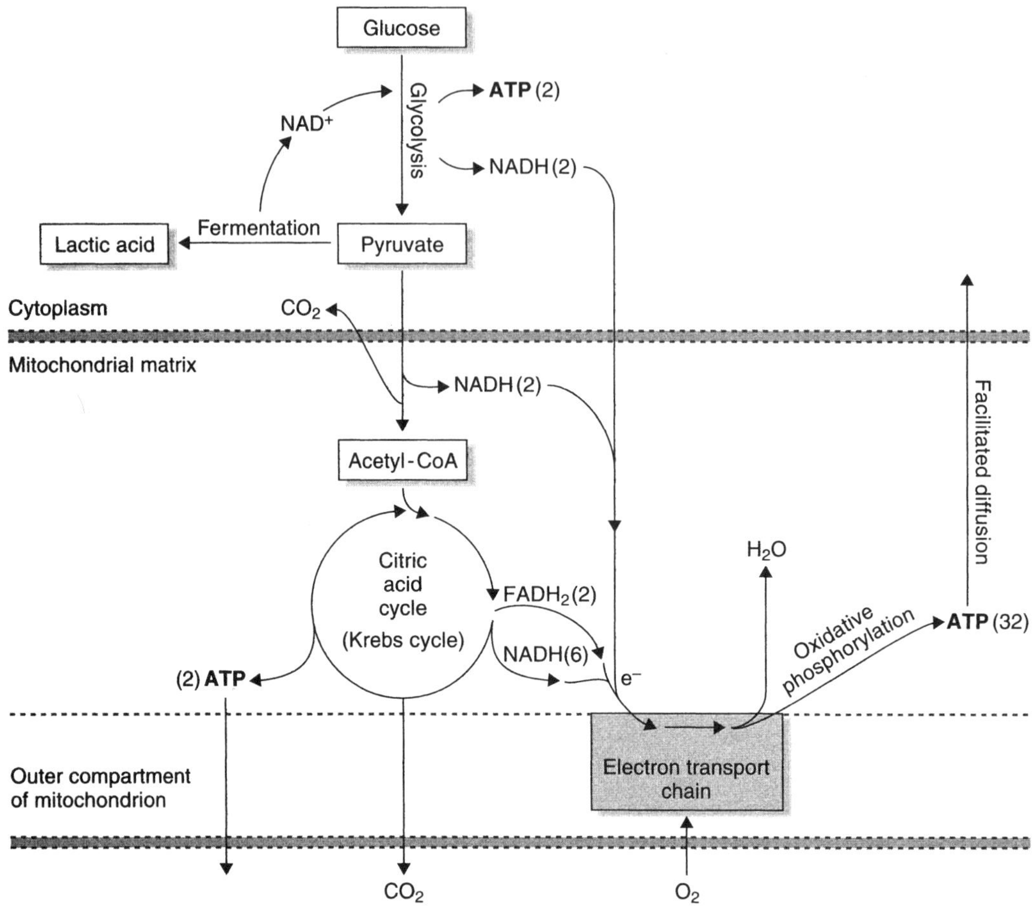

$$C_6H_{12}O_6 + 6H_2O + 6O_2 \longrightarrow 6CO_2 + 12H_2O + \text{Energy}$$
(Glucose)

ATP Balance Sheet

	Substrate-level Phosphorylation	Oxidative Phosphorylation
Glycolysis	2	4
Pyruvate to acetyl-CoA	0	6
Krebs cycle	2	22
Total	4	32

Total Yield = 36 ATP

Figure 2–46.
The process of eukaryotic cellular respiration, involving the oxidation of bio-organic molecules. The numbers of ATP and NADH molecules produced are indicated. *ATP* = adenosine triphosphate; *CO_2* = carbon dioxide; *CoA* = coenzyme A; e^- = negative electron; *$FADH_2$* = reduced form of flavin adenine dinucleotide; *H_2O* = water; *NAD^+* = oxidized form of nicotinamide adenine dinucleotide; *NADH* = reduced nicotinamide adenine dinucleotide; *O_2* = oxygen. (Reprinted with permission from Roth, D: *MCAT Essentials*, Baltimore, Williams & Wilkins, 1998, p 159.)

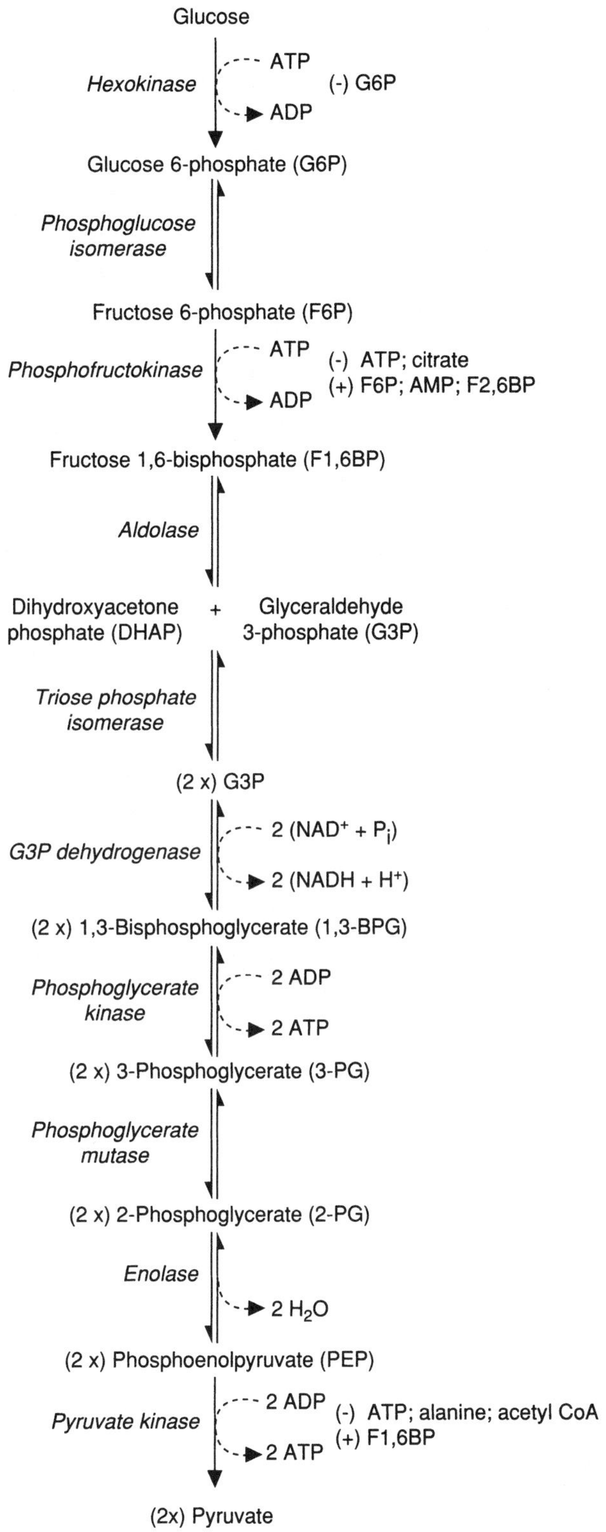

Figure 2-47.
The pathway of glycolysis. The signs (+) and (−) indicate the sites of action of allosteric positive and negative modulators of the activities of the key regulatory enzymes. *ADP* = adenosine diphosphate; *AMP* = adenosine monophosphate; *ATP* = adenosine triphosphate; *F2, 6BP* = fructose 2,6-bisphosphate; *NAD^+* = oxidized nicotinamide adenine dinucleotide; *NADH* = reduced NAD; P_i = inorganic phosphate. (Reprinted with permission from Davidson VL, Sittman DB: *NMS Biochemistry,* 3rd ed. Baltimore, Williams & Wilkins, 1994, p 340.)

an oxidized state relative to acetyl CoA. One ATP is generated per turn, three molecules of NAD^+ are reduced to NADH, and one molecule of FAD is reduced to $FADH_2$ (for use in the electron transport chain). Note: One turn of the Krebs cycle is required for each acetyl CoA, so two turns of the TCA cycle are required for each initial glucose molecule. See Figure 2-48 for details, but do not memorize it.

3. **Electron transport chain (ETC)/oxidative phosphorylation** occurs in the inner mitochondrial membrane. This stage of aerobic respiration requires oxygen. Most of the components of the electron transport chain are proteins that shift between oxidized and reduced states as they accept or release electrons. An important type of electron carrier is the **cytochrome**, which has a **heme** group that surrounds an iron atom. The electrons of NADH and $FADH_2$ are transferred to oxygen in an elegant series of reactions that produce energy and can in turn be used to phosphorylate ADP to ATP (Figure 2-49). For the MCAT, you need to know that before the ETC (as the electron transport chain is affectionately known), only four molecules of ATP have been produced (net production of 2 ATP because two are required for activation of reactants). During the ETC, another 34 molecules of ATP are produced (3

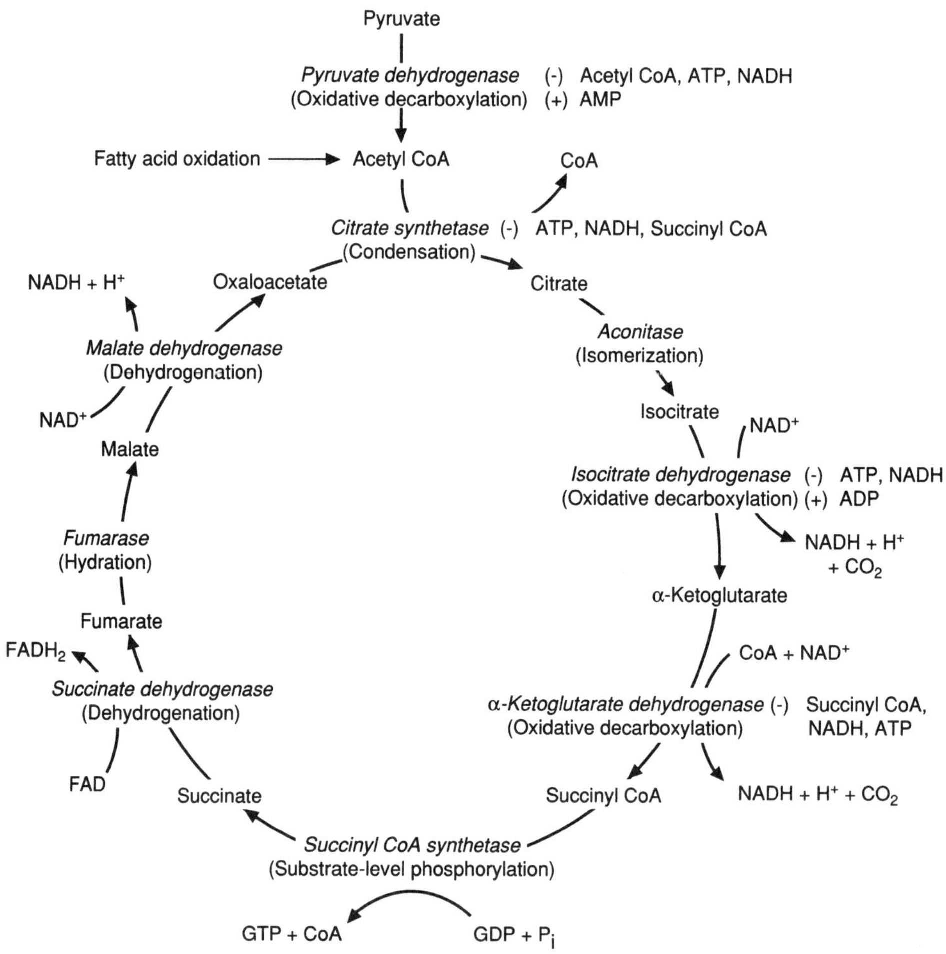

Figure 2-48. The reactions of pyruvate dehydrogenase and the Krebs cycle. The type of reaction that is catalyzed by each enzyme is indicated in *brackets* below the enzyme, which is indicated in *italic type*. Inhibitors and activators of regulatory enzymes are indicated by − and +, respectively. *ADP* = adenosine diphosphate; *AMP* = adenosine monophosphate; *ATP* = adenosine triphosphate; *CoA* = coenzyme A; *FAD* = flavin adenine dinucleotide; *$FADH_2$* = reduced FAD; *GDP* = guanosine diphosphate; *GTP* = guanosine triphosphate; *NAD^+* = oxidized nicotinamide adenine dinucleotide; *NADH* = reduced NAD; *P_i* = inorganic phosphate. (Reprinted with permission from Davidson VL, Sittman DB: *NMS Biochemistry,* 3rd ed. Baltimore, Williams & Wilkins, 1994, p 371.)

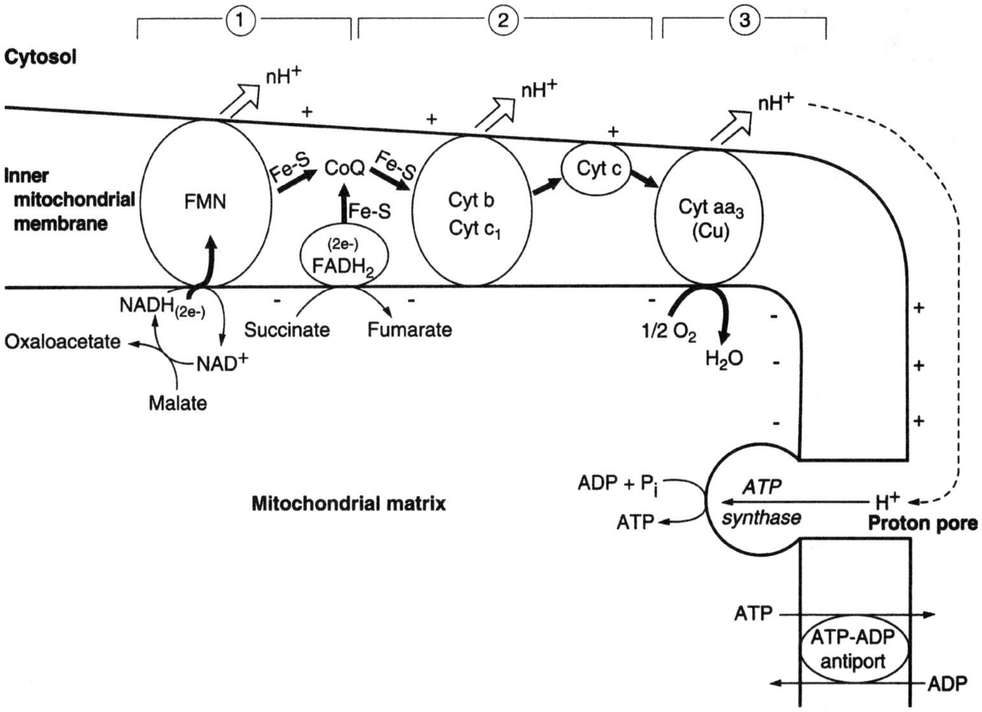

Figure 2-49. The electron transport chain and oxidative phosphorylation. *Heavy arrows* indicate the flow of electrons. *Fe-S* = iron-sulfur centers; *FMN* = flavin mononucleotide; *CoQ* = coenzyme Q (ubiquinone); *Cyt* = cytochrome. nH^+ indicates that an undetermined number of protons are pumped from the matrix to the cytosolic side. (Reprinted with permission from Marks DB: *BRS Biochemistry*, 2nd ed. Baltimore, Williams & Wilkins, 1994, p 118.)

ATP per NADH, 2 ATP per $FADH_2$) with a cost of 2 ATP, for a net gain of 32 ATP in this step and 36 ATP overall.

b. Aerobic versus Anaerobic Respiration

The series of reactions previously discussed are entitled aerobic respiration because they require oxygen (the ETC) to metabolize glucose to completion. Some bacteria cannot use oxygen, so what do they do? Or when eukaryotic cells run out of oxygen (e.g., muscle cells during strenuous exercise), what do they do?

Aerobic respiration yields 36 molecules of ATP, whereas anaerobic respiration yields only 2 molecules of ATP.

The answer is **anaerobic respiration** (the metabolism of glucose in the absence of oxygen). Whereas aerobic respiration consists of glycolysis, the Krebs cycle, and ETC/oxidative phosphorylation, anaerobic glycolysis involves glycolysis, then the conversion of pyruvate to lactic acid (or ethanol). Whereas aerobic respiration gives a net gain of 36 ATP, anaerobic respiration gives the cell only 2 ATP (no wonder eukaryotic cells choose aerobic respiration in the presence of oxygen). Unfortunately, not all bacteria have this luxury and have to subsist on anaerobic respiration, or fermentation, with an end product of either alcohol or lactic acid.

During strenuous exercise, muscle cells can run out of oxygen. Faced with no better option, these cells begin to anaerobically respire glucose to lactic acid, resulting in the buildup of an "oxygen debt." You can feel the "debt" when your muscles cramp and begin to burn as you work them hard. Once the muscles relax and again receive sufficient oxygen from the blood, the cells can "repay the oxygen debt" and convert the lactate back to pyruvate and continue with aerobic respiration.

6 ENZYME/HORMONE REGULATION

a. Definitions

1. **Covalent modification** usually involves the phosphorylation or dephosphorylation of specific enzymes and results in the activation or inactivation of that particular enzyme. For example, when insulin binds to its receptor, it triggers a series of events that lead first to the dephosphorylation of glycogen synthase and, as a result, to its activation, thereby promoting glycogen synthesis and decreasing blood glucose levels.

2. **Allosteric effects** constitute the major method of enzymatic regulation and usually proceed by an enzymatic reaction in which the product binds to the enzyme at a site other than its active site to inhibit further activity of the enzyme (this reaction is known as feedback inhibition). The allosteric enzyme oscillates between an active conformation (the enzyme is capable of catalyzing the reaction) and an inactive conformation (the enzyme is incapable of catalyzing the reaction).

   Characteristics of allosteric modification (Figure 2-50)

   - It always involves an allosteric enzyme.
   - It is very rapid (unlike transcriptional regulation of enzymes).
   - It can result in enzymatic inhibition or activation.
   - It provides an efficient method of conserving cellular energy and avoids the accumulation of metabolic intermediates.

Most hormones are regulated by negative feedback.

3. **Negative feedback** inhibition occurs when the end product of a pathway inhibits (i.e., negatively feeds back) an earlier enzyme/hormone on the pathway (Figure 2-51). It is the most common mechanism of hormone regulation.

Figure 2-51 shows a classic example of a system with negative feedback. The secretion of corticotropin-releasing hormone (CRH) by the hypothalamus stimulates the secretion of adrenocorticotropic hormone (ACTH) by the anterior pituitary; then ACTH stimulates the secretion of cortisol into the bloodstream by the adrenal cortex. If too much cortisol is present, it inhibits further CRH secretion by the hypothalamus. Cortisol can inhibit ACTH se-

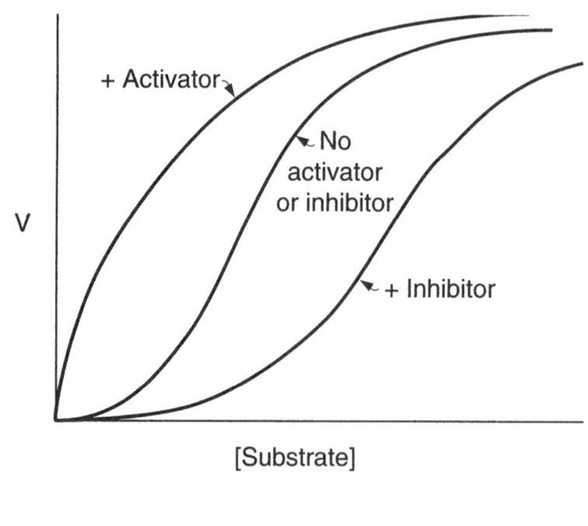

Figure 2-50. Effect of activators and inhibitors on an allosteric enzyme. (Reprinted with permission from Marks DB: *BRS Biochemistry,* 2nd ed. Baltimore, Williams & Wilkins, 1994, p 36.)

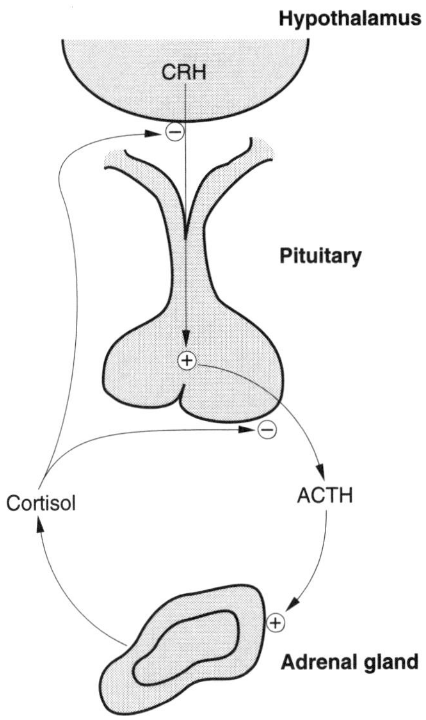

Figure 2-51. Hormone feedback regulation. *ACTH* = adrenocorticotropic hormone; CRH = corticortropin-releasing hormone; ⊕ = activates; ⊖ = inhibits. (Reprinted with permission from Marks DB: *BRS Biochemistry,* 2nd ed. Baltimore, Williams & Wilkins, 1994, p 285.)

cretion by the anterior pituitary if sufficient cortisol has already been secreted by the adrenal cortex in response to ACTH.

4. **Positive feedback** occurs when an end product stimulates the secretion or production of an earlier enzyme or hormone, which can lead to a continuous feedback cycle that escalates the levels of both chemicals. Positive feedback occurs during the menstrual cycle, when luteinizing hormone (LH) stimulates estrogen, which acts to further stimulate the secretion of LH, resulting in an **LH surge,** which triggers ovulation.

b. Transcriptional Regulation of Enzymes

1. **Prokaryotic gene regulation** is largely at the level of transcription. The two most common instances of prokaryotic gene regulation follow.

   (a) **Operons** are found in bacteria but have not been found in eukaryotes. The most common example of an operon is the *lac* operon, which codes for enzymes that regulate the transport and metabolism of lactose (Figure 2-52). The *lac* **repressor** is a protein that is continuously made by the *lac* operon. In the absence of lactose, the *lac* repressor can tightly bind to the **operator** sequence of the *lac* operon. If the repressor is bound to the operator, RNA polymerase cannot bind to the **promoter** sequence and initiate transcription. On the other hand, if lactose is present in the cell, a molecule of lactose can bind to the repressor and prevent the repressor from binding to the operator sequence. RNA polymerase can now bind to the repressor protein and can therefore transcribe the *lac* operon genes (which code for the transport and metabolization of lactose) in an example of **negative transcriptional regulation.** One

Gene regulation of enzymes occurs at the level of gene transcription and is therefore very slow to respond.

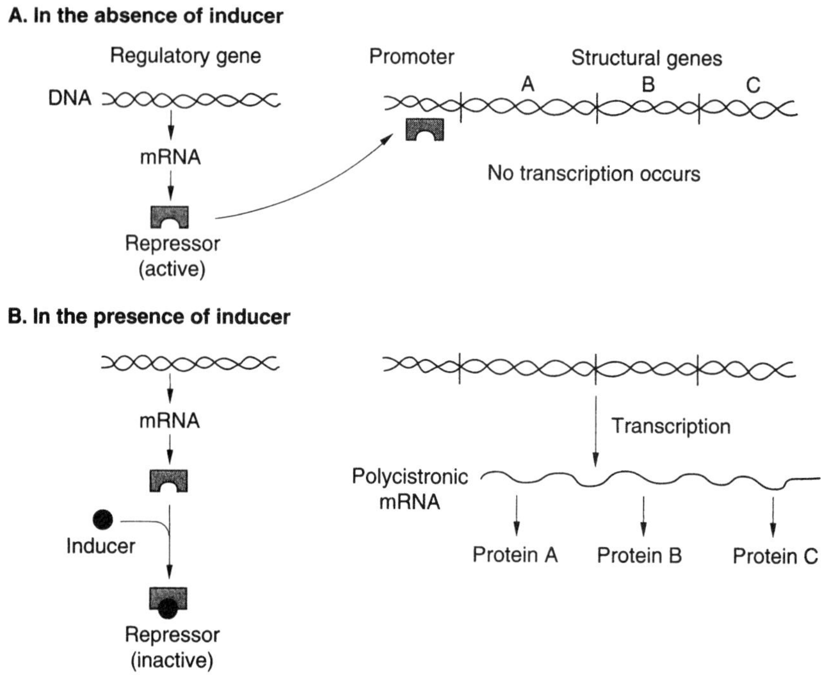

Figure 2-52.
An inducible operon (e.g., the *lac* operon). (Reprinted with permission from Marks DB: *BRS Biochemistry,* 2nd ed. Baltimore, Williams & Wilkins, 1994, p 75.)

can easily imagine the opposite process, called **positive transcriptional regulation,** where the inducible substance [e.g., cyclic AMP (cAMP)] can enhance RNA polymerase's ability to bind to the promoter sequence and initiate transcription.

(b) **Attenuation** is a much more complex process that uses the prokaryotic coupling of transcription and translation to regulate gene expression. The ribosome follows RNA polymerase closely; if it follows too closely, it will inhibit further transcription through the formation of a stem–loop complex. On the other hand, if it stalls because of lack of appropriate amino acid tRNA complexes to attach to the codons, the RNA polymerase can continue transcribing and the gene is turned on. This process is used to regulate the gene transcription necessary for the synthesis of amino acids; these genes are turned on only when amino acid levels are low and the ribosome stalls. The most common example of attenuation is the **tryptophan (trp) operon.**

2. **Eukaryotic gene regulation** is much more complex and less well understood. Proteins called **transcription factors** can enhance transcription by binding to any of the following types of sequences.

(a) **Promoters** are the sequence where the RNA polymerase binds. Many different transcription factors (TF) help RNA polymerase bind to the promoter, most notably TFIID (which binds to the upstream TATA box).

(b) **Proximal promoter elements** are additional sequences that are located upstream of the transcriptional start site and enhance transcription within 200 nucleotides of the promoter.

(c) **Enhancers** are sequences located far away from the transcriptional start site (greater than 200 nucleotides away, or even within or behind the gene) that increase transcriptional rates.

(d) **Steroid hormones** can regulate gene transcription of enzymes by binding to steroid receptor elements (SREs) on DNA, which affect transcriptional activity.

(e) **Chromatin structure** also affects gene transcription; genes within nucleosomes are not as likely to be transcribed as genes between nucleosomes.

QUESTION

In the disease congenital adrenal hyperplasia (CAH), the adrenal cortex is unable to make the hormone cortisol. Would the levels of ACTH be elevated or decreased in a patient with CAH?

ANSWER

ACTH levels would be **increased** in a patient with CAH owing to a lack of negative feedback caused by the absence of cortisol production.

7 MENDELIAN GENETICS

a. Locus

is a "gene," the smallest unit of hereditary information.

b. Allele

is one genetic variant at a particular locus (e.g., A or a).

c. Genotype

is the genetic constitution of an individual at a particular locus (e.g., Aa).

d. Phenotype

is the physical appearance of an individual (e.g., bald, tall).

e. Homozygote

is an individual who has two identical alleles at the same locus (e.g., AA or aa).

f. Heterozygote

is an individual who has two different alleles at the same locus in different chromosomes (e.g., Aa).

g. Dominant

is the allele whose phenotype is expressed in the heterozygote.

h. Recessive

is the allele whose phenotype is not expressed in the heterozygote.

The classic phenotypic ratio of a monohybrid cross (Aa × Aa) = 3:1 (dominant:recessive), as shown in Figure 2-53. The classic phenotypic ratio of a dihybrid cross (AaBb × AaBb) is 9:3:3:1 (dominant/dominant; dominant/recessive; recessive/dominant; recessive/recessive) [see Figure 2-53].

A

	A	a
A	AA	Aa
a	Aa	aa

B

	AB	Ab	aB	ab
AB	AABB	AABb	AaBB	AaBb
Ab	AABb	AAbb	AaBb	Aabb
aB	AaBB	AaBb	aaBB	aaBb
ab	AaBb	Aabb	aaBb	aabb

Figure 2-53.
(A) Monohybrid cross; *(B)* dihybrid cross.

i. A pedigree

is a flowchart depicting the transmission or inheritance of a particular trait or disease through a particular family. Males are written as squares, females as circles. Dead people are sometimes written with slashes through the circle or square, with the age inserted below. When examining a pedigree, keep in mind the following rules.

1. First, look at the number of males versus the number of females affected. If almost all of the people who are affected are males, the disorder is **X-linked recessive** (X-linked dominant disorders are very rare). If every single one of the people who have the disorder is male, it could be Y-linked (e.g., hairy ear rims). Y-linked conditions are extremely rare and probably will not be mentioned on the MCAT.
2. Then, look at the parents. **If two normal parents have an affected child, the disorder is most likely autosomal recessive.** If an affected parent married to a nonaffected parent has 50% or more children who receive the trait in question, the disease is probably autosomal dominant.

QUESTION

A man with a family history of red–green color blindness has the following pedigree:

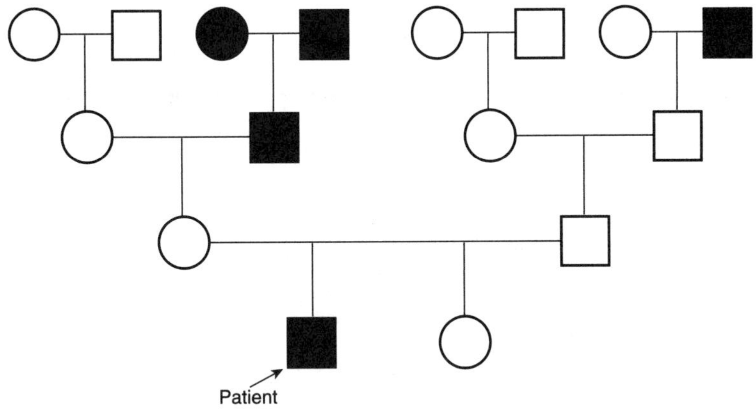

a) What is the most likely mode of inheritance of red–green color blindness that reflects this patient's pedigree?

(b) What is the probability that the patient's sister is a carrier of the red–green color blindness trait?

(c) If the patient's sister marries a man who does *not* have red–green color blindness, what is the probability that their child will be color-blind?

ANSWER

(a) Because four males are affected and only one female is affected, and because two normal parents can have an affected child, the trait is most likely X-linked recessive.

(b) Using Punnett squares (X^a = color-blindness gene)

Patient's grandmother on mother's side (X^A, X^A) × Patient's grandfather on mother's side (X^a, Y):

	X^a	Y
X^A	X^AX^a	X^AY
X^A	X^AX^a	X^AY

∴ Patient's mother's genotype is X^AX^a (carrier)

Patient's mother (X^A, X^a) × Patient's father (X^A, Y):

	X^A	Y
X^A	X^AX^A	X^AY
X^a	X^AX^a	X^aY

∴ Probability that daughter is a carrier = 50%

(c) The probability that their child will be color-blind

$= P$ (daughter is a carrier) × P ($X^AX^a \times X^AY$ results in a color-blind child)

50% [see (b)] ×

	X^A	Y
X^A	X^AX^A	X^AY
X^a	X^AX^a	X^aY → color-blind

25%

Therefore, the probability that their child will be color-blind

$= 50\% \times 25\% = 12.5\% = 1/8$

QUESTION

If a person with blood group O marries a person with blood group AB, what is the probability that their baby will have blood group O?

ANSWER

ABO blood grouping is an example of a **codominant trait:** Blood groups A and B are both dominant, and blood group O is recessive.

Genotype	Phenotype
I^Ai or I^AI^A	A
I^Bi or I^BI^B	B
I^AI^B	AB
ii	O

Therefore, when the Punnett square for this problem is:

	I^A	I^B
i	I^Ai	I^Bi
i	I^Ai	I^Bi

the probability that their baby will be blood group O is 0%.

8 POPULATION GENETICS: HARDY-WEINBERG EQUILIBRIUM

a. Hardy-Weinberg equilibrium

describes the genotype frequencies (called PIC values) and phenotype frequencies of a large population that has reached an equilibrium state.

$$p + q = 1$$

p = frequency of the dominant allele
q = frequency of the recessive allele

Squaring this equation results in the **Hardy-Weinberg equation:**

$$(p + q)^2 = p^2 + 2pq + q^2 = 1$$

p^2 = frequency of dominant homozygotes
2pq = frequency of heterozygotes
q^2 = frequency of recessive homozygotes

p = frequency of the dominant allele
q = frequency of the recessive allele

b. Assumptions of Hardy-Weinberg equilibrium

- **Large population** is necessary to minimize the effects of "**genetic drift**" (the random elimination of low-frequency alleles owing to the small size of a population).

- **Random mating** is assumed: No natural selection or preferential mating to ensure that organisms with the preferred genotype are more likely to leave greater numbers of offspring.
- **No immigration or emigration** is assumed: Within the population, even a small amount of gene flow can affect a Hardy-Weinberg equilibrium.
- **No spontaneous mutations**

QUESTION

Cystic fibrosis is an autosomal recessive disease that affects 16% of the people in a given population. Assuming that the population is in Hardy-Weinberg equilibrium, what percentage of heterozygous carriers has the cystic fibrosis gene?

ANSWER

$$q^2 = 0.16$$

$$q = 0.4$$

Since

$$p + q = 1$$

$$p = 0.6$$

Using the Hardy-Weinberg equation:

$$p^2 + 2pq + q^2 = 1$$

where $2pq$ = number of heterozygous carriers, the answer is $2(0.6)(0.4) = 48\%$

9 MOLECULAR BIOLOGY OF DNA AND RNA

a. DNA (Deoxyribonucleic Acid)

A = T has 2 H-bonds

G ≡ C has 3 H-bonds

In 1953, Watson and Crick worked out the structure of DNA and RNA using x-ray crystallography. DNA is composed of a 2′-deoxyribose and base pairs A–T, C–G (A = adenine, T = thymine, C = cytosine, G = guanine, and U = uracil; **uracil is found only in RNA, and thymine is found only in DNA**). It is arranged into a double helix, with the nucleic acid–base pairs in the center, which are connected to the sugar–phosphate backbone (Figure 2-54). The three types of DNA are A, B, and Z; most DNA in eukaryotic nuclei is in the B–DNA conformation. B–DNA has approximately 10 base pairs per turn of the double helix, and the helix has major and minor grooves (in B–DNA). The major grooves are bigger than the minor grooves.

Adenine and guanine are double-ringed purines, whereas cytosine, uracil, and thymine are single-ringed pyrimidines.

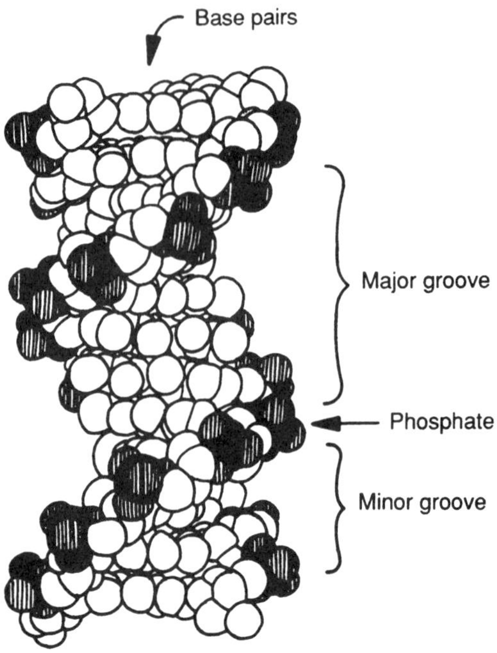

Figure 2-54.
The DNA double helix. (Reprinted with permission from Marks DB: *BRS Biochemistry,* 2nd ed. Baltimore, Williams & Wilkins, 1994, p 52.)

The leading strand of DNA is synthesized in a continuous fashion, whereas the lagging strand is synthesized in a discontinuous fashion involving the synthesis and ligation of multiple Okazaki fragments.

The DNA replication process is catalyzed by the enzyme DNA polymerase. The process has been duplicated in vivo and is well understood. **DNA replication is semiconservative,** as this was demonstrated by the Meselson-Stahl labeling experiment. The parent DNA breaks into two separate single strands, which can then serve as templates for DNA polymerase to add nucleotides and make two new daughter strands (each of which has half of the parent strand). DNA synthesis occurs in the $5' \rightarrow 3'$ direction (these directions are defined by the directionality of the deoxyribose–phosphate bond). One daughter strand is replicated continuously, but the other daughter strand must be synthesized in a series of **Okazaki segments.** In addition to DNA polymerase, a number of enzymes contribute to DNA replication, including DNA ligase, which connects Okazaki segments. DNA replication begins at specific sites with the formation of **replication forks.**

TEST CORRELATION

AZT (azidothymidine), an antiviral drug used to combat HIV, is a thymidine analog that prevents the synthesis of viral DNA from an RNA template test correlation (reverse transcription). AZT is a nucleoside (ribose sugar and nitrogenous base) analog that is converted into a nucleotide (ribose sugar and nitrogenous base and phosphate group) and then incorporated into the newly sythesized viral DNA strand. AZT then subsequently acts as a DNA chain terminator, preventing the addition of subsequent nucleotides onto the growing viral DNA strand, thus preventing viral DNA replication. Since HIV and AIDS is a popular medical topic with widespread and growing public awareness, studying this material as it relates to the MCAT is very high yield.

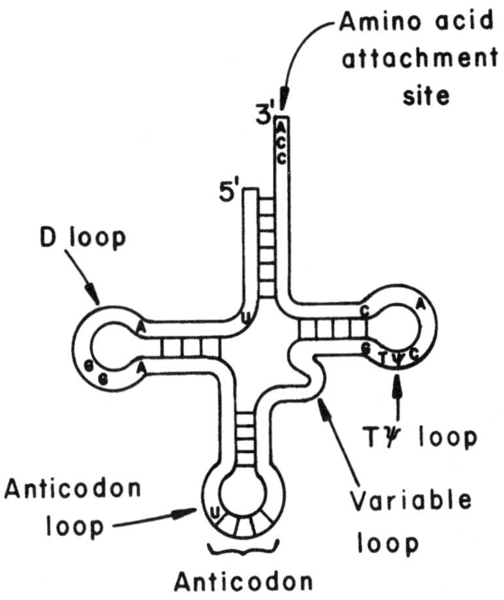

Figure 2-55.
The cloverleaf structure of tRNA. Bases that commonly occur in a particular position are indicated by *letters.* Base-pairing in stem regions is indicated by *lines* between strands. Ψ = pseudouridine; *T* = ribothymidine; *D* = dihydrouridine. (Reprinted with permission from Marks DB: *BRS Biochemistry,* 2nd ed. Baltimore, Williams & Wilkins, 1994, p 55.)

b. RNA (ribonucleic acid)

is composed of a ribose sugar, phosphate, and base pairs **A–U** (instead of A–T), C–G. Unlike DNA, **RNA is single-stranded** and very unstable. The three major types of RNA are:

1. **rRNA**—ribosomal RNA. This type of RNA makes up ribosomes and is the most abundant form of RNA in vivo.
2. **mRNA**—messenger RNA. This type is transcribed from DNA in the nucleus and translated into proteins in ribosomes in the cytoplasm. Heterogeneous nuclear RNA (hnRNA) is a predecessor that is modified to form mRNA by intron splicing. mRNA is the largest type of RNA in vivo.
3. **tRNA**—transfer RNA (Figure 2-55). tRNA are small RNA molecules that can match specific amino acids to specific mRNA triplet nucleotide sequences (codons). Specificity is the basis for the genetic code. It is important to remember that there are three termination (stop) codons (UAA, UAG, UGA), one initiation codon (AUG = methionine), and 60 other codons. Therefore, **more than one codon can be present for a particular amino acid;** most of the degeneracy in the genetic code is in the third nucleotide of the codon. tRNA is the smallest type of RNA in vivo.

c. Central Dogma (Figure 2-56)

All genetic information is stored as DNA (mostly in the nucleus; mitochondria and chloroplasts have their own DNA). The "central premise" elucidates the process of genetic information transfer in all known organisms, from little *Escherichia*

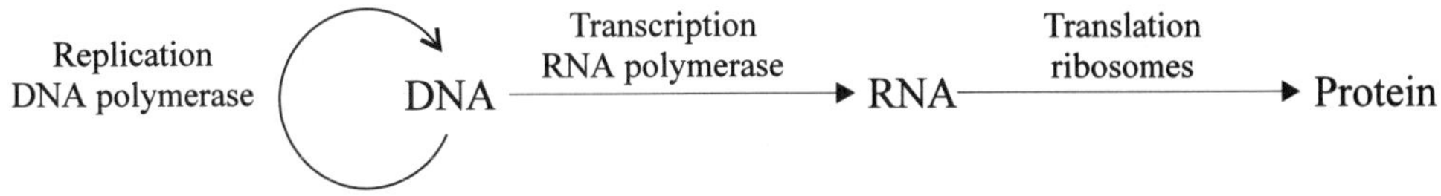

Figure 2-56.
The central premise of molecular biology.

Eukaryotic transcription occurs in the nucleus, whereas translation occurs in the cytosol on ribosomes.

coli to the biggest eukaryotic organisms. DNA must first be transcribed to mRNA by RNA polymerase (specifically by RNA polymerase II) within the nucleus. The mRNA then leaves the nucleus (in eukaryotes) and travels to the ribosomes, where it is translated to protein. The ribosome subunits recruit the proper tRNAs, which can bond to the mRNA codons and carry the proper amino acids. The amino acids are joined via peptide bonds to create a protein. As a result, all genetic information is transmitted through the formation of proteins, which catalyze reactions, form structural macromolecules, and initiate all other important cellular functions.

The central premise has two important exceptions.

- One occurs in **retroviruses,** which carry their information as RNA, which can then reverse-transcribe to DNA via the enzyme **reverse transcriptase** (the DNA is then transcribed as normal). Molecular biologists have used reverse transcriptase to make complementary DNA (cDNA) from eukaryotic mRNA, which has the genes without the promoters, introns, and so forth (which makes them easier to manipulate in bacterial systems).
- Other RNA viruses can use RNA-dependent RNA polymerases to turn their RNA information directly into translatable mRNA.

In eukaryotes, transcription occurs in the nucleus and translation occurs in the cytoplasm on ribosomes. Because prokaryotes do not have a nuclear membrane, the processes of transcription and translation are coupled and occur simultaneously.

QUESTION

Look at the following nucleotide:

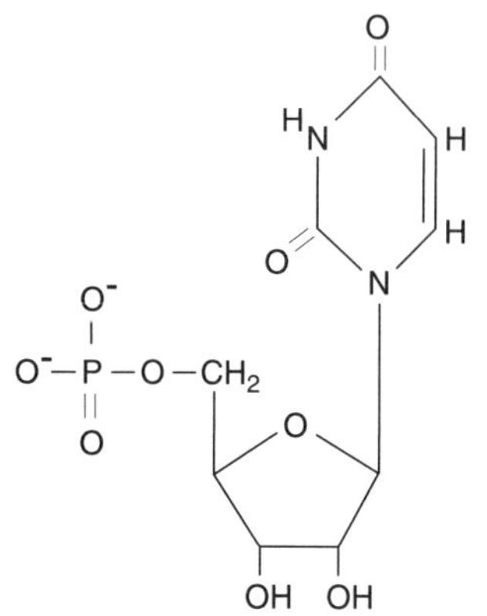

(a) Is this nucleotide found in DNA or RNA?
(b) This nucleotide contains all of the following organic functional groups EXCEPT:
    (1) Alkene
    (2) Alcohol
    (3) Ether
    (4) Ester
    (5) Amide
(c) If the content of adenine in a piece of double-stranded DNA is 30% of the total nitrogenous bases, what is the percentage of guanine?

ANSWER

((a) Because an -OH group is present on the 2′ position of the ribose sugar (see below), this nucleotide is only present in RNA.

(b) The answer is **4.** The functional groups are outlined in the figure below:

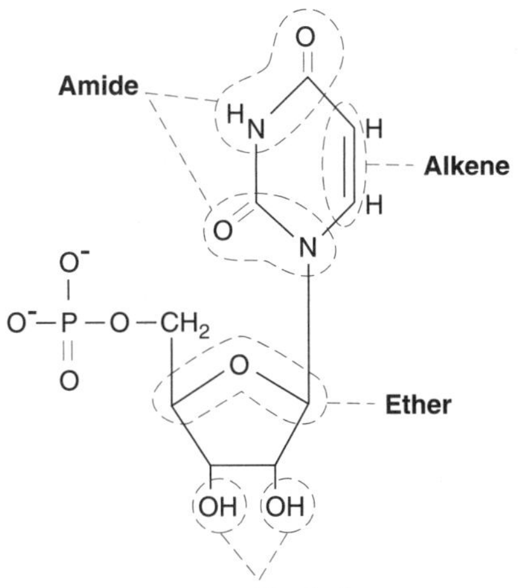

(c) In a piece of double-stranded DNA, adenine base pairs with thymine and cytosine base pairs with guanine. The percentage of adenine (i.e., 30%) is equal to the percentage of thymine. If the percentage of adenine plus thymine equals 60%, then the percentage of guanine plus cytosine equals 40%. The percentage of guanine (i.e., 20%) is equal to the percentage of cytosine.

10 AMINO ACIDS AND PROTEIN STRUCTURE

Table 2-15 lists amino acids and the group to which each belongs. Structures of the amino acids are shown in Figure 2-57.

a. Amino Acids: Distinguishing Characteristics

- Arginine is the most alkaline (basic) amino acid.
- Glycine is the only achiral amino acid. All other amino acids are optically active.
- Glycine and proline are "helix busters." They disrupt the secondary structure of proteins.
- Cysteine can bind with other cysteines via an oxidative reaction to form a disulfide bond (R–S–S–R).

b. Protein Structures

- **Primary structure** refers to the specific amino acid sequence.
- **Secondary structure** refers to the presence of regularly repeated three-dimensional structures, notably α-helices (especially in membrane-spanning proteins) and β-pleated sheets (e.g., keratin).
- **Tertiary structure** is the total three-dimensional structure of a peptide.

Positively charged amino acids (lysine, histidine) can be found on histone proteins, allowing the histones to interact with DNA. DNA carries an enormous negative charge because of its phosphate backbone.

TABLE 2-15. Amino acid groups

Group	Amino Acids
Acidic [Negatively charged: R-COO$^-$]	Aspartate (Asp) Glutamate (Glu)
Basic [Positively charged: R-NH$_3^+$]	Arginine (Arg) Lysine (Lys) Histidine (His)
Alipathic side chain	Glycine (Gly) Alanine (Ala) *Valine (Val) *Leucine (Leu) *Isoleucine (Ile)
Aromatic side chain	Tyrosine (Tyr) *Phenylalanine (Phe) Tryptophan (Trp)
Amide-containing	Asparagine (Asn) Glutamine (Gln)
Sulfur-containing	Cysteine (Cys) *Methionine (Met)
-OH-containing alipathic	Serine (Ser) Threonine (Thr)
Cyclic imino acid (C=N link)	Proline (Pro)

*These hydrophobic amino acids are typically found on the inside of the protein (away from the periphery, which is usually in contact with water).

- **Quaternary structure** is the structure of a protein made of multiple peptides, such as the four subunits of hemoglobin that bind around the central iron ion.

QUESTION

Which amino acids are likely to be found inside the protein?

ANSWER

As mentioned previously, the hydrophobic amino acids are most likely to be found inside the protein because this part of the protein is not usually in contact with water. The hydrophobic amino acids are valine, leucine, isoleucine, phenylalanine, and methionine (see Table 2-15).

QUESTION

Which amino acids are likely to be found on the outside of the protein?

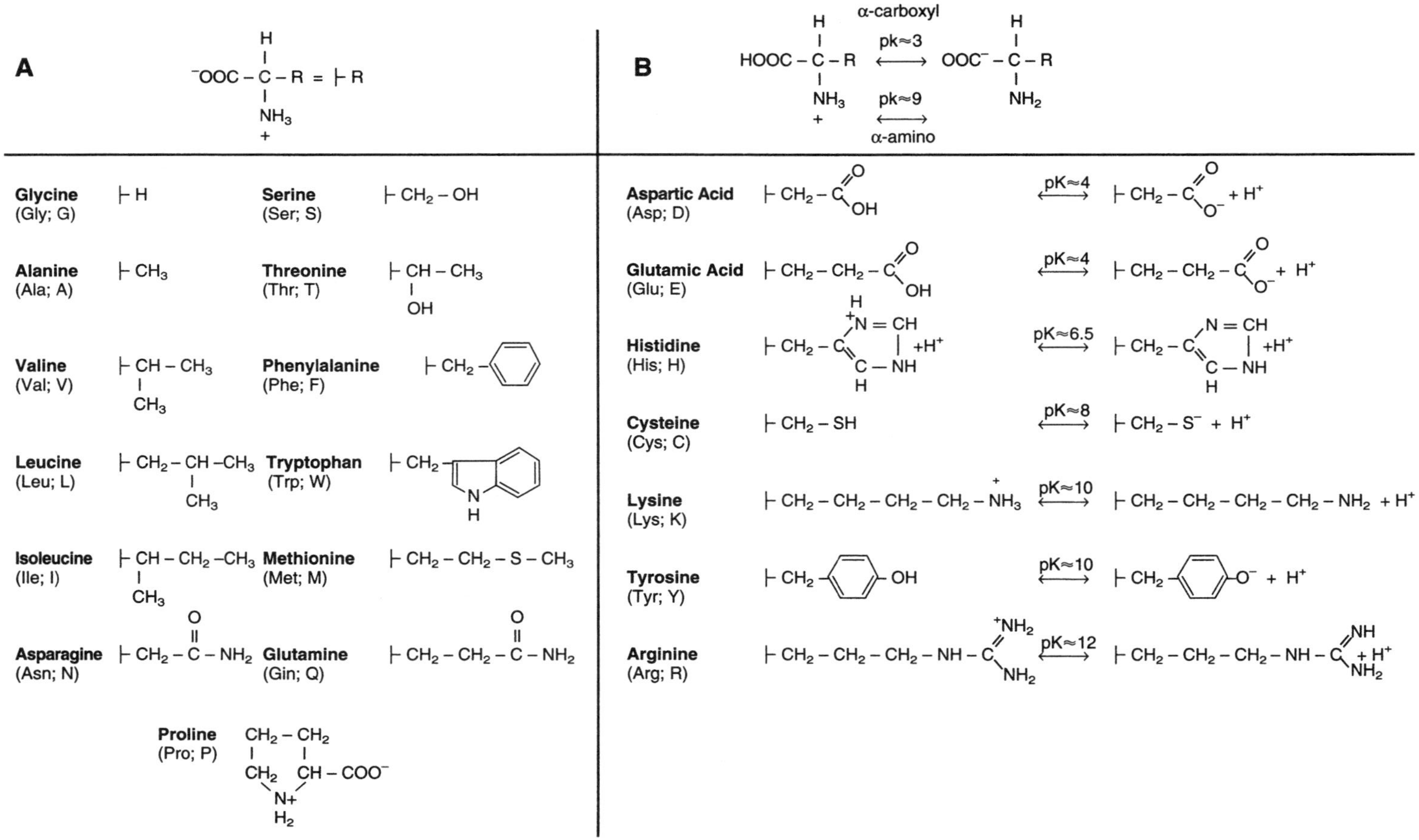

Figure 2-57.
Structures of the amino acids. Abbreviations are given for all amino acids. *(A)* shows amino acids that do not have ionizable side chains. *(B)* shows side chains that are ionizable. In *(B)*, for each amino acid, the species that predominates at a pH below the pK is shown on the *left;* the species that predominates at a pH above the pK is shown on the *right*. Note that the charge changes from 0 to − or from + to 0. At the pK, equal amounts of both species are present. (Reprinted with permission from Marks DB: *BRS Biochemistry,* 2nd ed. Baltimore, Williams & Wilkins, 1994, p 24.)

ANSWER

Along the same lines as the preceding answer, any amino acid other than hydrophobic amino acids are likely to be found on the outside of the protein, which is in contact with the hydrophilic, aqueous intra- and extracellular fluid.

QUESTION

Which amino acids are most likely to be found at the active site of the protein?

ANSWER

Which amino acids are present at the active site depends on the chemical nature of the substrate. If the substrate is positively charged, an acidic amino acid that is negatively charged ($R–COO^-$), such as aspartate or glutamate, would most likely be found in the active site, attracting and holding onto the cationic substrate. Conversely, a negatively charged substrate would require the presence of a positively charged basic amino acid ($R–NH_3^+$), such as lysine, arginine, or histidine, to form an electrostatic interaction with the anionic substrate.

QUESTION

Which amino acids are most likely to be found on histone proteins?

ANSWER

Positively charged amino acids (e.g., lysine, arginine, histidine) found in histone proteins enable them to interact with DNA, which is highly negatively charged because of its phosphate backbone.

11 AUTONOMIC NERVOUS SYSTEM

a. Sympathetic Nervous System

Often referred to as the **"fight or flight"** component, the sympathetic nervous system ganglia are all in the spinal cord; therefore, the preganglionic neurons are short and the postganglionic neurons are long (Figure 2-58). The sympathetic nervous system increases energy expenditure, accelerates the heart, increases metabolism, inhibits digestion, and diverts blood flow to the muscles. In other words, it prepares the organism for action (Table 2-16).

b. Parasympathetic Nervous System

Often called the **"rest and digest"** component, the parasympathetic nervous system ganglia are near the organs themselves; that is, the preganglionic neurons are long and postganglionic neurons are short (see Figure 2-58). The parasympathetic

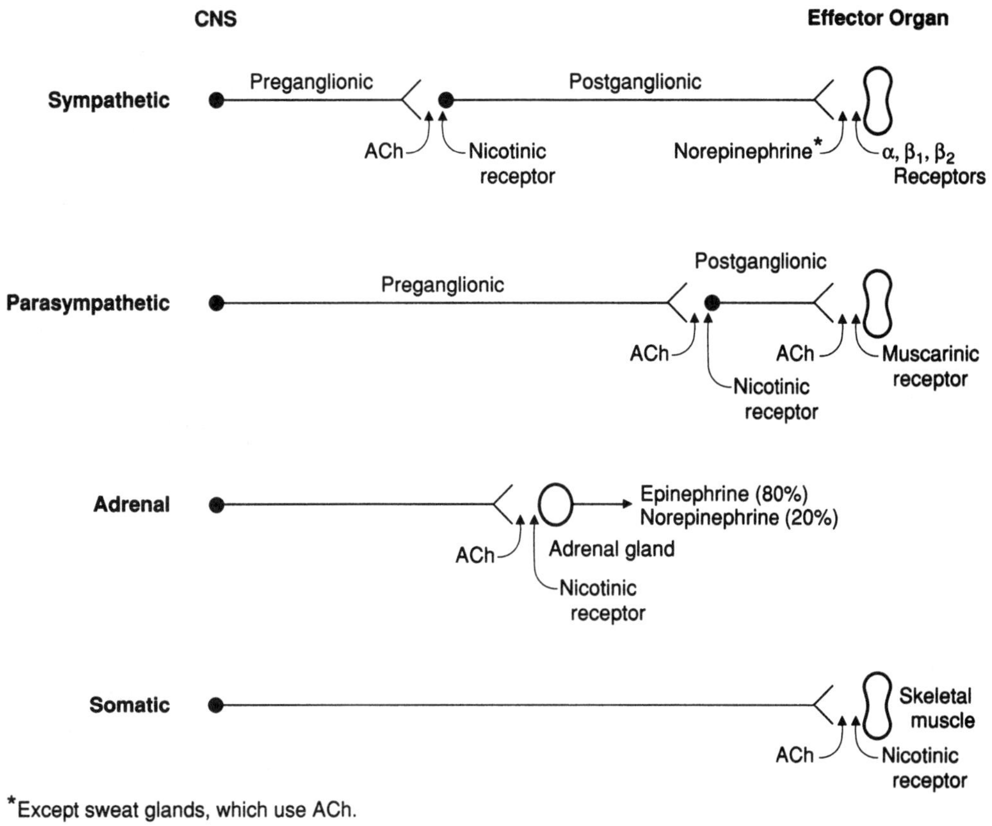

Figure 2-58. Organization of the autonomic nervous system. (Reprinted with permission from Marks DB: *BRS Biochemistry,* 2nd ed. Baltimore, Williams & Wilkins, 1994, p 30.)

nervous system enhances activities that conserve and gain energy, such as decreased heart rate, decreased metabolism, increased digestive action, and increased blood flow to the gut (see Table 2-16 for further details).

c. Renin–Angiotensin System (Figure 2-59)

1. **Angiotensinogen** is a plasma protein that is produced by the liver. The majority of plasma proteins are produced by the liver, with the exception of antibodies, which are produced by specialized B cells (plasma cells).
2. **Renin** is produced by the juxtaglomerular cells of the kidney. These cells are also responsible for producing **erythropoietin**, which stimulates the bone

TABLE 2-16. System function and response

System Function	Sympathetic Response	Parasympathetic Response
Heart rate and contractility	Increased	Decreased
Pupillary reaction	Dilation	Constriction
Respiratory system action	Bronchodilation	Bronchoconstriction
Gastrointestinal motility and blood flow	Decreased	Increased
Glycogen metabolism	Breakdown (catabolic)	Synthesis (anabolic)
Blood flow to skeletal muscle	Increased	Decreased

marrow to produce red blood cells. In addition to regulating blood pressure through the renin–angiotensin system, the kidneys also play an important role in regulating acid/base balance, controlling excretion nitrogenous wastes (as a result of urea formation in the liver secondary to protein breakdown), and the hormone-regulated maintenance of water and electrolyte balance (e.g., sodium, potassium, calcium) via antidiuretic hormone (ADH) aldosterone, and parathyroid hormone (PTH) receptors.

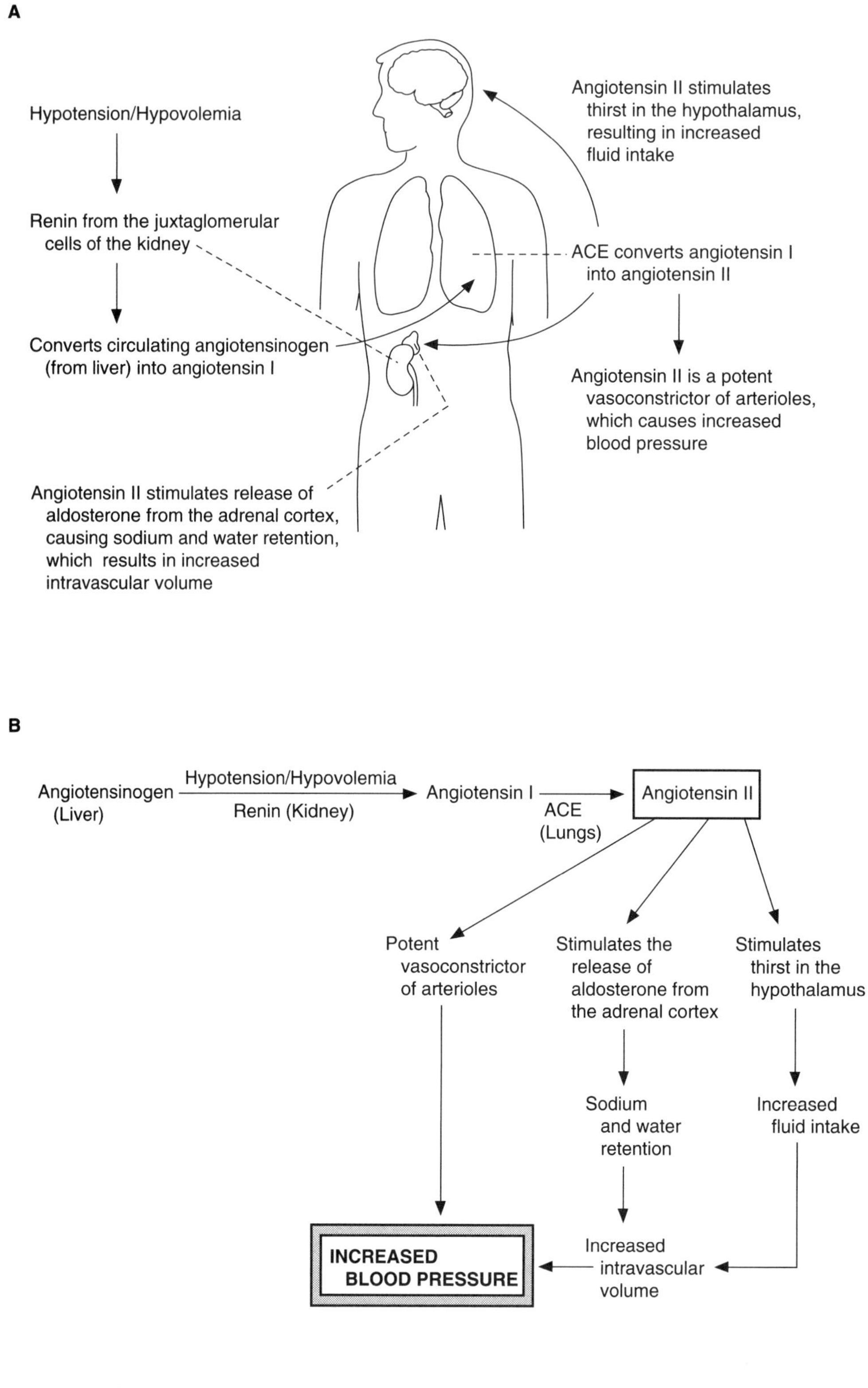

Figure 2-59. Renin–angiotensin system. *(A)* Physiologic responses to hypotension/hypovolemia. *(B)* Flow chart showing the mechanisms by which the renin–angiotensin system increases blood pressure. *ACE* = angiotensin-converting enzyme.

TABLE 2-17. Summary of effects of exercise

Heart rate	↑↑	
Stroke volume	↑	
Cardiac output	↑↑	
Arterial pressure	↑	(slight)
Pulse pressure	↑	(due to increased stroke volume)
TPR	↓↓	(due to vasodilation of skeletal muscle beds)
AV O_2 difference	↑↑	(due to increased O_2 consumption)

AV = atrioventricular; *TPR* = total peripheral resistance.
Reprinted with permission from Costanzo LS: *BRS Physiology*, Baltimore, Williams & Wilkins, 1995, p 94.

d. Baroreceptor Reflex

This phenomenon occurs when hypotension (low blood pressure) stimulates the release of catecholamines (epinephrine and norepinephrine) from the sympathetic nervous system, causing an increased heart rate and thus preserving cardiac output. Remember:

$$\text{Cardiac output} = \text{heart rate} \times \text{stroke volume}$$

e. Cardiovascular

responses to exercise and hemorrhage (Tables 2-17 and 2-18).

12 ENDOCRINE REGULATION

a. Peptide hormones

(Table 2-19) cannot pass through the cell membrane because they are hydrophobic (the largely lipid plasma membrane is lipophilic). Instead, these hormones **bind**

Peptide hormones are released more quickly and have more rapid effects than steroid hormones, making them the more rapid response system. It takes longer for steroid hormones to act because they work at the level of DNA, subsequently altering protein synthesis, thereby creating a longer term effect.

TABLE 2-18. Summary of responses to hemorrhage

Heart rate	↑
TPR	↑
Contractility	↑
Unstressed volume	↓ (↑ stressed volume)
Renin	↑
Angiotensin II	↑
Aldosterone	↑
Circulating epinephrine and norepinephrine	↑
ADH	↑

ADH = antidiuretic hormone; *TPR* = total peripheral resistance.
Reprinted with permission from Costanzo LS: *BRS Physiology*, Baltimore, Williams & Wilkins, 1995, p 94.

TABLE 2-19. Hormones and their functions

Hormone	Type of Hormone	Source	Target	Function
ADH (vasopressin)	Peptide	Hypothalamus (synthesis) Posterior pituitary (secretion)	Kidney (collecting ducts)	Stimulates retention of water in the kidney by increasing the collecting ducts' permeability to water. Alcohol consumption suppresses ADH secretion.
Oxytocin	Peptide	Hypothalamus (synthesis) Posterior pituitary (secretion)	Uterus	Induces labor by stimulating uterine contraction; also causes breast to eject milk
***Growth hormone (GH)**	Protein	Anterior pituitary	Many organs, including liver	Stimulates growth of bone, muscle, and other tissues
Adrenocortico-tropic hormone (ACTH)	Protein	Anterior pituitary	Adrenal cortex	Stimulates synthesis and secretion of cortisol from adrenal cortex
Luteinizing hormone (LH)	Protein	Anterior pituitary	Testes Ovaries	Stimulates secretion of testosterone by testes Stimulates ovulation and formation of corpus luteum in females
Follicle-stim-ulating hormone (FSH)	Protein	Anterior pituitary	Testes Ovaries	Stimulates spermatogenesis in testes Stimulates development of follicle in ovary
Thyroid-stim-ulating hormone (TSH)	Protein	Anterior pituitary	Thyroid	Stimulates production and secretion of thyroid hormones
Prolactin	Protein	Anterior pituitary	Breast tissue	Stimulates production of milk by breast
T_3 and thyroxine (T_4)	Peptide (cytoplasmic receptor)	Thyroid gland	Many organs, including heart	Increases basal metabolic activity in many tissues and sensitizes heart to catecholamines
Parathyroid hormone (PTH)	Peptide	Parathyroid gland	Bone, kidney	Increases serum calcium by causing bone resorption (stimulates osteoclast activity) and decreases calcium excretion by the kidney
Calcitonin	Peptide	Thyroid gland	Bone	Decreases serum calcium by causing calcium deposition in bone. Also inhibits bone resorption by inhibiting osteoclasts
***Glucocorticoids (e.g., cortisol)**	Steroid	Adrenal cortex	Many organs, including liver	Many effects, including increasing blood glucose levels and reducing inflammatory response
Mineralocorticoids (e.g., aldosterone)	Steroid	Adrenal cortex	Kidney (distal tubule)	Causes sodium and water retention by distal tubule, as well as potassium excretion into the urine
***Catecholamines (e.g., epinephrine and norepinephrine)**	Peptides	Adrenal medulla	Many organs, including heart, pupil, and blood vessels	Coordinates all fight-or-flight responses (see Table 2-16)

Continued

TABLE 2-19. Hormones and their functions—Cont.

Hormone	Type of Hormone	Source	Target	Function
†Insulin (antagonistic to glucagon, cortisol, epinephrine, norepinephrine & GH)	Protein	Beta-islet cells of pancreas	Many organs, including liver, muscle, and adipose tissue	Anabolic hormone: decreases blood glucose by stimulating synthesis of glycogen from glucagon; also stimulates lipid and protein biosynthesis
***Glucagon (antagonistic to insulin)**	Protein	Alpha-islet cells of pancreas	Many organs, including liver, muscle, and adipose tissue	Catabolic hormone: increases blood glucose by stimulating glycogen breakdown; also stimulates lipid and protein degradation
Progesterone	Steroid	Ovaries Placenta	Endometrium	Promotes growth of uterine endometrium and decreases contraction of myometrium
Estrogen	Steroid	Ovaries Placenta	Many organs, including bone	Many functions, including maintaining bone density and developing and maintaining female secondary sexual characteristics
Testosterone	Steroid	Leydig cells of testes	Many organs	Many functions, including development of muscle and bone and development of male secondary sexual characteristics

*These hormones are hyperglycemic (raise blood glucose concentrations); they stimulate both the breakdown of glycogen to glucose and gluconeogenesis (catabolic).
†Insulin is the only hypoglycemic hormone (lowers blood glucose concentrations); it stimulates the synthesis of glycogen from glucose and inhibits glycogenolysis (anabolic).

to cell membrane receptors and activate **second messengers.** The best-known second messenger is **cAMP** (Figure 2-60). A peptide hormone binds to a receptor, which then activates a **G protein,** which in turn activates the enzyme adenylate cyclase. Adenylate cyclase subsequently catalyzes the transformation of ATP to cAMP. An increase in intracellular cAMP can then mediate many different biologic reactions, often via the action of a **cAMP-dependent protein kinase** that phosphorylates proteins and changes their activity.

b. Steroid hormones

(see Table 2-19; Figures 2-61 and 2-62) are much more hydrophobic and therefore can pass right through the plasma membrane. They reach the nucleus and **bind to nuclear receptors, cytoplasmic receptors,** or both. These steroid receptors, once bound to the incoming steroid hormone, then bind to DNA and directly influence DNA transcription. This occurs via binding to specific enhancer sequences that recognize the steroid receptor's DNA-binding domain.

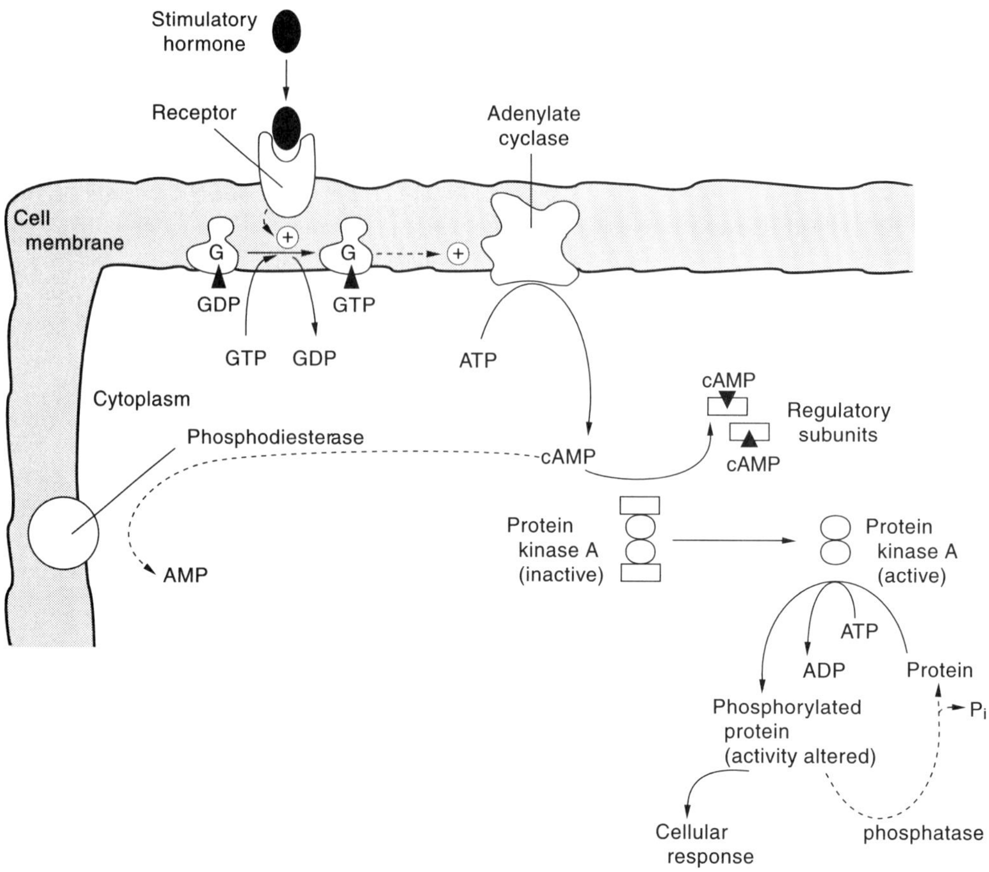

Figure 2-60.
The production and action of cyclic AMP (cAMP). *G* = G protein (G proteins function when GTP is bound); ○ = free catalytic subunits; ▭ = regulatory subunits of protein kinase A; ⊕ = stimulates. (Reprinted with permission from Marks DB: *BRS Biochemistry,* 2nd ed. Baltimore, Williams & Wilkins, 1994, p 280.)

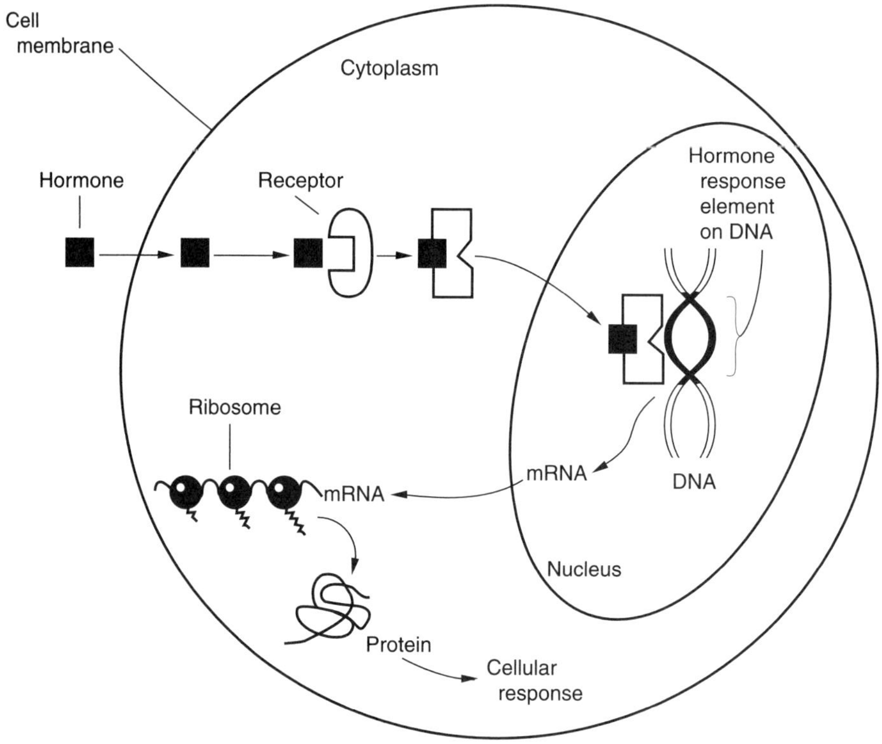

Figure 2-61.
The mechanism of action of hormones of the steroid–thyroid family. (Reprinted with permission from Marks DB: *BRS Biochemistry,* 2nd ed. Baltimore, Williams & Wilkins, 1994, p 284.)

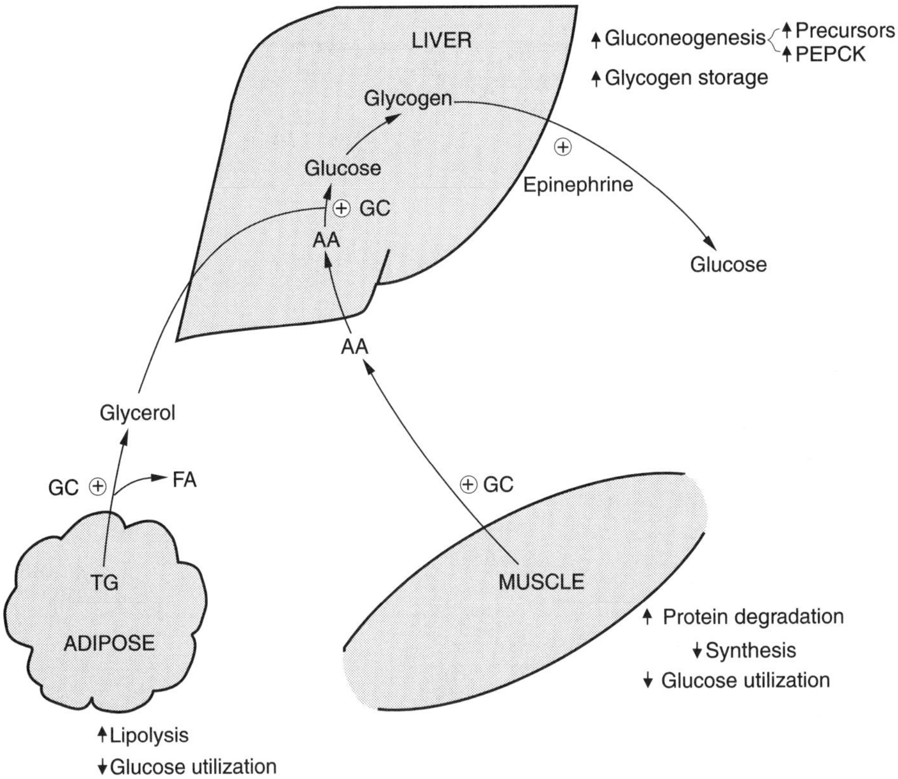

Figure 2-62. The effects of glucocorticoids *(GC)* and epinephrine on fuel metabolism. (Reprinted with permission from Marks DB: *BRS Biochemistry,* 2nd ed. Baltimore, Williams & Wilkins, 1994, p 288.)

TABLE 2-20. Digestion and absorption of carbohydrates, proteins, and lipids

Nutrient	Enzyme	Site of Production	Site of Function	Function
Carbohydrates	Ptyalin (Salivary amylase)	Salivary glands	Mouth	Starch → maltose
	Lactase	Intestinal glands	Small intestine	Lactose → glucose and galactose
	Sucrase	Intestinal glands	Small intestine	Sucrose → glucose and fructose
	Maltase	Intestinal glands	Small intestine	Maltose → 2 glucose
	Pancreatic amylase	Pancreas	Small intestine	Starch → maltose
Proteins	Pepsin†	Gastric glands	Stomach	Hydrolyzes certain peptide bonds
	Trypsin†	Pancreas	Small intestine	Hydrolyzes certain peptide bonds
	Chymotrypsin†	Pancreas	Small intestine	Hydrolyzes peptide bonds
	Carboxypeptidase	Pancreas	Small intestine	Hydrolyzes terminal carboxyl peptide bond
	Aminopeptidase	Intestinal glands	Small intestine	Hydrolyzes terminal amino peptide bond
	Dipeptidases (e.g., lactase)	Intestinal glands	Small intestine	Hydrolyzes amino acid pairs
	Enteropeptidase	Intestinal glands	Small intestine	Converts trypsinogen to trypsin
Lipids	Bile*	Liver	Small intestine	Emulsifies fats and fat-soluble vitamins (A, D, E, K)
	Lipase	Pancreas	Small intestine	Hydrolyzes lipids

*Bile is not an enzyme. It emulsifies fat globules, making it easier for pancreatic lipase to break down fats.
†Trypsin, pepsin, and chymotrypsin are initially secreted in their inactive forms (known as zymogens: trypsinogen, pepsinogen, and chymotrypsinogen), then activated when they reach their final site of action. Trypsinogen is converted to trypsin by the enzyme enteropeptidase; trypsin in turn converts chymotrypsinogen to chymotrypsin and activates aminopeptidases and carboxypeptidases. Pepsinogen is converted to pepsin by the low pH of the stomach.

13 DIGESTION AND ABSORPTION

The bulleted items and Tables 2-20 and 2-21 outline nutrient transport for digestion and absorption.

The liver is the first organ to receive digested food from protein- and lipid-rich blood and lymph.

- Fatty acids and triacylglycerides (TAGs) are packaged as chylomicrons and are carried in the lacteals (part of the lymphatic system), which drain into the liver (Figure 2–63).
- All other materials, such as carbohydrates and amino acids, are carried in the bloodstream via the portal circulation to the liver.
- Therefore, digested food **first** makes its way to the liver, which distributes its metabolites to all the other organs of the body.
- Bile salts emulsify fats and fat-soluble vitamins (vitamins A, D, E, and K) and are absorbed in the ileum of the small intestine (Figures 2-64 and 2-65). Therefore, if a good portion of the ileum is resected for any reason (e.g., can-

TABLE 2-21. Summary of digestion and absorption

Nutrient	Digestion	Site of Absorption	Mechanism of Absorption
Carbohydrates	To monosaccharides (glucose, galactose, fructose)	Small intestine	Na^+-dependent cotransport (glucose, galactose) Facilitated diffusion (fructose)
Proteins	To amino acids, dipeptides, tripeptides	Small intestine	Na^+-dependent cotransport
Lipids	To fatty acids, monoglycerides, cholesterol	Small intestine	Micelles form with bile salts in intestinal lumen Diffusion of fatty acids, monoglycerides, and cholesterol into cell Reesterification in the cell to triglycerides and phospholipids Chylomicrons form in the cell (requires apoprotein) and are transferred to lymph
Fat-soluble vitamins		Small intestine	Micelles with bile salts
Water-soluble vitamins		Small intestine	Na^+-dependent cotransport
Vitamin B_{12}		Ileum of small intestine	Intrinsic factor
Bile acids		Ileum of small intestine	Na^+-dependent cotransport; recirculated back to the liver
Ca^{2+}		Small intestine	Vitamin D-dependent Ca^{2+}-binding protein
Fe^{2+}	Fe^{3+} is reduced to Fe^{2+}	Small intestine	Binds to apoferritin in the cell Circulates in blood bound to transferrin

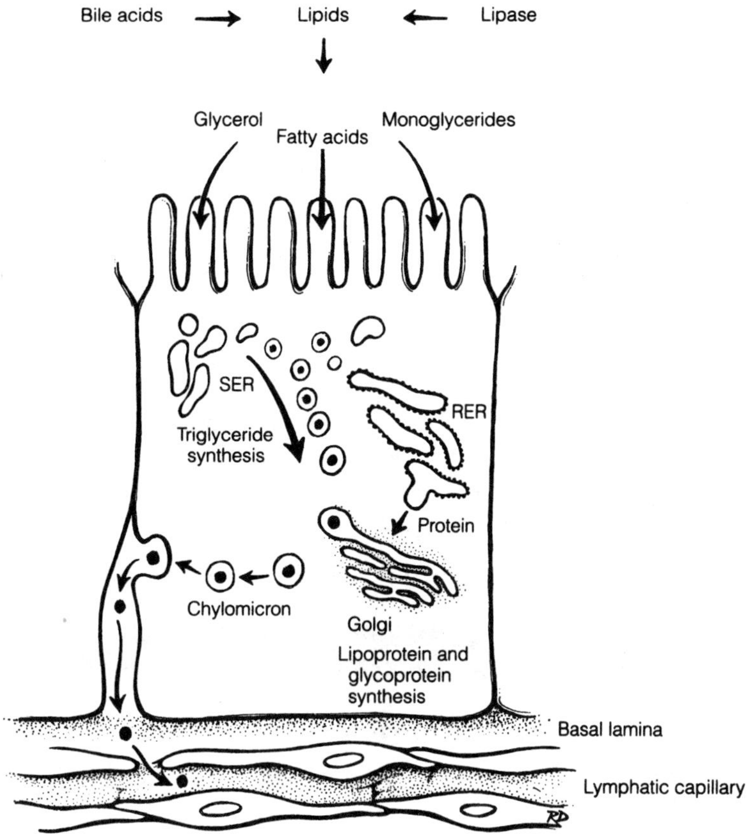

Figure 2-63.
Diagram of the absorption of lipids by surface absorptive cells of the small intestine and the formation of chylomicrons. *RER* = rough endoplasmic reticulum; *SER* = smooth endoplasmic reticulum. (Reprinted with permission from Gartner, LP, Hiatt, JL, Strum JM: *BRS Cell Biology and Histology*, 3rd ed. Baltimore, Williams & Wilkins, 1998, p 249.)

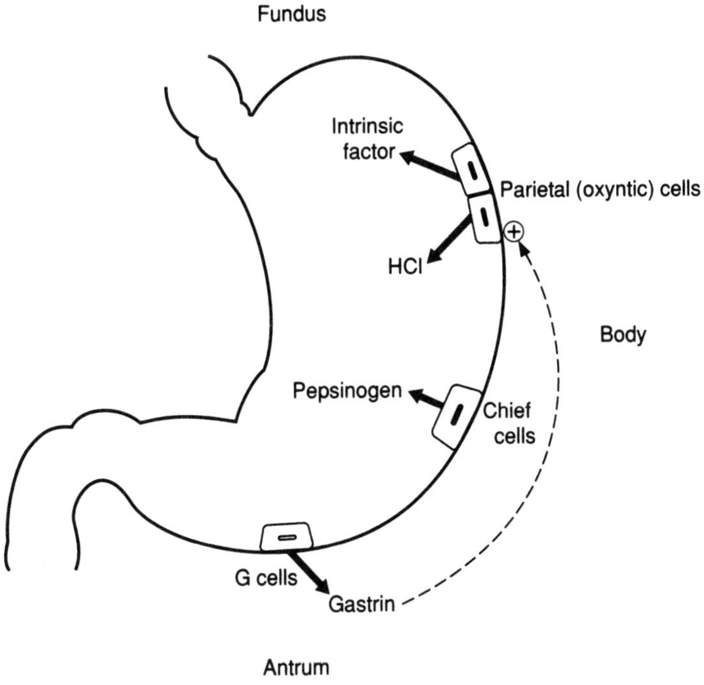

Figure 2-64.
Gastric cell types and their functions. (Reprinted with permission from Costanzo LS: *BRS Physiology*, Baltimore, Williams & Wilkins, 1995, p 193.)

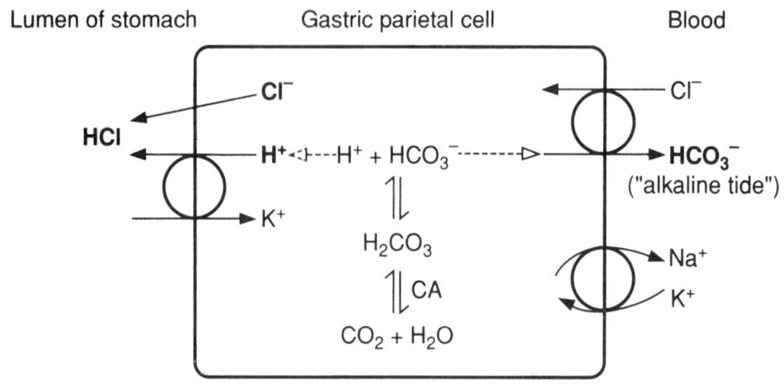

Figure 2-65. Simplified mechanism of secretion of H^+ by gastric parietal cells. (Reprinted with permission from Costanzo LS: *BRS Physiology*, Baltimore, Williams & Wilkins, 1995, p 193.)

cer), this loss of absorptive surface could result in fat malabsorption, resulting in deficiencies of fat-soluble vitamins (A, D, E, K) as well as vitamin B_{12} deficiency (because vitamin B_{12} is bound to intrinsic factors and absorbed in the ileum), which causes anemia and neurologic problems.

- **Cholesterol** is the precursor of bile and steroid hormones.

14 THE PANCREAS AND THE LIVER

a. Pancreas

The pancreas is both an exocrine and an endocrine organ.

- Exocrine functions of the pancreas include secretion of digestive enzymes (e.g., pancreatic lipase, amylase, trypsin, chymotrypsin).
- Endocrine functions of the pancreas include hormone secretion of insulin and glucagon.

Because the pancreas is both an endocrine and exocrine organ, destruction of the pancreas (e.g., chronic pancreatitis) can result in diabetes mellitus (endocrine dysfunction) as well as protein, fat, and vitamin A, D, E, and K (fat-soluble vitamins) malabsorption (exocrine dysfunction).

b. Liver

The liver performs many functions.

- Synthesis of bile from cholesterol
- Synthesis of many serum proteins, including albumin and clotting factors
- Drug detoxification (e.g., alcohol)
- Storage of vitamins and minerals (e.g., vitamin A, vitamin E, vitamin B_{12}, iron, copper)

It is a major site of metabolism, including:

- **Gluconeogenesis** (conversion of lactic acid to glucose)
- **Interconversion of carbohydrates**
- **Fatty acid degradation,** resulting in the formation of ketone bodies

Along with the spleen, the liver contributes to the destruction and removal of old erythrocytes and circulating immune complexes. The **Kupffer cells,** specialized macrophages in the liver, remove old erythrocytes and circulating immune complexes from the bloodstream.

15 OXYGEN TRANSPORT IN THE BODY

a. Hemoglobin

is a complex polypeptide protein that has four subunits (two α subunits and two β subunits) bonded together around an iron ion. This complex can reversibly bind four oxygen molecules, making it an ideal oxygen carrier for the circulatory system, allowing the red blood cells to deliver oxygen to all the cells in the organism. The structure of hemoglobin is highly conserved through evolution, and hemoglobin protein sequence homology can be used to delineate recency of ancestry. In addition, fetal hemoglobin (expressed before birth) is slightly different from adult hemoglobin (expressed after birth).

Fetal hemoglobin has an increased oxygen affinity because it cannot bind 2,3-BPG as well as adult hemoglobin can.

Figure 2-66 charts how well hemoglobin within the blood binds to oxygen. The sigmoid-shaped oxygen dissociation curve increases rapidly at moderate oxygen partial tension (oxygen concentration) and increases more slowly at very low or very high oxygen partial tension. This is caused by positive cooperativity as a result of interaction between the four protein subunits in the hemoglobin molecule.

b. Myoglobin

is similar to hemoglobin found in mammalian muscular tissue; but unlike hemoglobin, myoglobin binds oxygen at very low oxygen tensions (see Figure 2-66). Active muscle cells can deplete the surroundings of oxygen and therefore depend on myoglobin for oxygen transport and supply. In a low oxygen tension environment, hemoglobin has very little oxygen to release to the muscle. Diving mammals, who must adapt to an oxygen-depleted environment, have a high blood concentration of myoglobin, which allows them to transport oxygen in their blood even when oxygen levels drop to dramatic lows. And unlike hemoglobin, which is composed of four subunits, myoglobin is a single subunit protein that exhibits a hyperbolic- (not sigmoid) shaped oxygen dissociation curve (see Figure 2-66).

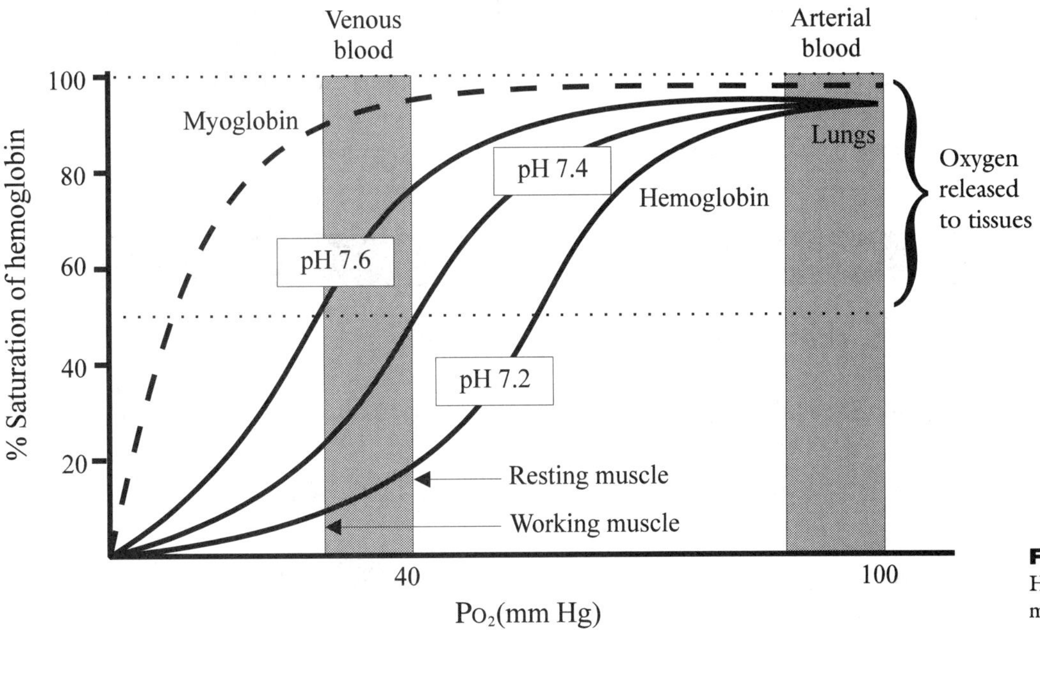

Figure 2-66. Hemoglobin and myoglobin binding curve.

c. High Altitudes

People physiologically adapt to living at high altitudes by producing more erythrocytes, a process that takes approximately 30 days and is stimulated by erythropoietin.

At high altitudes, the low atmospheric pressure means that the partial pressure of oxygen is lower than the pressure at sea level. This means that we move **along the curve** to a lower partial oxygen pressure (PO_2), corresponding to a lower oxygen saturation in the blood, which causes you to feel tired at high altitudes. However, if you live at high altitudes, your cardiovascular system cannot adapt quickly to this higher altitude because it takes approximately 1 month to make new red blood cells. However, other species can produce a hemoglobin molecule with a higher affinity for oxygen under conditions of low atmospheric pressure, which means that the oxygen dissociation curve shifts to the left (for a given PO_2 there is a higher oxygen saturation percent) owing to the increased ability of hemoglobin to bind and transport oxygen in oxygen-depleted surroundings. At high altitudes, the body initially compensates for the lower oxygen saturation in the blood by producing 2,3-BPG (see Part II, H 15 e).

d. Erythropoietin

Red blood cell production is stimulated by the hormone erythropoietin, which is made by the juxtaglomerular cells of the kidney (also the site of renin production) in response to a low arterial blood oxygen concentration (PaO_2). These cells sense the low concentration of oxygen in the blood under certain conditions (e.g., high altitudes, lung disease) and secrete erythropoietin, which stimulates the bone marrow to make more oxygen-carrying red blood cells.

e. Bohr Effect

Higher temperatures, acidity, and 2,3-BPG increase the unloading of oxygen from red blood cells.

Under different environmental conditions, the hemoglobin dissociation curve changes through a phenomenon called the **Bohr effect,** which shifts the oxygen curve to the right. The Bohr effect occurs during conditions of acidity, elevated carbon dioxide levels, increased temperature, and increased 2,3-BPG. When these conditions occur, cells can increase their ability to pick up oxygen from the blood by increasing the extracellular pH of its surroundings, which induces hemoglobin to give up more of its oxygen to the oxygen-starved cells in the peripheral tissues. The Bohr effect is important because it facilitates the offloading and delivery of oxygen to the hypoxic target organs (leg muscles anaerobically producing lactic acid). At high altitudes, the body produces 2,3-BPG, which facilitates the unloading of oxygen to its target organs. This action compensates for the lack of oxygen content in the air.

16 BIOLOGY OF MUSCLE CONTRACTION

a. Muscle Types

- **Skeletal muscle** is voluntary and includes the muscles of the hand, arm, and leg. This muscle has striations.
- **Smooth muscle** is involuntary. It is found in the stomach, arteries, bladder, and other locations.
- **Cardiac muscle** is involuntary and is found exclusively in the heart. It has striations and intercalated disks.

b. Sarcoplasmic reticulum

is a specialized type of smooth endoplasmic reticulum found in all types of muscle cells that sequester calcium ions. The sarcoplasmic reticulum has voltage-dependent calcium channels. When the muscle cell is depolarized by neuronal stimulation, these channels open, releasing calcium ions from the sarcoplasmic reticulum and stimulating muscle contraction.

c. Actin

is a globular protein with one heavy and two light chains (the light chains wrap around the heavy chain). The head of the actin molecule can bind to myosin and make muscles contract in the presence of ATP by forming **cross-bridges**. The actin molecules make up the thin filaments of the sarcomere. Muscle contraction occurs as a result of hydrolysis of the actin-myosin-ATP cross-bridges. Neither actin nor myosin is broken down during muscle contraction (see Figure 2–67).

d. Myosin

is a type of globular protein that provides a binding site for the head group of the actin molecule. It forms the thick filaments of the sarcomere (Figure 2-68).

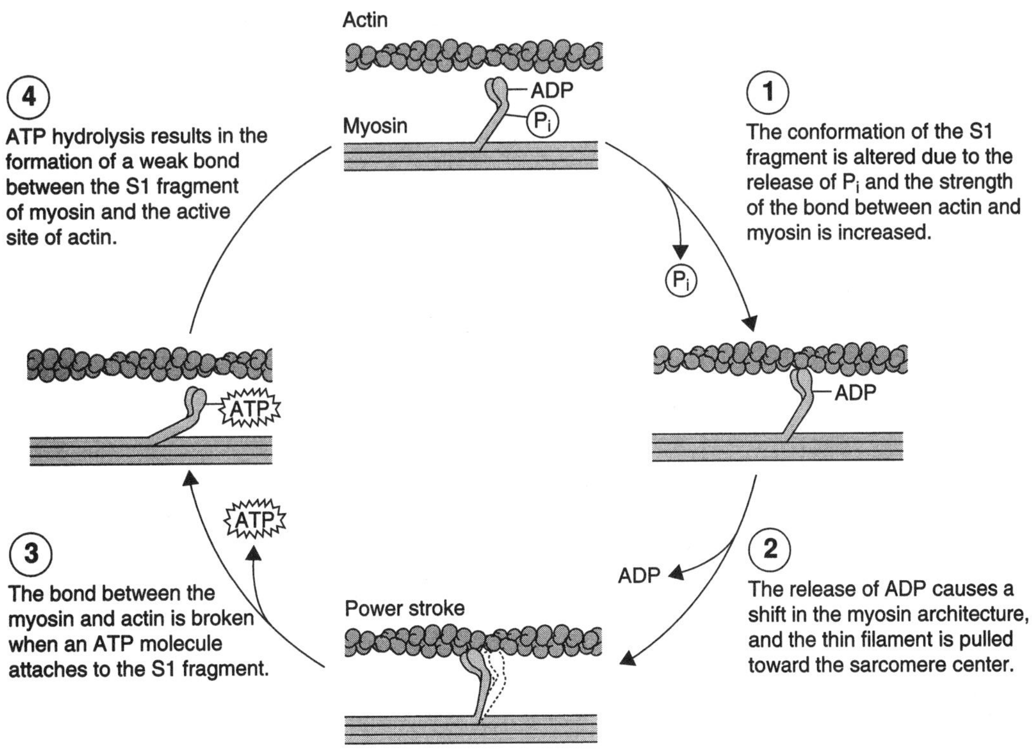

Figure 2–67.
Contraction cycle in skeletal muscle cells. This sequence of steps is repeated many times, leading to extensive overlay of thick and thin filaments which shortens the sarcomere and consequently the entire skeletal muscle fiber. (Adapted with permission from Alberts B, Bray D, Lewis J, et al: *Molecular Biology of the Cell,* 3rd ed. New York, Garland Publishing, 1994, p 852.)

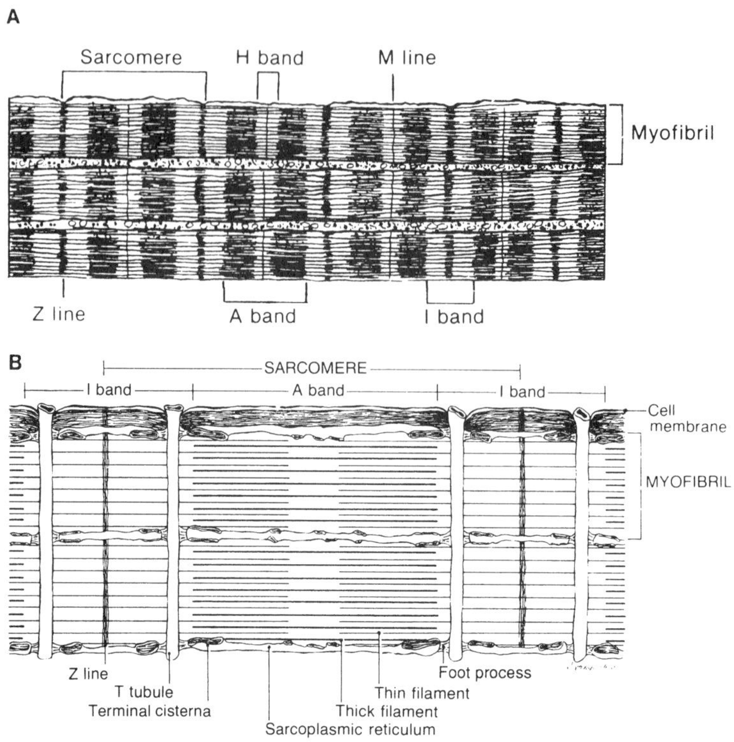

Figure 2-68. The sarcomere: thick and thin filaments. *A band* = length of one thick filament (does not change during contraction); *H band* = area with only thick filaments (shortens during contraction); *I band* = area with only thin filaments (shortens during contraction); *thick band* = myosin filaments; *thin band* = actin filaments; *Z line* = distance of one sarcomere (shortens during contraction). (Reprinted with permission from Bullock J, Boyle J, Wang MB: *NMS Physiology,* 2nd ed. Baltimore, Williams & Wilkins, 1991, p 29.)

17 BONE GROWTH AND REMODELING

a. Osteoclasts

are cells responsible for bone resorption (breakdown of bone).

b. Osteoblasts

are cells responsible for laying down the protein matrix of the bone. The process of bone formation is coupled with bone resorption; that is, osteoclasts and osteoblast actions must be coordinated.

c. Parathyroid hormone (PTH)

Osteoclasts have been found to have estrogen receptors on their surface; when activated by estrogen, these receptors inhibit osteoclast activity and therefore prevent osteoporosis.

stimulates the breakdown of bone, mostly through the action of osteocytes and some osteoclasts (Figure 2-69 and Table 2-22). This resorption of bone increases serum calcium levels (in fact, PTH is the most important regulator of serum calcium levels) by decreasing the amount of calcium that is secreted by the kidneys. PTH also stimulates the renal enzyme that converts vitamin D to a more active form that can increase intestinal uptake of calcium and renal reabsorption of calcium. PTH stimulates the renal excretion of serum phosphate (a product of bone resorption) into the urine.

d. Calcitonin

decreases serum calcium levels by stimulating the movement of serum calcium into bone, resulting in bone formation. It also inhibits osteoclastic activity, thereby inhibiting bone resorption. Calcitonin increases the level of calcium and phosphorus

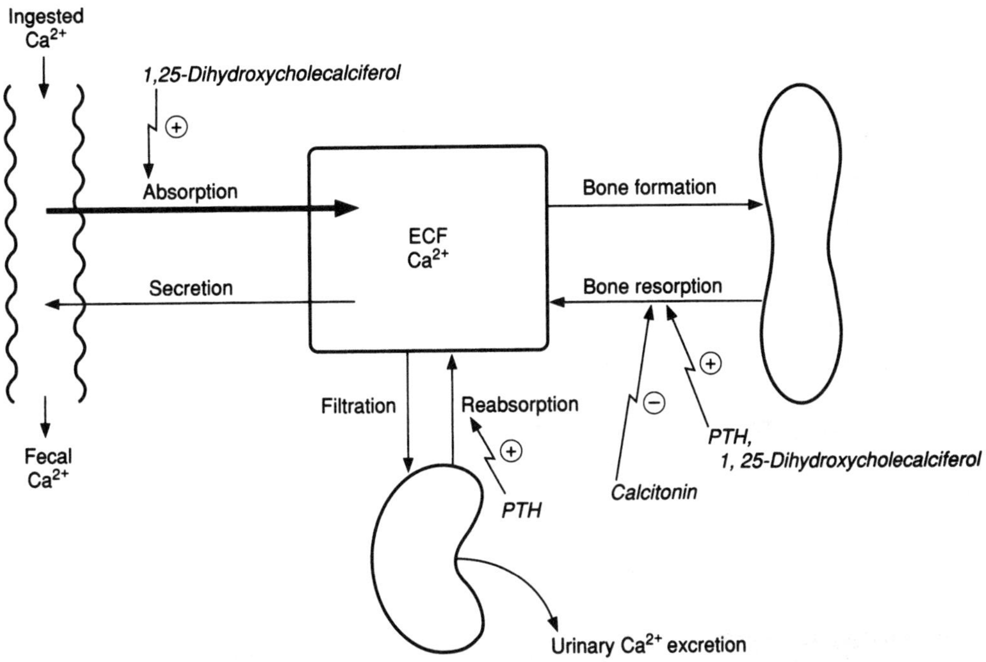

Figure 2-69. Hormonal regulation of Ca^{2+} metabolism. *ECF* = extracellular fluid; *PTH* = parathyroid hormone. (Reprinted with permission from Costanzo LS: *BRS Physiology*, Baltimore, Williams & Wilkins, 1995, p 236.)

TABLE 2-22. Summary of hormones regulating Ca^{2+}

	PTH	Vitamin D	Calcitonin
Stimulus for secretion	↓ serum [Ca^{2+}]	↓ serum [Ca^{2+}] ↑ PTH ↓ serum [phosphate]	↑ serum [Ca^{2+}]
Actions on:			
Bone	↑ resorption	↑ resorption	↓ resorption
Kidney	↓ P reabsorption (↑ urinary cyclic AMP) ↑ Ca^{2+} reabsorption	↑ P reabsorption ↑ Ca^{2+} reabsorption	
Intestine	↑ Ca^{2+} absorption (via vitamin D)	↑ Ca^{2+} absorption (vitamin D-dependent Ca^{2+}-binding protein) ↑ P absorption	
Overall effect on:			
Serum [Ca^{2+}]	↑	↑	↓
Serum [phosphate]	↓	↑	

P = phosphate; PTH = parathyroid
Reprinted with permission from Costanzo LS: *BRS Physiology*, Baltimore, Williams & Wilkins, 1995, p 235.

in urinary excretion. Levels of calcitonin may rise right after a meal in response to gastrin secretion.

e. Vitamin D

in the active form causes increased absorption of dietary calcium from the gut as well as increased calcium reabsorption in the kidney. Vitamin D is ingested in an inactive form that is modified in the liver and in the kidney, which activate this molecule's ability to influence the digestive system and renal system. PTH acts on the kidney to stimulate conversion of vitamin D into its active form.

MNEMONIC

> "Calcitonin" rhymes with **"bone in"** (it puts calcium in bone by stimulating osteoblasts and inhibiting osteoclasts). Osteo**b**lasts are **b**uilders whereas osteo**c**lasts are **c**arvers of bone.

18 IMMUNOLOGY

a. Antigen

is any foreign molecule that stimulates a specific immune response; proteins are the most effective antigens.

B cells are responsible for humoral (antibody-mediated) immunity, whereas T cells are responsible for cell-mediated immunity.

b. Antibody

is an immunoglobulin that is secreted by plasma cells and can function as an antibody receptor on a B cell (see Fig. 2–70). The antibody reacts with the antigen (which originally stimulated its production) to neutralize it or make it more ingestible for phagocytic cells; this process is called **opsonization**.

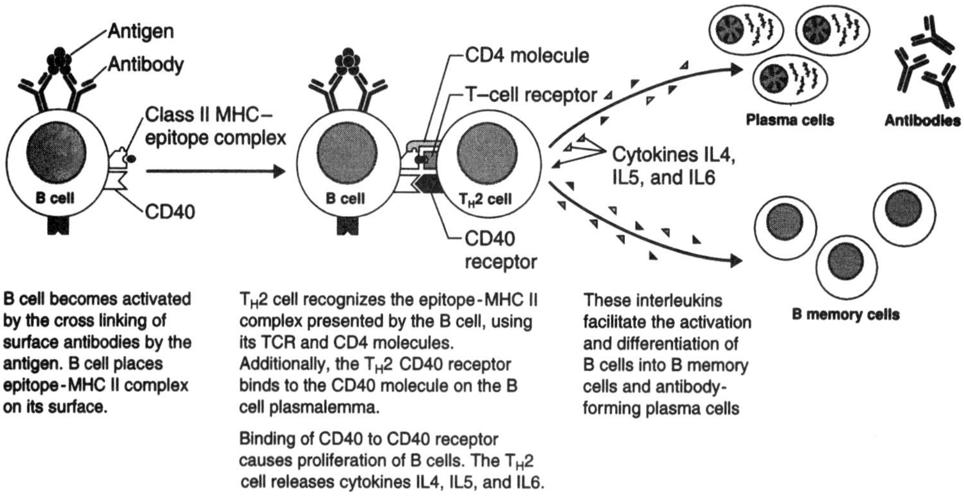

Figure 2-70. Thymic-dependent antigen-induced B-memory and plasma-cell formation. (Adapted with permission from Gartner LP and Hiatt JL: *Color Textbook of Histology.* Philadelphia, WB Saunders, 1997, p 236–237.)

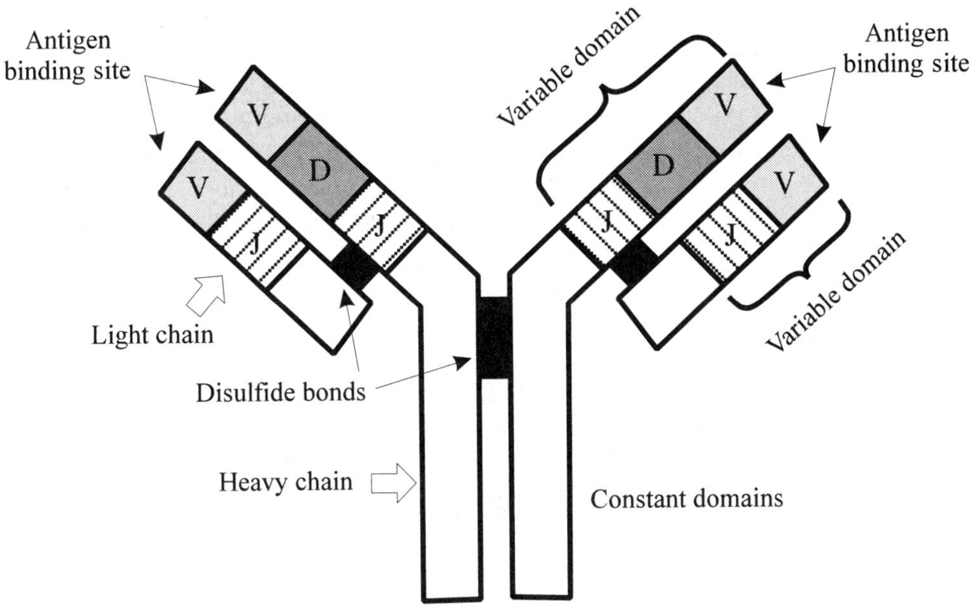

Figure 2-71.
Immunoglobulin.

1. An **immunoglobulin** (Figure 2-71) is another term for antibody; the five classes of immunoglobulins are as follows:

   (a) **IgA,** monomer or dimer. IgA is the antibody secreted by the cells of the different "tracts" (e.g., gastrointestinal, respiratory). IgA is found in bodily secretions and is the major antibody given to infants in their mothers' milk right after birth. Secretory IgA protects the mucous membranes from bacteria and viruses. It binds with antigens, and the invading antigen–antibody complex is then swept from the body's mucosal surfaces.

   (b) **IgM,** pentamer. IgM is the largest and most abundant immunoglobulin produced during the initial (primary) response to an invading microorganism. It is restricted to the bloodstream, where it can cluster (agglutinate) antigens and activate the complement immune response.

   (c) **IgG,** monomer. IgG is the most abundant of the circulating antibodies (IgG constitutes more than 80% of all antibodies in the plasma). It can cross capillary molecules easily and can also cross the placenta. An organism must be exposed to high antigen concentrations before a specific IgG is made. These antibodies destroy cells by activating complement. IgG is produced in the secondary immune response to a previously encountered antigen.

   (d) **IgD,** monomer. IgD is bound to the plasma membrane of B cells. It is the primary antigen receptor of immunocompetent B cells.

   (e) **IgE,** monomer. This antibody is associated with some of the body's immune responses and is found in increased numbers in people with allergies. IgE can bind to mast cells, which release histamine as part of the allergic response.

2. Antibodies, like any other protein, are encoded by genes. **Antibody diversity** is generated by the recombination and rearrangement of DNA segments coding for the V, D, and J segments of the heavy chain as well as the V and J segments of the light chain (i.e., gene shuffling) [Figure 2-72]. When a specific combination is produced to generate an antibody that is capable of binding to a specific antigen, interleukins as well as other cytokines are produced by helper T cells, which stimulate the differentiation of B cells to antibody-producing plasma cells.

Bone marrow precursors mature into red blood cells, white blood cells (granulocytes and lymphocytes), and platelets, and are very sensitive to radiation.

c. Bone marrow

is the source of all blood cells and other blood components (e.g., red blood cells, B and T lymphocytes, platelets, macrophages, neutrophils). Radiation can kill the rapidly dividing stem cells of the bone marrow, thereby causing immunosuppression (by killing lymphocyte precursors) and anemia (by killing red blood cell precursors).

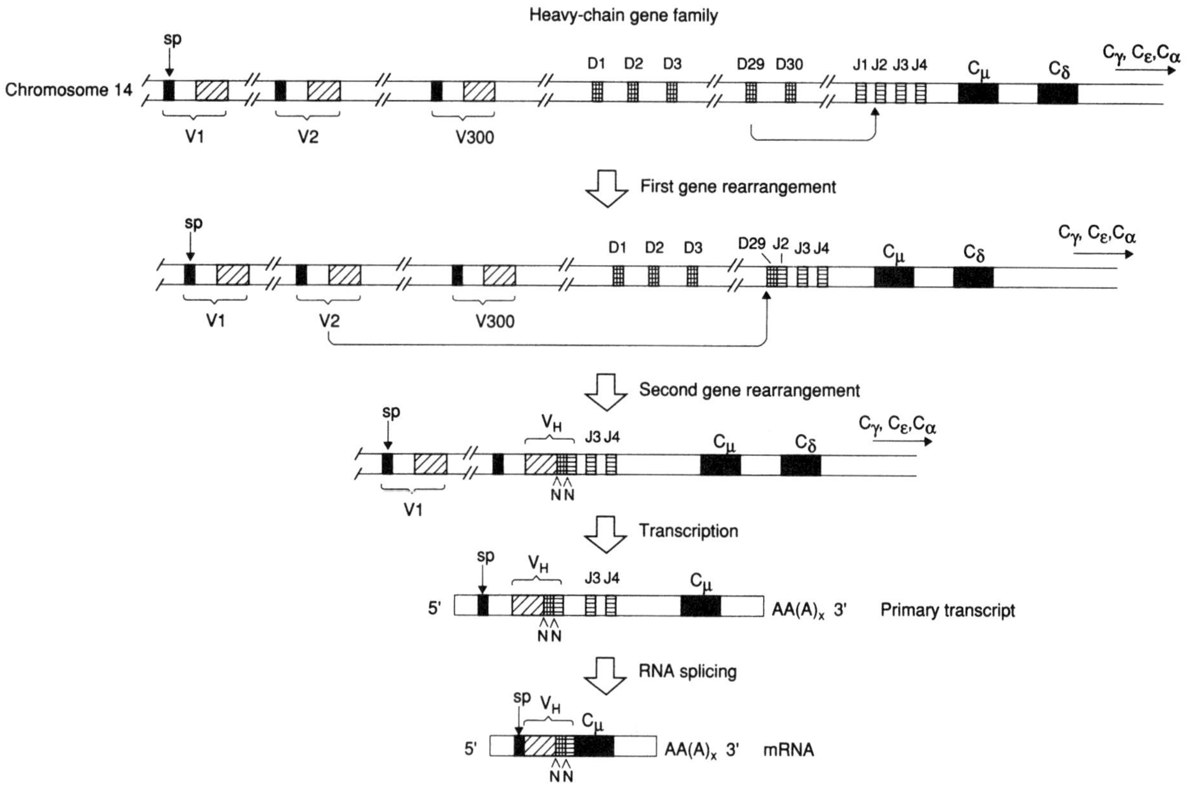

Figure 2-72.
Example of the formation of a heavy-chain (*H*) immunoglobulin-gene. Heavy-chain formation takes place by joining a partial variable region of the heavy chain (V_H), the diversity region (*D*), and the joining region of the heavy chain (J_H), which requires two DNA rearrangements. In the *first gene rearrangement,* one of about thirty D segments *(D29)* is moved immediately upstream of one of four J_H genes *(J2)*. The *second gene rearrangement* moves one of about three hundred partial V_H genes *(V2)* immediately upstream of the newly joined D and J segments *(D29-J2)* to form a complete exon that codes for the V_H domain. During these DNA rearrangements, up to 30 nucleotides *(N)* may be added between the V and D and the D and J segments by terminal deoxynucleotidyl transferase. Splicing of the primary transcript of this newly formed heavy-chain gene removes the intron between the V_H exon and the exon that codes for the constant *(C)* domain for immunoglobulin M (i.e., C_u). The intron between the exon that codes for the signal peptide *(sp)* and the V_H exon is also removed by splicing. Translation of this messenger RNA *(mRNA)* is directed to the endoplasmic reticulum (*ER*). (Reprinted with permission from Davidson VL, Sittman DB: *NMS Biochemistry,* 3rd ed. Baltimore, Williams & Wilkins, 1994, p 273.)

19 EMBRYOLOGICAL DERIVATIVES OF GERM LAYERS (TABLE 2-23)

TABLE 2-23. Embryological derivatives of germ layers

Primary Germ Layer	Resulting Structures
Ectoderm	Skin (including hair and the lens of the eye) Nervous system (including the brain, spinal cord, and peripheral nerves)
Endoderm	Epithelium of digestive system (e.g., esophagus, stomach, intestines) Epithelium of respiratory system (e.g., trachea, lungs) Inner linings of visceral organs (e.g., lungs, heart, gastrointestinal tract)
Mesoderm	Everything else (e.g., muscles, bone, kidneys, gonads, spleen, and the circulatory system)
Notochord	Vertebral column and annulus fibrosus

20 MEIOSIS VERSUS MITOSIS

Figure 2-73 shows the process of mitosis and meiosis.

Interphase comprises the majority of the cell life cycle (Figure 2–74), and consists of cell growth, DNA replication, as well as organelle replication (G_1, S, and G_2 phases of the cell cycle).

Prophase is the first stage of mitosis/meiosis, and is characterized by chromosome coiling (condensation) around histone proteins and disappearance/dissolution of the nuclear membrane.

Metaphase is characterized by alignment of the paired chromosomes at the equator of the cell, with the spindle fibers attached to the chromosomes at the centromeres.

Anaphase is characterized by segregation of the sister chromatids toward the poles of the dividing cells.

Telophase is characterized by the reformation of the nuclear membrane as well as the uncoiling of chromosomes into chromatin. Replication of centrioles also occurs. This is the final stage of mitosis, and is followed by division of the cell cytoplasm (cytokinesis).

21 NERVE CONDUCTION

- The nerve cell relies on conduction of electrical charges to transmit information. In order to propagate current along nerve cells, ions must move in and out of the cell, changing the electrical charges.

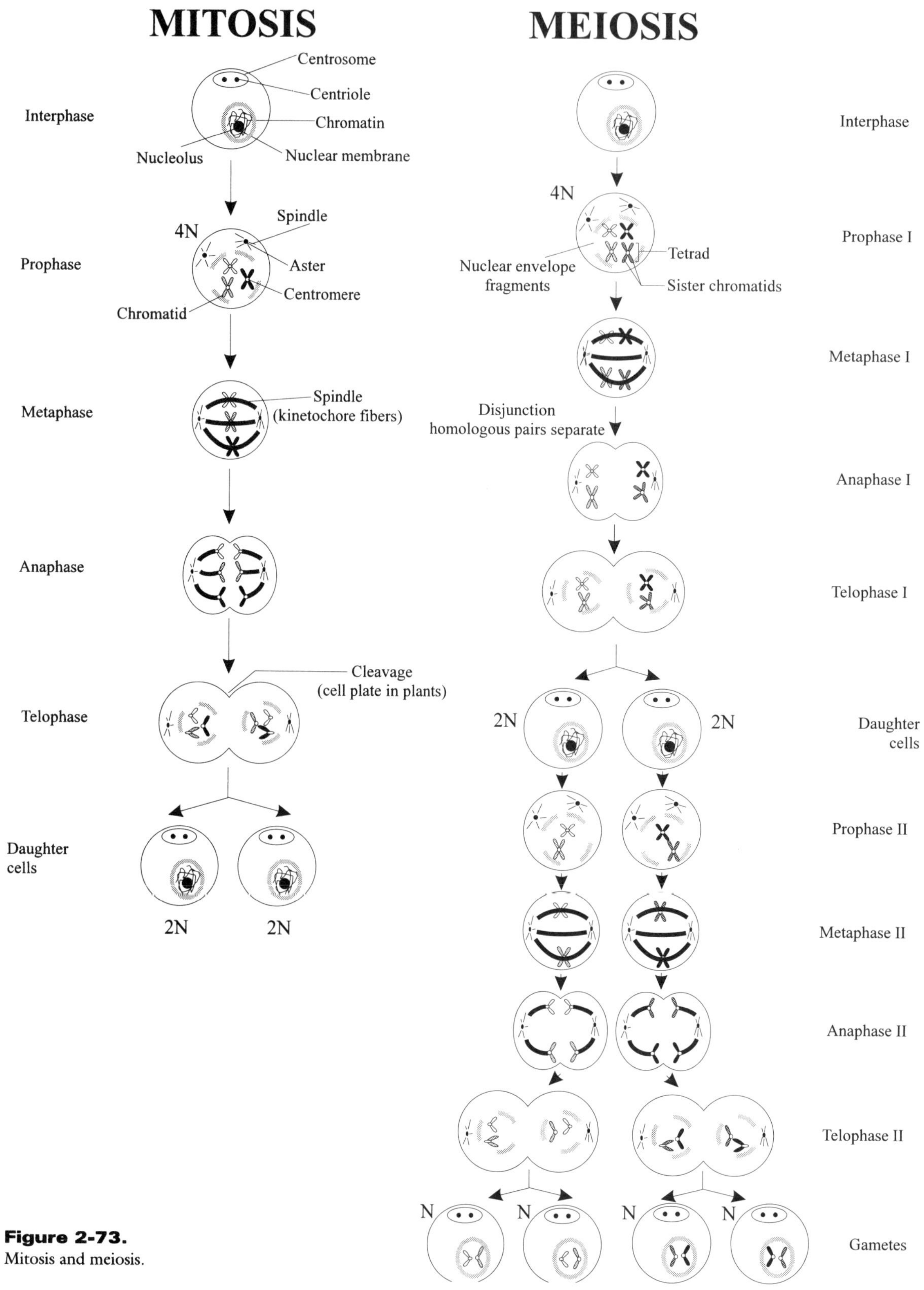

Figure 2-73.
Mitosis and meiosis.

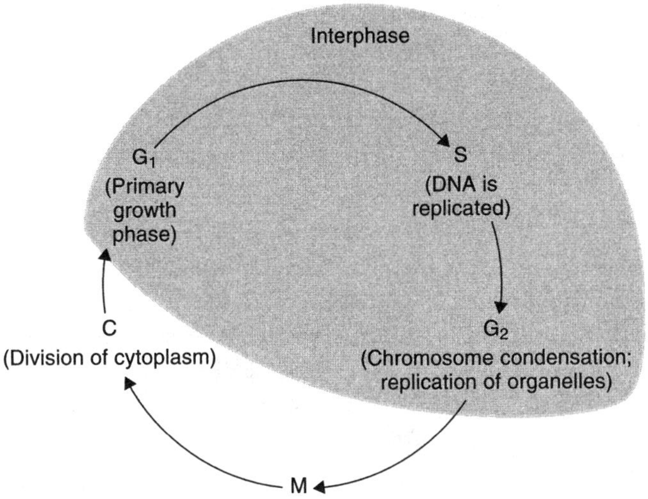

Figure 2-74.
The cell life cycle. G_1 = presynthetic gap; G_2 = postsynthetic gap; C = cytokinesis; M = mitosis; S = synthesis phase. (Reprinted with permission from Roth, D: *MCAT Essentials*, Baltimore, Williams & Wilkins, 1998, p 160.)

◆ The nerve cell is shown in Figure 2–75. In respect to the conduction of electrical charge in the nerve cell, there are two main ions: sodium (Na^+) and potassium (K^+). When the nerve cell is at rest, the concentration of Na^+ inside the cell is much lower than the concentration outside the cell. Vice versa, at rest, the concentration of K^+ inside the cell is much higher than K^+ outside the cell. Therefore, there exists a concentration gradient of Na^+ directed into the cell and a concentration gradient of K^+ directed out of the cell.

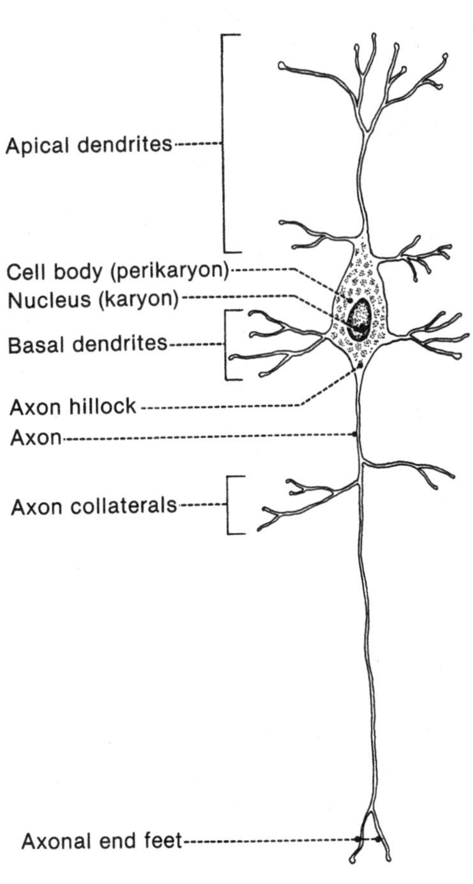

Figure 2-75.
Typical components of a multipolar neuron. (Reprinted with permission from DeMyer, W: *NMS Neuroanatomy*, 2nd ed., Baltimore, Williams & Wilkins, 1998, p. 18.)

- These two ions travel across the membrane of the cell along their concentration gradients. There exist protein channels that allow their passage through the membrane. At rest, the K^+ channel is "more leaky" than the Na^+ channel. Therefore, more K^+ exits the cell than Na^+ entering the cell (remember, the ions travel along their gradient). That means more positive charges are leaving the cell than entering. This leaves us with an overall negative charge inside the cell. To be exact, -70mV.
- The stage is set for the action potential to occur. Remember, we said only two ions are really involved, Na^+ and K^+. When the nerve gets excited by a mechanical, electrical, or chemical stimulus, it triggers the opening of both Na^+ and K^+ channels. The key point to remember is that the Na^+ channels open faster than the K^+ channels. Please follow along Figure 2–76 as the progress of the action potential is explained.
- If the Na^+ channels open first, then the Na^+ will come rushing into the cell along its gradient. This will give an overall positive charge to the cell. This is called depolarization and is seen in the upstroke in Figure 2–72. At this point, the conductance of the Na^+ ions across the membrane is greater than the K^+ conductance.
- Eventually the Na^+ channels close (become inactivated) and the K^+ channels begin to open. As the Na^+ channels close, less positive charges are entering the cells, and as the K^+ channels open, more positive charges are leaving the cell. This combined effect results in the cell becoming more negative. This is called repolarization.
- At the end, the K^+ channels are also slow to close, causing the cell to become more negative than it originally started out with. This is called hyperpolarization.
- During the action potential, there are two phases called the absolute refractory period and the relative refractory period. These terms refer to the cells ability to become restimulated after the initial stimulus.

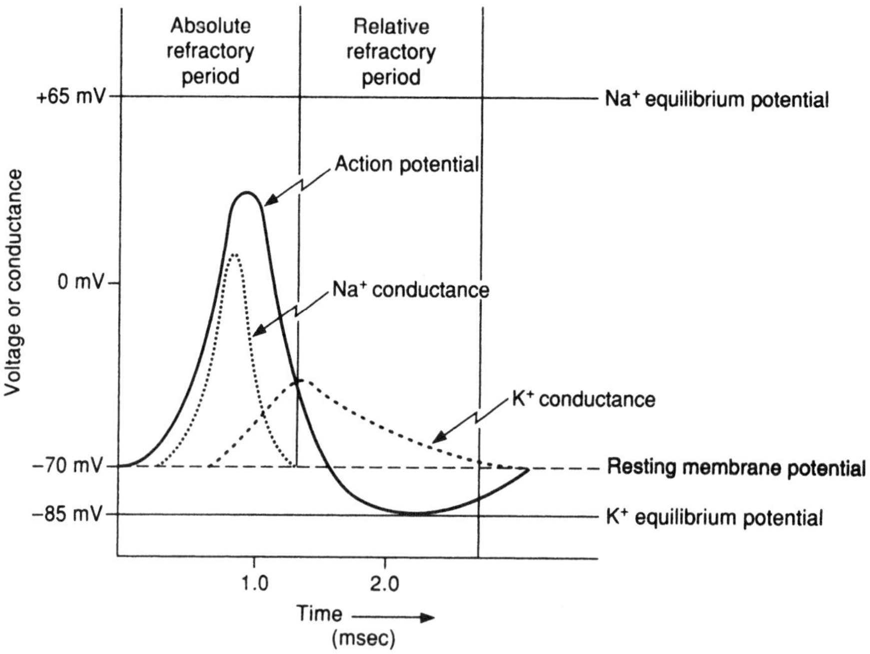

Figure 2–76.
Nerve action potential and associated changes in Na^+ and K^+ conductance. (Reprinted with permission from Costanzo, LS: *BRS Physiology*, 2nd ed. Baltimore, Willliams & Wilkins, 1998, p. 12.)

- **Absolute refractory period:** The cell is completely unable to transmit another action potential. This period lasts almost the entire time of the action potential. It cannot be restimulated because the Na^+ channels were inactivated. They do not become reactivated until the cell is repolarized.
- **Relative refractory period:** This period consists of the later half of the action potential when the cell is returning to resting levels. An action potential may occur again, but a stronger stimulus is needed. The Na^+ channels are open now, but so are the K^+ channels, making their conductance higher. This means that the cell is at a more negative level, making it harder to start another depolarization.
- The Na^+/K^+ pump restores the levels of Na^+ and K^+ inside and outside the cell to prepare for another action potential.

PART III

mcat review books

A Word About Review Books ...

THIS SECTION PROVIDES information on the MCAT books and study aids that are currently available. Each publication has been assigned a letter grade based on factors such as content, usability, and price. These ratings reflect the experience and opinions of many premed students who used the resources listed below. We invite your opinions and ratings (see How to Contribute).

Rating

A = Excellent resource—a "must-buy"
B = Very good—gets the job done
C = Adequate, but better resources are available
N = No rating given

For each book we provide the address and phone number for ordering directly from the publisher. We also give you the scoop on the books with overviews and "bottom line" evaluations. Before you buy anything, make sure you think about your available study time and your willingness to study independently.

A+ MCAT PRACTICE TEST II AND MCAT PRACTICE ITEMS

Author: Association of American Medical Colleges (AAMC)

Price: $20.00

Format: Test

Questions: 220 [*MCAT Practice Test II*]
685 [*MCAT Practice Items*]

Pages: 290 (both booklets)

Edition: 1st ed.

Publisher: Association of American Medical Colleges (AAMC)
Membership and Publication Orders
2450 N Street, NW
Washington, DC 20037-1126
(800) 828-0416

The *MCAT Practice Test II* (220 questions) is a reprint of the actual April 1991 MCAT. The *MCAT Practice Items* consists of 265 verbal reasoning and 420 physical/biological sciences passage-based questions, with letter answers only. These two booklets were written by the Association of American Medical Colleges (AAMC), the same friendly folks who bring you the MCAT. Therefore, the questions in these booklets have the same format, level of difficulty, detail, and content emphasis as do the MCAT questions.

Bottom line. This set of booklets is a "must-buy" and very high yield. The *MCAT Practice Test II* is a useful full-length diagnostic exam to take a week or two before the actual MCAT under simulated testing conditions. The *MCAT Practice Items* are an excellent source of practice questions and are indispensable as a study aid. Student experience shows that the topics and content covered in these questions are a very reliable predictor of many topics that are tested on the actual MCAT.

A+ MCAT PRACTICE TEST III

Author: Association of American Medical Colleges (AAMC)

Price: $20.00

Format: Test

Questions: 220

Pages: 134

Edition: 1st ed.

Publisher: Association of American Medical Colleges (AAMC)
Membership and Publication Orders
2450 N Street, NW
Washington, DC 20037-1126
(800) 828-0416

Like the *MCAT Practice Tests I* and *II,* this book contains sample test questions from past MCATs. Many of these questions are from the 1994 MCAT. There is one full-length practice test, which includes a writing sample. Letter answers are provided only for multiple-choice components of the test. However, sample essays with a critique are included for evaluating the writing sample.

Bottom line. As the most recent of the released AAMC MCAT practice tests, *MCAT Practice Test III* does the best job of simulating the current MCAT. This is also a "must-buy"!

A+ MCAT STUDENT MANUAL AND MCAT PRACTICE TEST I

Author: Association of American Medical Colleges (AAMC)

Price: $20.00

Format: Orientation/Test

Questions: 315

Edition: 1st ed.

Publisher: Association of American Medical Colleges (AAMC)
Membership and Publication Orders
2450 N Street, NW
Washington, DC 20037-1126
(800) 828-0416

The *MCAT Student Manual* includes an orientation chapter written by the test makers. This section covers the format and content of the MCAT as well as a description of how the MCAT is scored. In addition, the *MCAT Student Manual* includes a fairly descriptive and detailed outline of the science content on the MCAT, which can be used as a study guideline. According to the AAMC, this outline contains all the possible topics that are tested on the MCAT. Finally, the *MCAT Student Manual* provides 95 sample questions with answers and detailed explanations.

The *MCAT Practice Test I* is a full-length diagnostic exam with 220 questions. This practice test was used as the template for the new MCAT examination. Unfortunately, there are no explanations to the answers (only letter answers are given).

Bottom line. You should purchase these books. The *MCAT Student Manual* is the official (although probably not the best) guide to the MCAT. In addition, it provides useful study and test-taking advice. The practice test may be a little dated, but it is still close to the real MCAT. Consider using this as a diagnostic tool as you begin your MCAT preparation.

A– COLUMBIA REVIEW: INTENSIVE PREPARATION FOR THE MCAT

Author: Stephen D. Bresnick

Price: $43.95

Format: Review/Test

Questions: 829

Pages: 825

Edition: 1st ed.

Copyright: 1996

Publisher: Williams & Wilkins
351 West Camden St.
Baltimore, MD 21201-2436
(800) 638-0672
Website: http://lww.com

ISBN: 0683010271

Columbia Review presents its own review text that features a comprehensive review of biology, organic chemistry, physics, and inorganic chemistry in an outline format. Students can test their progress with the sample problems throughout the text and with the 120 passage-based questions at the end of each science section. Also, two practice verbal reasoning tests and a full-length sample MCAT are included. In addition, a 40-page guide introduces the student to the MCAT and provides study and test-taking strategies.

Bottom line. Columbia Review does an excellent job of providing the reader with a concise yet exhaustive content review that can be read in less then six weeks. The easy-to-read outline format provides appropriate coverage of MCAT topics without straying into needless detail. The text is complemented by useful and easy-to-understand tables and diagrams. Practice MCAT-style questions at the end of each section closely simulate the real MCAT. Helpful explanations to the practice questions are a major plus. Overall, students have found this book to be extremely useful as a comprehensive MCAT review.

A– COLUMBIA REVIEW MCAT PRACTICE TESTS

Author: Stephen D. Bresnick, William H. Bresnick
Price: $24.95
Format: Test
Questions: 657
Pages: 288
Edition: 1st ed.
Copyright: 1997
Publisher: Williams & Wilkins
351 West Camden St.
Baltimore, MD 21201-2436
(800) 638-0672
Website: http://lww.com
ISBN: 0683180991

Columbia review presents three full-length practice MCATs with answers and explanations to every question and a score conversion scale. Included is a brief overview on how to approach passages with test-taking techniques.

Bottom line. Students have found these practice tests to be very helpful and representative of the actual MCAT in both content and level of difficulty. The tests are different than those that are given in the full-length review so students can buy both and get their money's worth. The passage lengths are appropriate and the types of questions are also appropriate. This is an excellent source of practice tests that is good to use after one has completed the AAMC sample tests and practice items. However, the writing sample offers no sample essays with critiques and suggestions. Overall this is a good source of review questions.

B+ FLOWERS & SILVER MCAT

Author: James L. Flowers, Theodore Silver
Price: $50.00
Format: Review/Test
Questions: 1000+
Pages: 985 + CD-ROM
Edition: 4st ed.
Copyright: 1998
Publisher: The Princeton Review
Random House, Inc.
2315 Broadway
New York, NY 10024
ISBN: 0-375-75003-7

This book provides a comprehensive topic review of the material tested on the MCAT. Numerous chapters are devoted to the biological and physical sciences. Also provided is a section on mathematics review for the MCAT. Questions with detailed explanations are interspersed at the end of each section. In addition, this book contains nine sample verbal reasoning passages with questions and detailed explanations as well as six essay exercises. The new edition of the book also includes a CD-ROM with over 1000 practice MCAT questions.

Bottom line. This book is about as big as it gets! Although big in size, this book is surprisingly easy-to-read and well organized. The questions at the end of each section are passage-based with detailed explanations. This book is a good starting point for those who may be weak in the physical and biological sciences. However, students have stated that this book does require an extensive time commitment to complete. The CD-ROM contains two full-length diagnostic exams that do an excellent job of simulating the actual MCAT examination. Because of the length of the book, we recommend that students who are considering using this book allow 2–3 months time to complete it. Students with a strong background in the physical and biological sciences may find this book to be too bulky and may be better off with a more concise review.

B+ COLUMBIA REVIEW MCAT VERBAL REASONING POWERBUILDER

Author: Stephen D. Bresnick, William H. Bresnick
Price: $14.95
Format: Review/Test
Questions: 250
Pages: 238
Edition: 1st ed.
Copyright: 1997
Publisher: Williams & Wilkins
351 West Camden St.
Baltimore, MD 21201-2436
(800) 638-0672
Website: http://lww.com
ISBN: 0683300733

This book focuses on the verbal reasoning section of the MCAT, containing general strategies, reading and skimming techniques, and verbal test-taking skills. The book also has three full-length verbal reasoning practice exams with explanations.

Bottom line. This book provides a comprehensive review of various techniques on how to approach verbal reasoning passages. There is a little bit of something for everyone in this book. Students are able to pick and choose what techniques are best suited for them. Not every method on how to approach the passage will cater to everyone's style. Be cautious not to focus too much on utilizing every technique discussed. Overall we feel this book contains a solid summary of methods on how to approach the verbal section. The passages and practice exams are of similar length and difficulty to the actual MCAT. If you feel you are especially weak in the verbal section, this may be a good book for you.

B+ ARCO MCAT SUPERCOURSE (4TH ED)/ MCAT SAMPLE EXAMS (3RD ED)

Author: Stefan Bosworth (Editor), et al.

Price: \$39.95 [*Arco MCAT Supercourse*]
\$13.95 [*Arco MCAT Sample Exams*]

Format: Review/Test

Questions: 900+ (657 in the three full-length tests plus many review questions)

Pages: 697 *[Arco MCAT Supercourse]*
226 *[Arco MCAT Sample Exams]*

Edition: 4th ed. *[Arco MCAT Supercourse]*
3rd ed. *[Arco MCAT Sample Exams]*

Copyright: 1997 *[Arco MCAT Supercourse]*
1998 *[Arco MCAT Sample Exams]*

Publisher: Arco-Macmillan
Simon & Schuster Macmillan Company
1633 Broadway
New York, NY 10019-6785

ISBN: 0-02-861711-8 *[Arco MCAT Supercourse]*
0-02-862501-3 *[Arco MCAT Sample Exams]*

ARCO's MCAT SuperCourse contains comprehensive reviews of the four components of the MCAT. Each review unit is peppered with plenty of practice problems and is followed by a full-length subject-specific practice test with answers and explanations. Three full-length practice exams are also sold separately as *ARCO MCAT Sample Exams.* For this reason, do not buy the *ARCO MCAT Sample Exams* if you plan on purchasing the SuperCourse. In addition to a basic orientation to the MCAT, SuperCourse also provides a brief description of medical school and residency training, which was excerpted from the book, *Getting into Medical School: Strategies for the 90s* (Plantz, S., Lorenzo, N., and Cole, J., Arco-Macmillan 1993).

Bottom line. This book offers a good combination of content review and practice tests. The comprehensive science review provides an adequate coverage of MCAT covered topics, but is spotty in certain sections (cardiovascular and endocrine systems, organic chemistry). Subject-specific practice tests are given at the end of each section. The practice exams are of a similar level of difficulty as the actual MCAT, but the physical and biological science passages are shorter than those of the actual exam. Overall, students who have used this book have found it to be a good review source when used in conjunction with other review books.

B+ HIGH YIELD SERIES: GENERAL CHEMISTY (COLUMBIA REVIEW)

Author: Stephen Bresnick

Price: \$12.95

Format: Review
Questions: ~200
Pages: 141
Edition: 1st ed.
Copyright: 1996
Publisher: Williams & Wilkins
351 West Camden St.
Baltimore, MD 21201-2436
(800) 638-0672
Website: http://lww.com
ISBN: 068318072

Columbia Review provides a quick review of general chemisty presented in a high-yield format. This book covers the essential topics that would be covered in a college-level class in three different sections. It is not solely meant for MCAT preparation, but is intended to be a general review for all science pre-graduate school exams. It provides review questions at the end of the book for each of the three sections, along with answers and explanations.

Bottom line. The High-Yield series is a good series for those who want to see the "basics" of what they need to know for the MCAT. Although this book is not intended solely for the MCAT, it does a good job of covering the basics that are needed for the MCAT. This book is written in a text format explaining the topic at a conceptual level. Students have found that this book does a good job of making complex concepts easy to understand. The questions are not like the MCAT because it is testing your knowledge of the material and not the application of it. In general, this book should be used in conjunction with other more detailed books that are geared specifically for the MCAT. Overall, this book is a good source to give a foundation for your studying, but should not be the only source you use.

B+ HIGH-YIELD SERIES: PHYSICS (COLUMBIA REVIEW)

Author: Stephen Bresnick
Price: $12.95
Format: Review
Questions: ~250
Pages: 244
Edition: 1st ed.
Copyright: 1996
Publisher: Williams & Wilkins
351 West Camden St.
Baltimore, MD 21201-2436
(800) 638-0672
Website: http://lww.com
ISBN: 068318069

Columbia Review provides a quick review of non-calculus based general physics presented in a high-yield format. This book covers the essential topics that would be covered in a college level class. It is not solely meant for MCAT preparation, but is intended to be a general review for all science pre-graduate school exams. It is divided into three sections corresponding to topics that would normally appear in a college level physics class.

Bottom line. The high-yield series is a good series for those who want to see the "basics" of what they need to know for the MCAT. Although this book is not intended solely for the MCAT, it does a good job of covering the basics that are needed for the MCAT. The physics book of the series does an excellent job of presenting the basics of physics. Students have found that the book teaches conceptually what is helpful for MCAT preparation and that the numberous examples are an added benefit to help comprehension. The questions are not like the passage-based MCAT questions, but are review questions that test your knowledge of the material and not the application of it. Students have found that this book should be used in conjunction with other more detailed books that are geared specifically for the MCAT, but that this book does the most complete job of all the high-yield books in covering and presenting the material in a helpful manner. Overall, this book is a good source to give a foundation for your studying, but should not be the only source you use.

B KAPLAN MCAT ALL-IN-ONE

Author: R. Rothstein (editor), et al.

Price: $34.95

Format: Orientation/Review/Test + Software disk

Questions: 328 (two-thirds in book and one-third on disk)

Pages: 275

Edition: 1st ed.

Copyright:

Publisher: Bantam Doubleday Dell Publishing Group
1540 Broadway
New York, NY 10036
(800) 323-9872

ISBN: 038531633X

This new book (updated in 1996) is a comprehensive but not overwhelming source of information for the entire medical school application process. It is divided into four components: medical school admissions, which provides basic information and strategy for developing an application, deciding where to apply, and interviewing; MCAT review, which briefly discusses general strategies and test-taking mentality and briefly provides section-specific reviews containing strategies and sample questions with answers and explanations; a full-length practice MCAT exam; and a half-length practice exam on disk (Mac/Win). Plugs for Kaplan's test preparation course are scattered throughout the text.

Bottom line. *Kaplan MCAT All-in-One* has a little something for everyone, but not everything for anybody. The admissions section is useful, but short compared with other books that dedicate themselves entirely to the admissions process. The MCAT advice is also helpful and humorous but not complete. The full-length practice MCAT with answers and explanations (yes!) is an adequate simulation of the real MCAT. The computer software is user friendly and provides questions with answers and explanations, data about your performance, and information on your test-taking habits. This book can get you started, but it won't take you all the way.

B HIGH YIELD SERIES: BIOLOGY (COLUMBIA REVIEW)

Author: Stephen Bresnick
Price: $12.95
Format: Review
Questions: ~250
Pages: 244
Edition: 1st ed.
Copyright: 1996
Publisher: Williams & Wilkins
351 West Camden St.
Baltimore, MD 21201-2436
(800) 638-0672
Website: http://lww.com
ISBN: 068318069

Columbia Review provides a quick review of general biology presented in a high-yield format. This book covers the essential topics that would be covered in a college level class. It is not solely meant for MCAT preparation, but is intended to be a general review for all science pre-graduate school exams. The facts are presented in an outline format with review questions and answer explanations at the end of the book.

Bottom line. The High-Yield series is a good series for those who want to see the "basics" of what they need to know for the MCAT. Although this book is not intended solely for the MCAT, it does a good job of covering the basics that are needed for the MCAT. The outline presentation is easy to read and comprehend. The questions are not like the MCAT because it is testing your knowledge of the material and not the application of it. Students have found that this book should be used in conjunction with other more detailed books that are geared specifically for the MCAT. Overall, this book is a good source to give a foundation for your studying, but should not be the only source you use.

B UNDERGROUND MCAT ANSWERS

Authors: Vikas Bhushan, Chirag Amin, Tao Le
Price: $39.95
Format: Explanation/Review
Questions: None
Pages: 356
Edition: 1st ed.

Copyright: 1997

Publisher: Student to Student (S2S) Medical Publishing
(800) 247-6553
Website: www.s2smed.com

ISBN: 1-890061-02-6

This book provides original explanations to the 1345 officially released questions from the AAMC publications (Practice Items, Practice I-III that are sold separately). This content review is designed to be read with or without the questions to aid students in preparing for the verbal reasoning, physical sciences, and biological sciences examinations. The book is very hard to find in college bookstores, but can be obtained mail-order using the toll-free number listed above.

Bottom line. This guide serves as a unique MCAT study tool that focuses on the concepts explicitly tested by the AAMC. Because the originally published AAMC questions do not come with explanations (letter answers only), this book serves as a valuable companion to the AAMC publications. The explanations are detailed and are good in quality, explaining not only the correct answer but also the incorrect choices with a brief review of the topic being tested. Although some review courses may have a similar publication, this is the only book available outside of a commercial review course that provides detailed explanations to these questions. The conceptual material found in these explanations is extremely high-yield, making this book a useful content review that can be used either with or without the AAMC questions. Overall, students have found this to be a useful companion to the AAMC publications.

B FLOWERS & SILVER ANNOTATED PRACTICE MCATs

Author: The Princeton Review

Price: \$20.00 (\$34.95 with diagnostic test disk)

Format: Orientation/Test

Questions: 219 in the book, 657 on disk

Pages: 210

Edition: 1st ed.

Copyright: 1996

Publisher Random House Publishing
400 Hahn Road
Westminster, MD 21157
(800) 733-3000

ISBN: 0679771271, 0679771050 (CD-ROM), 0679771042 (3.5″ disk)

Formerly titled *Cracking the MCAT*, this book is divided into three sections: orientation, diagnostic test, and diagnostic explanations to answers. The orientation section provides information about the format of the MCAT. Following the Princeton Review philosophy (i.e., the "Joe Bloggs approach"), the suggested strategies are based on intuition and common sense. The full-length diagnostic test includes detailed explanations to answers. The optional disk (Mac/Win) provides two additional sample tests. These tests are timed, generating scores automatically and providing letter answers after each question you finish.

Bottom line. The one full-length diagnostic test is a dandy. It is one of the best non-AAMC practice tests available. Reprinting the questions next to the answers and explanations is a great idea! Use the diagnostic test as one of your final practice exams (along with the AAMC *MCAT Practice Test III*). The additional tests on disk provide great practice, but they have no explanations. The orientation guide to the MCAT is not very helpful. It is less of a strategy guide to the MCAT than a lead-in for Princeton Review's test preparation course.

B KAPLAN MCAT 1997-1998

Author: Rochelle Rothstein (Editor), et al.

Price: $20.00

Format: Overview/Diagnostic Test

Questions: 219

Edition: 1st ed.

Copyright: 1996

Publisher: Kaplan Educational Centers and Simon & Schuster
1230 Avenue of the Americas
New York, NY 10020

ISBN: 0-684-83673-4

This is the 1997–98 version of the KAPLAN preparation for the MCAT. The information presented in this text is purely preparational in the logistics sense. There is no science content review. It is a comprehensive source for information about the MCAT and medical school application process. There are four parts to this book: 1. An introduction to the MCAT, breaking down the test into the big picture and showing what each section and the MCAT is all about. 2. The KAPLAN stress management section. 3. A full-length exam with detailed explanations for each answer. 4. The medical school admissions section that provides information and strategy for how, where, and when to apply and how to organize your applications. Plugs for the KAPLAN test preparation course are seen throughout the book.

Bottom line. The KAPLAN MCAT preparation book is a good introduction to the MCAT and the medical school admissions process. The strongest point of this book is the full-length exam and the explanations (a definite plus!). The other information is good and informative but not complete. The medical school admissions section does a good job of getting you started, but there are many more books that are more exhaustive. The organizational tips for the application process, however, are a definite plus. The MCAT advice and information are good, but very brief and not complete. If you have no idea what the MCAT and medical school are all about, this may be the book for you to get started, but you will need additional material.

B THE GOLD STANDARD FOR MEDICAL SCHOOL ADMISSION: MCAT

Author: B. Ferdinand

Price: $24.95

Format: Review

Questions: None

Pages: 397

Edition: 1st ed.

Copyright: 1994

Publisher: RevenueCo Inc., Publications
1641 Place Victor Hugo
Montreal, P.Q., Canada H3C 4P1

ISBN: 0-9696863-0-7

This book begins with an introductory section that discusses the medical school admissions process, and provides a directory of the medical schools in North America. The next section discusses the format of the MCAT examination, with brief chapters on how to prepare for the verbal reasoning and writing sample. The majority of the book is devoted to a detailed content review of physics, general chemistry, biology, and organic chemistry. A mathematics review is also provided.

Bottom line. This book provides the student with a good review of the physical and biological sciences. The science chapters are well-organized and easy-to-read, providing the student with a conceptual review of the MCAT science disciplines. The scope of the science topics discussed in this book is good, but not overdone, covering the concepts tested on the MCAT. The book also provides the student with helpful advice on the medical school admissions process as well as the medical school interview. However, this book does not provide any practice questions. There are also very few example problems in the text. The verbal reasoning section of this book is very brief, only two pages long. The writing sample section also is very brief, only six pages long. Despite these shortcomings, this book provides the student with an above-average conceptual review for the science disciplines tested on the MCAT.

B MCAT PRE-TEST A AND MCAT: PRE-TEST B (SOLD SEPARATELY)

Author: Dr. Eftekar Jahan (Editor)

Price: $15.00

Format: Test

Questions: 219

Pages: 78

Edition: 1st ed.

Copyright: 1997

Publisher: Maval Publishing, Inc.
567 Harrison St.
Denver, Co 80206

ISBN: 1884083951 *[MCAT: Pre-Test A]*
1884083978 *[MCAT: Pre-Test B]*

These books each contain a mock MCAT exam provided for the student who wants to see what a simulated MCAT exam looks like. One sample MCAT is provided in the correct format and length for students to practice with.

Bottom line. These two books provide a fairly accurate representation of the actual MCAT. These tests come close enough to the real thing that it would be useful to take if your are looking for tests to practice with. The level of difficulty is appropriate for the MCAT. There are very brief explanations for the science sections but the verbal section answers do not give explanations so you are left wondering why you got the answers wrong. Overall, these two books are a good source for full-length tests and should be used in addition to the *AAMC Practice Tests.*

B BEST TEST PREPARATION AND REVIEW FOR THE MCAT: MEDICAL COLLEGE ADMISSION TEST

Author: Joseph A. Alvarez, et al.
Price: $52.95
Format: Review/Test
Questions: 1314
Pages: 1002 + Software Disk
Edition: 4th ed.
Copyright: 1996
Publisher: Research & Education Association (REA)
61 Ethel Road West
Piscataway, NJ 08854

ISBN: 0-87891-807-8

Best Test Preparation and Review for the MCAT consists of comprehensive reviews of the subjects tested on the MCAT (including a mathematics review), along with six full-length practice tests with detailed explanations. The reviews are organized to parallel the content outline in the *MCAT Student Manual.* The introductory section in this book discusses MCAT format and scoring and general test-taking strategies. This book also includes *MCAT TESTware* interactive software (Windows and Macintosh), which provides the student with two, timed, full-length exams, as well as an on-screen tutorial and computer analysis and feedback.

Bottom line. This book offers a large amount of practice questions for preparation. Although the questions are similar in both length and format to the MCAT, the scope in coverage of the topics tested does not necessarily reflect the concepts emphasized on the actual MCAT exam. The detailed explanations to the test questions are very helpful. The science reviews are well written and easy-to-read, but may not be adequate as a primary review source for students. Review questions are interspersed at the end of each review section, which is helpful. The software is a computerized version of practice tests #5 and #6 in this book, and provides helpful computerized analysis and feedback. Overall, students have found this book to be a good source of practice questions with an above average content review.

B- HIGH YIELD SERIES: ORGANIC CHEMISTRY (COLUMBIA REVIEW)

Author: Stephen Bresnick

Price: $12.95

Format: Review

Questions: ~200

Pages: 186

Edition: 1st ed.

Copyright: 1996

Publisher: Williams & Wilkins
351 West Camden St.
Baltimore, MD 21201-2436
(800) 638-0672
Website: http://lww.com

ISBN: 068318071

Columbia Review provides a quick review of organic chemistry presented in a high-yield format. This book covers the essential topics that would be covered in a college-level class. It is not solely meant for MCAT preparation, but is intended to be a general review for all science pre-graduate school exams. The facts are presented in a text format with review questions and answer explanations at the end of the book.

Bottom line. The High-Yield series usually does a good job on the "basics" of what a student needs to know for the MCAT. Although this book is not intended solely for the MCAT, the material is still applicable. However, students have found that the organic chemistry portion of the series leaves out too many facts that need to be covered for the MCAT. It does provide a conceptual basis for the topics it does cover, but again, the book is not exhaustive. Students have also found that this text lacks depth, even for a high-yield book, in some areas. The questions are not like the passage-based MCAT questions, but are review questions that test your knowledge of the material and not the application of it. Students have found that this book should be used in conjunction with other more detailed books that are geared specifically for the MCAT. Overall, this book is lacking in depth and is not exhaustive enough but it still provides high-yield review of most of the major topics in organic chemistry.

B- COMPLETE PREPARATION FOR THE MCAT, 1999

Author: Williams & Wilkins

Price: $49.50

Format: Review/Test

Questions: >1000 (136 in MCAT format)

Pages: 779

Edition: 1st ed.

Copyright: 1998

Publisher: Williams & Wilkins
351 West Camden St.
Baltimore, MD 21201-2436
(800) 638-0672
Website: http://lww.com

ISBN: 0683305220

Formerly known as the Betz guide, this book is now known as the *Complete Preparation for the MCAT, 1999.* Most of the book's questions are content-review questions that appear at the end of each chapter, testing your knowledge of the specific information presented. There are no full-length exams, but it includes MCAT-style passages. There is a verbal section of 61 questions that is written in a passage-based format in the beginning of the book.

Bottom line. Although revised numerous times under its former title and publisher, this text still remains full of detail and complexity. This book is too verbose and detailed in many areas, especially the biological and physical sciences. Even though there have been promises of change, the unneeded detail still remains and can slow you down significantly in your MCAT studies. The content review questions asked at the end of each chapter are not typical of MCAT questions. From our discussions with numerous premedical students, many that have used this book were unable to complete it. Because this book is so detailed and long, it is only recommended for the highly motivated student.

B– THE MCAT BIOLOGY BOOK

Author: Nancy Morvillo, Matthew Schmidt

Price: $19.95

Format: Review/Questions

Questions: 150+

Pages: 424

Edition: 1st ed.

Copyright: 1998

Publisher: Nova Press
11659 Mayfield Ave., Suite 1
Los Angeles, CA 90049
(800) 949-6175

ISBN: 1-889057-08-8

This book attempts to review both the verbal and the biology section, even though the name says only biology. The book is easy to read, but done in a bullet format to define key words. Paragraphs are written about the words that tie them together. The organization is more narrative than outline and most of the diagrams appear hand-drawn. Questions are presented at the end of each chapter. The verbal section gives lots of questions to practice on.

Bottom line. This book presents a content review of the biology section of the biological sciences and provides strategy on how to approach the verbal section. Students have found the verbal review to be more comprehensive than the biology review, but not as adequate as other verbal reviews available. Also students found the biology review to be inadequate due to the hard-to-follow organization and questions that are not reflective of the actual MCAT. Overall, this book does not provide a comprehensive review for either subject and does not adequately prepare the student for either section.

B– PETERSON'S MCAT SUCCESS

Author: Beryl Packer, et al.
Price: $24.95
Format: Tests
Questions: 657+ (3 Full-length practice exams)
Pages: 352 + Software Disk
Edition: 1st ed.
Copyright: 1996
Publisher: Peterson's
202 Carnegie Center
Princeton, NJ 08540
Website: www.petersons.com
ISBN: 1-56079-689-8

The *Peterson's MCAT Success* preparation book is a completely question-based review with complete detailed explanations for every answer. There is no content review. It contains in effect 3 full-length exams (1 diagnostic and 2 sample tests). Also included are extra questions for every section of the MCAT, as well as general strategies to the verbal reasoning and essay sections, as well as a mathematics review. The book also comes with a software disk that contains 2 full-length, interactive, sample MCAT examinations with computerized analysis and feedback.

Bottom line. If you are looking for review material to understand concepts for the MCAT, this book may not be for you. It attempts to teach concepts through a question-only format, which may not be sufficient for students who need to "learn" for the MCAT. This format promotes memorization and problem-solving skill, and does not help the student to think conceptually. Also, the questions that are presented in this book do not completely reflect those on the actual exam in terms of format and level of difficulty. The verbal passages are too long and the science passages are too short as compared with the actual exam. This book is not adequate as a sole study source and should be used after other question sources have been exhausted.

B– MCAT PHYSICS BOOK

Author: Garrett Biehle
Price: $19.95
Format: Review/Questions
Questions: 500+
Pages: 424
Edition: 1st ed.
Copyright: 1997
Publisher: Nova Press
11659 Mayfield Ave., Suite 1
Los Angeles, CA 90049
(800) 949-6175
ISBN: 1-889057-00-2

This book is a comprehensive subject review of physics topics for the MCAT. The material is presented in a textbook format with review and passage-based MCAT-style questions at the end of each chapter.

Bottom line. This book is written in an easy-to-read manner that allows for comprehension. This book emphasizes conceptual material specific to the MCAT exam and places the necessary equations in the context of the concepts. Many examples are given to illustrate these concepts. The types of questions are reflective of the MCAT, but more passage-based questions could be given instead of the plethora of objective questions. This book may serve as a good physics review for those weak in the subject, but is long and requires a significant time commitment. It may not be helpful for students strong in this discipline.

B– MCAT STUDY CARDS

Author: Elizabeth R. Burchard
Price: $9.95
Format: Question and Answer
Pages: 384 cards
Edition: 1st ed.
Copyright: 1997
Publisher: Ace Academics, Inc.
ISBN: 1881374815

This unique study tool puts common concepts and terms that show up on the MCAT in a flash-card format. These cards cover the four science sections: organic chemistry, general chemistry, biology, and physics. It is a memorization-intensive study tool geared toward helping the student remember facts about each subject.

Bottom line. The MCAT study cards present the science information on the MCAT in a unique manner. This type of studying lends itself to rote memorization rather than conceptual processing. Students have found these cards to be most helpful with the biology section, since that requires the most memorization of facts. These cards may be a good way to review all of your studying once the material has been covered. Overall, these cards are not a good way to study initially, but may be used to help review. It is not adequate as a sole review source.

C+ BARRON'S HOW TO PREPARE FOR THE MEDICAL COLLEGE ADMISSION TEST: MCAT

Author: Hugo R. Seibel (Editor), et al.

Price: $13.95

Format: Review/Test

Questions: 876

Edition: 8th ed.

Copyright: 1997

Publisher: Barron's Educational Series, Inc.
250 Wireless Blvd.
Hauppage, NY 11788

ISBN: 0-8120-9730-0

This book is divided into three major sections. The first is an overview of the MCAT, including test-taking strategies and preparation hints. The second is an overall review of biology, chemistry, and physics. The third section has four full-length exams with answers and explanations. This book also has sections on strategies for the verbal reasoning and essay portions of the MCAT, as well as a mathematics review.

Bottom line. Students that have used this book for MCAT preparation have found the book to be inadequate in terms of content review and somewhat disappointing as compared with other review books on the market. The introduction does provide some help with test-taking and study strategies. The science review section provides spotty topic coverage with information presented in a text format with poor readability. At times you feel like you are reading a textbook and not a test preparation book (biology), whereas other sections feel like you are hitting and missing important concepts and the material is incomplete (chemistry). There is very little conceptual emphasis on basic science topics that are crucial for MCAT preparation.

The four practice exams do not adequately represent the topic coverage or format of the MCAT. The tests are condensed on the page making it hard to read. The verbal passages are much too long, whereas the science passages are much too short. The physical science questions are excessively math-oriented as is the review section for the physical sciences. This "plug-and-chug" style of testing is less often seen than the conceptual style of testing on the MCAT. Overall, students felt that better sources exist for MCAT review. Nevertheless, this book is one of the most inexpensive books out there for MCAT review, and this may be a consideration for those students who do not have adequate financial resources to devote to MCAT preparation.

C+ CADUCEUS SOFTWARE FOR THE MCAT

Price: $135.00
Format: Review
Questions: 800 (non-MCAT style)
Pages: N/A
Edition: 1st ed.
Copyright: 1996
Publisher: Scientia
657A Summerville Ave.
Summerville, MA 02143
(800) 453-4725
ISBN: 1885727003 (Mac), 1885727011 (PC), 1885727046 (CD-ROM)

Caduceus MCAT Review is a multimedia software review that covers physics, biology, inorganic chemistry, and organic chemistry. The software presents lessons that cover basic science topics. Concepts are brought to life with color animation clips and illustrations. You can test your comprehension of the topic with the click of a button at anytime. Convenient options include the ability to print out topics on paper and to place "bookmarkers" at topics that need extra attention.

Bottom line. Caduceus is a well-written piece of software that may be better suited for remedial science review than for MCAT preparation. The visuals and animated graphics are outstanding, and the user interface is very intuitive. However, the questions are not MCAT style and do not test your ability to apply information under test conditions. Use this tool only in conjunction with other review books.

C+ GUIDE TO MEDICAL SCHOOL AND THE MCAT

Author: David A. Hacker, Kenneth Ibsen
Price: $19.95
Format: Review
Questions: 219
Pages: 298
Edition: 1st ed.
Copyright: 1997
Publisher: Williams & Wilkins
351 West Camden St.
Baltimore, MD 21201-2436
(800) 638-0672
Website: http://lww.com
ISBN: 0683006797

This book contains information on how to get into medical school and the medical school application process, as well as advice on letters of recommendation and specific information about medical schools. In addition, the book provides general advice about the MCAT, accompanied by a full-length practice examination.

Bottom line. This book does a good job of covering every aspect that needs to be addressed when considering medical school. The information regarding MCAT scores and GPAs is helpful. It provides a solid timeline and good advice regarding the application process and specific aspects, such as obtaining letters of recommendation. However, in regard to MCAT preparation, this book is grossly inadequate. General guidelines and test-taking advice are provided. The practice examination is not a good reflection of the actual MCAT. Overall, this book provides solid information for the application process, but, by itself, is inadequate as an MCAT review source.

C BETZ MCAT DIAGNOSTIC EXAMS (PRACTICE TESTS 4, 5, AND 6)

Author: Betz Publishing

Price: $29.95

Format: Test

Questions: 219

Pages: 78

Edition: 1st ed.

Publisher: Williams & Wilkins
351 West Camden Street
Baltimore, MD 21201-2436
(800) 638-0672
Website: http://lww.com

ISBN: 0941406644

These publications each contain a full-length MCAT simulation that you mail for free computer scoring and analysis. The test itself does a good job of simulating the form and content of the current MCAT. An answer key without explanations is included in a sealed envelope. After taking the practice exam under test conditions, you send the scoring sheet and writing sample essays to the computer-scoring center. Two weeks later, you receive a 6-page report that identifies your weaknesses in MCAT skills and content. You can opt for express scoring service (3 working days), but it will cost you another $20.

Bottom line. The report is of limited benefit. You receive grades for your writing samples, but no written critique. To fully understand the report, you must have *A Complete Preparation for the MCAT: The Betz Guide* to explain the problem-solving skills that are evaluated. The lack of explanations for questions that are answered incorrectly also limits the usefulness of the analysis. Finally, the 2-week turnaround for scoring and analysis is too long to be useful; by the time you get your results, your preparation may be at a completely different stage. In addition, you may have forgotten most of that exam. Express scoring service, which costs you extra money, is a must if you want to maximize the utility of the report.

C AAMC MCAT VIDEOTAPE: PREPARING FOR THE MCAT

Author: Association of American Medical Colleges (AAMC)

Price: $12.00

Format: Orientation

Questions: None

Pages: 25-minute videotape

Edition: 1st ed.

Publisher: Association of American Medical Colleges (AAMC)
Membership and Publication Orders
2450 N Street, NW
Washington, DC 20037-1126
(202) 828-0416

This 25-minute video produced by the AAMC is an introduction to preparation for the MCAT. It briefly discusses the format and structure of the MCAT, and it provides basic study tips and suggestions.

Bottom line. Unfortunately, this videotape plays like a long "infomercial" for the MCAT. All of the information provided is similar to that in the *MCAT Student Manual,* but without all of the useful tips. If you're a student who likes a little visual motivation to get started, you may want to borrow the video if your university or career center has a copy.

C– FUTURE TEST MCAT

Price: $69.95

Format: Review Software

Questions: 3500+

Pages: N/A (Software)

Edition: 1st ed.

Publisher: National Learning Corporation
212 Michael Drive
Syosset, NY 11791
(516) 921-8888

ISBN: 0837394279

Future Test MCAT is an interactive, self-paced software program available for both Macintosh® and MS-DOS computers. The review covers basic science information in six sections through terms with definitions and questions with answers. The final exam can be custom tailored to contain a specific number of questions under specific time restrictions. Most questions on the exams are direct recall. There are neither problem-solving nor passage-based questions. After quizzes and exams, *Future Test* provides a "report card" to track your progress.

Bottom line. The material is very basic, almost remedial, and the questions, which are not in an MCAT style, provide little practice for the actual exam. In addition, there is no organization of the topics covered. This software review is expensive and has minimal preparatory value for the MCAT.

C– NEW RUDMAN'S QUESTIONS AND ANSWERS ON THE MCAT

Author: Jack Rudman
Price: $23.95
Format: Test
Questions: 2000+
Pages: 375
Edition: 1st ed.
Copyright: 1997
Publisher: National Learning Corporation
212 Michael Drive
Syosset, NY 11791
(516) 921-8888
ISBN: 0837350115

This book contains about 2000 MCAT-style questions with letter answers only. Explanations are not provided. It includes a brief 5-page introduction about study and test-taking strategies.

Bottom linc. This book has many poorly written, outdated questions. Most questions are not passaged-based and test knowledge rather than the ability to interpret and apply concepts. Also, the questions are not organized in the standard MCAT format. In addition, the production quality is mediocre; it looks like it was created on a typewriter. Don't spend too much time on these practice questions.

C– MCAT ESSENTIALS

Author: Daniel Roth
Price: $14.95
Format: Review
Questions: None
Pages: 183
Edition: 1st ed.
Copyright: 1998

Publisher: Williams & Wilkins
351 West Camden St.
Baltimore, MD 21201-2436
(800) 638-0672
Website: http://lww.com

ISBN: 0683301055

This book serves as a dictionary of frequently used MCAT terms providing definitions and illustrations of these alphabetically listed concepts. It does not contain any practice questions.

Bottom line. This book is organized as a glossary of MCAT terms, with no subject or topic organization by scientific discipline. Topics are covered from A to Z in that order, making this a very difficult book to use for MCAT preparation. Like reading a dictionary, this book does not provide any orderly flow of related information. Overall, students have not found this book to be very useful as an MCAT review source.

C- GRE-LSAT-GMAT-MCAT READING COMPREHENSION WORKBOOK

Author: Mark Alan Stewart

Price: $10.95

Format: Review

Questions: 100+

Pages: 196

Edition: 1st ed.

Copyright: 1995

Publisher: Arco-Macmillan
Simon & Schuster Macmillan Company
1633 Broadway
New York, NY 10019-6785

ISBN: 0-02-860349-4

This book contains reading comprehension strategy for standardized tests of various disciplines. It is formatted in a workbook style with 18 practice passages devoted to all four professional and graduate school exams.

Bottom line. This book does not adequately focus on approaching the MCAT verbal reasoning passages. Although reading comprehension is included in all of the above mentioned tests, there are definitely differences in format and types of questions. For example, the MCAT passages are typically longer with characteristic question types. Over half of the book is used to describe material about the GRE, GMAT, and LSAT. The LSAT, GMAT, and GRE are produced and administered by a different testing company than the MCAT, thus the techniques cannot be generalized across all these exams. The book only has three verbal passages devoted to the MCAT alone. Overall, student experience has stated that there are other books better suited for the MCAT verbal reasoning section.

C– MCAT PREPARATION GUIDE

Author: Miriam S. Willey, Barbara M. Jarecky
Price: $15.95
Format: Overview
Questions: None
Pages: 137
Edition: 1st ed.
Copyright: 1995
Publisher: University Press of Kentucky
663 South Limestone St.
Lexington, KY 40508–4008
(800) 839–6855
ISBN: 0-8131-0847-0

The *MCAT Preparation Guide* is a book designed to be a companion to the AAMC *MCAT Student Manual.* The guide first discusses some basic test-taking techniques for the multiple-choice sections of the exam and offers a stepwise strategy to approaching the writing sample. It then provides a series of tables keyed to *MCAT Practice Test I.* These tables help you identify your weaknesses in each section of *MCAT Practice Test I.*

Bottom line. *MCAT Preparation Guide* has an interesting approach to the MCAT, but it doesn't provide much MCAT "enlightenment." Because the analysis is derived from only one practice test (as opposed to an analysis based on performance over several practice tests, which can reveal true trends and weaknesses), this book neither reviews any topics nor provides explanations to questions. In addition, many of the test-taking strategies and techniques are too basic and nonspecific.

N GETTING INTO MEDICAL SCHOOL: A PLANNING GUIDE FOR MINORITY STUDENTS

Author: Edward J. James
Price: $12.50
Format: Admissions Guide
Questions: None
Pages: 198
Edition: 1st ed.
Copyright: 1996
Publisher: Williams & Wilkins
351 West Camden St.
Baltimore, MD 21201-2436
(800) 638-0672
Website: http://lww.com
ISBN: 0941406512

Like all other admissions guides, half of the text is filled with program names. What this book does beyond the other books, however, is to not only list the medical schools, but also the post-bac programs available. The general advice given in the first half of the book is good. It starts from the very basics of if medical school is even for me. This is a great book even for non-minority students because the advice given here is solid and very applicable to one's journey toward medical school. It addresses every aspect from grades, to the MCAT, to the application process. If you have no idea about what it takes to get into medical school, this book will give you a good overview of what you are getting yourself into.

N CAREER PLANNING GUIDE FOR THE ALLIED HEALTH PROFESSIONS

Author: Zubie Metcalf

Price: $14.95

Format: Admissions Guide

Questions: None

Pages: 176

Edition: 1st ed.

Copyright: 1997

Publisher: Williams & Wilkins
351 West Camden St.
Baltimore, MD 21201-2436
(800) 638-0672
Website: http://lww.com

ISBN: 0683301667

This book provides a general overview with descriptions of over 30 allied health professions. It not only provides the student with addresses of the various college- and university-based allied health programs across the country, but also gives a brief overview of a typical allied health curriculum. This book provides excellent information on choosing a specific allied health profession, and discusses the overall admissions process. The book also provides valuable information regarding the interview, as well as financial aid. This book is useful for any student interested in the medical field and considering an alternative to medical school.

PART IV

mcat course reviews

A Word About Review Courses ...

MORE AND MORE students preparing for the MCAT are turning to review courses. The competition for admission to medical school has heated up, and students are looking to others for help in getting an edge on the MCAT. Commercial review courses can be effective in organizing material and guiding a student who is overwhelmed by the "MCAT experience." In response to the demand, new review courses continue to appear. Ten years ago, there were only one or two choices, but now there are at least five, and the list grows annually. The two national courses are Kaplan and Princeton Review. Berkeley Review and Columbia Review are regional review courses that are largely based on the West Coast.

Although many students are satisfied with their review course experience, commercial review courses are not a "magic pill" for everyone's MCAT woes. Many cited cost as a major issue; at around $800 for each review course, the concern is well founded. One comment of almost all students, regardless of the review course they took, was that studying for the MCAT didn't become quite as "easy, fast, and fun" as promised. Some students said that they had fallen for the advertising hype.

On the next few pages is some information on the major review courses. This information is intended to supplement your decision on whether to attend a review course. The following are some tips for evaluating a review course:

- Ask yourself what you are looking for in an MCAT review course (e.g., discipline, organization, specialized study materials) and if the time and financial commitments are worth it.
- Find out if the course fits your schedule and your style of learning. Some classes are offered on evenings and weekends.
- Tour the learning center, look at the review materials, ask about the qualifications of the instructors, and sit in on a class if possible.
- Talk to friends and classmates who have taken review courses.

Don't expect that paying for a review course will motivate you to study. Only *you* can motivate yourself to study! We welcome your opinions on review courses, so we can include evaluations in future editions. Note that review courses evolve continually and prices, format, and availability are subject to change. We recommend that you call each commercial review course for the latest available information.

National Review Courses

THE PRINCETON REVIEW

2315 Broadway, 3rd Floor
New York, NY 10024-4332
(800) 995-5565 or (800) 2 REVIEW
Website: www.review.com

Cost: \$895–\$1000 (regional costs may vary; ask about financial aid)

Classroom hours: 90

Class size: No more than 24 students per instructor

Length: 9 weeks

The Princeton Review course emphasizes strategies and concepts rather than memorization techniques. The course extends approximately 9 weeks, with 4 meetings per week, each lasting about $2^1/_2$ hours. Its small classes are interactive. The Princeton Review course includes five full-length proctored mock MCAT exams (8 hours each), and up to 20 hours of free tutoring is available. The Princeton Review course also provides study materials to use at home, including a comprehensive science review covering biology, organic chemistry, physics, and general chemistry and three sample MCAT exams.

STANLEY H. KAPLAN EDUCATIONAL CENTER

810 Seventh Avenue, 26th Floor
New York, NY 10019
(800) KAP-TEST (in the U.S.) or 01-212-262-4980 (outside the U.S.)
Website: www.kaplan.com

Cost: \$949–1049 (regional costs may vary; ask about financial aid and alumni and campus discounts)

Classroom hours: Approximately 72 hrs. (24 three-hour sessions)

Class size: Up to 25 students per instructor

Length: 4–6 months

Course location: Over 160 Kaplan review centers and over 1000 classroom sites worldwide

The course begins with the student taking two different types of MCAT diagnostic tests. The student receives a 10–15 page computer analysis that provides the student with a performance feedback as well as a personal study plan, which guides the student with regard to what to specifically focus on for efficient exam preparation. The Kaplan course includes classroom instruction, problem-solving workshops, and comprehensive review materials. Review material contains approximately 3700 MCAT practice questions with explanations. Kaplan also provides the student access to its toll-free national MCAT hotline. The course includes seven review books, Kaplan MCAT flashcards, computer software (Kaplan's "Digital Test Booklet"), as well as six full-length, proctored, simulated MCAT exams, with computerized feedback reports. Furthermore, Kaplan provides the student with video lectures, entitled *The Inside Scoop on Med School Admissions*, as well as Kaplan's *Medical School Admissions Workbook*, which provides the student with advice on the entire medical school application and admissions process.

Regional Review Courses

THE BERKELEY REVIEW

P.O. Box 40140
Berkeley, CA 94704
(800) 622-8827
Website: www.berkeley-review.com

Cost: $895 (included in the cost of tuition is a $125 non-refundable administrative fee) (work–study program available for students with financial need)

Hours: 100 in-class lecture hours (50 two-hour lectures with 4 lectures per week) and 300–500 office hours

Class size: No more than 25 students per classroom

Length: 15 weeks

Course Locations: Davis, Berkeley, Stanford, Westwood, Irvine, San Diego (all California locations)

The Berkeley Review course provides an intensive four-point system that includes classroom instruction, comprehensive review books, practice exams, and office hours. The classroom instruction is for 15 weeks, four 2-hour sessions per week. These sessions usually involve thorough discussion of MCAT passages and questions, including multiple timesaving strategies and approaches. Writing techniques for the essay are also reviewed. Ten comprehensive review books that cover all MCAT subjects, consisting of approximately 2600 pages of material and more than 550 MCAT-style passages, and 10 full-length exams that students may complete at home are provided. Office hours are offered for the verbal reasoning section, including one-on-one essay and verbal reasoning analysis. Practice exams test each of the various subjects, one full-length exam assesses progress in the middle of the course, and two mirror the MCAT under simulated conditions at the very end of the course. The Berkeley Review also sells their course review materials for home study separately through their website, at a price of $50 for a set of two coursebooks and $20 for each full-length exam.

THE COLUMBIA REVIEW

220 Madison Avenue
San Francisco, CA 94134
(800) 300-PREP
(415) 337-2009
Website: www.columbiareview.com

Cost: $795 (included in the cost of tuition is a $200 non-refundable administrative fee) (regional costs may vary; ask about financial aid and alumni and campus discounts) The MCAT Intensive Home Study Course is $325.00

Classroom hours: 100+ (over 25 class sessions) lecture/classroom hours, and over 50 hours of small-group sessions

Class size: 20–25 per classroom

Length: 9 weeks (summer course), 13 weeks (spring MCAT course)

The Columbia Review course emphasizes concepts and passage analysis rather than memorization of facts. It is an intensive MCAT preparation course that combines many hours of class time with lots of practice tests and home-study materials. A home-study program is available at a cost of $325 for students who do not live near a Columbia Review center. The home-study program consists of over 2500 pages of material, complete lecture notes, over 110 MCAT practice questions with explanations, and 8 full-length MCAT exams with detailed solutions. The course for the April MCAT begins in January and lasts 13 weeks (meeting twice weekly plus small-group study sessions). The course for the August MCAT begins in June and lasts 9 weeks (meeting three times weekly plus small-group study sessions). The course reviews first the physical sciences, then the biological sciences, with a review of verbal reasoning and essay writing throughout. The course includes more than 50 hours of small-group study sessions devoted to helping students who have specific weaknesses. Individual tutorials are also available. The Columbia Review supplements its 100 hours of classroom instruction with an array of home-study materials, including review notes, formula sheets, problem sets, practice tests, and all MCAT material currently available from the AAMC. The primary course instructors are academic MDs, MD–PhD candidates, and graduate students.

PART V

beyond the mcat:

the medical school application process

A GREAT RELIEF comes from having completed the MCAT successfully. However, you should not celebrate too long and ignore other aspects of the application process. The American Medical College Application Service (AMCAS) begins to accept applications in mid-June. You would be well advised to submit your application as early as possible (e.g., by mid-July). Both the AMCAS and medical schools process applications on a rolling basis. Therefore, your file is evaluated in the order received. Medical schools do not wait to evaluate all the applicants before interviewing or even accepting students. This aspect is especially important for students who are borderline applicants; medical schools are more likely to grant interviews in the earlier months because of space availability. For example, a student with a 3.4 grade-point average (GPA) and a score of 10 on each section of the MCAT may be granted an interview at a school if 150 spaces are available but may not be when only 20 or fewer spaces are available later in the year. The same logic applies to competitive students who want to be accepted into competitive programs.

Submit your application as early as possible.

The Application

DO NOT BE INTIMIDATED. Just do it. Apply. For unknown reasons, some applicants cannot seem to get started with their applications. Remember: With the exception of the personal statement, this application is like most others. Writing your personal statement is, however, more complicated. Before you consult anyone, write out a few general topics that most admission committees want to know, for example, (1) why you want to become a doctor, (2) what your motivations are, (3) what significant events have occurred in your life, (4) your experience in a medical setting, (5) your research experience, and (6) your future goals. Initially, go for quantity, not quality. You may be surprised at how many pages you can fill. Next, hunt for personal statements from medical students, interns, residents, and others who may still have a copy of their application. Most people are happy to share them, and reading personal statements of successful applicants may be tremendously beneficial. Note, too, that not everything you wrote on your rough draft will fit on your final one-page application. But do not throw anything away; in a few weeks to months, you will be receiving secondary applications from medical schools requesting more information—in which case the additional thoughts on your rough drafts may be useful. Then, begin the most important task: edit, edit, and edit. Show the drafts to many people ahead of you in the game: advisors, medical students, residents, and a professional editor or English professor. Balance and integrate their feedback into something that reflects your personal strengths. Also remember that your personal statement reflects directly on you; therefore, it should be error-free. If you cannot make your page error-free, get it professionally typed.

Choosing Where to Apply

CHOOSING THE SCHOOLS to which you will apply can be a difficult task. In general, applicants know their top few choices. However, you may not know how to choose the next group of schools (assuming you are applying to 30 schools). As mentioned earlier, this process is relatively expensive; therefore, you should take a few hours and go through the most recent *Medical School Admissions Requirements* book and *Curriculum Directory*, both published by AAMC. These two publications will give you a general idea about your chances for admission at specific schools (e.g., they will indicate that it is not wise to apply to a school in another state that accepts only its own students even if your GPA and MCAT score exceed their average). How many medical schools you should apply to depends on your goals and credentials, but applying to at least ten is reasonable.

Some candidates think that because they are strong applicants, they need apply only to the most competitive schools. This attitude is a mistake, because many "strong" applicants do not get into medical school for just this reason. Apply to some of the less competitive schools as "safe schools." Medical school admission committees are influenced by your acceptances to other schools. Besides, being accepted into even one medical school may give you a sense of relief, security, and self-confidence.

If you have been accepted by a medical school but you prefer another, let them know.

If you have been accepted to a medical school but you would prefer another, let that school know. Writing letters and making phone calls may be very useful. Remind the school of your existence and interest. If the school is nearby, it may be beneficial to visit. Remember: If you do not get accepted, you are no worse off than if you had not tried. If you are accepted, you may be in a better program or you may save thousands of dollars in the long run.

Letters of Recommendation

IN GENERAL, THE most important aspect of this part of the application process is to not let these letters delay the completion of your application. Letters of recommendation are usually similar. Some, however, make a student stand out for unique reasons (e.g., "This student is in the top 1% of all the students I have been associated with"); others are less than enthusiastic about a candidate (e.g., "He/she was a good student"). In such cases, the committee usually takes notice.

It may be difficult at the last moment to determine whom you want to write letters for you. You should plan ahead, even up to 1 to 3 years. It is important to get letters from people who know you well. Letters are usually obtained from research professors, hospital volunteer coordinators, instructors for classes in which you have done exceptionally well, leaders of other volunteer programs, and sometimes athletic directors.

Letters of recommendation should be requested several months in advance.

Requests for letters of recommendations should be made several months in advance of applying to medical schools. Generally, people writing these letters are even more busy than you are. Periodic reminders are helpful; however, there is a fine line between being persistent and being pushy. Do not rest until you know that your letters have been received either by the central processing agency at your university or by the programs that you have applied to. Applications have been known to be delayed several weeks to months because one or more letters had not been submitted (e.g., the professor went on vacation or letters were lost in the mail or at the medical school admissions office). The bottom line is to plan ahead and keep on top of it.

The Interview

A few days before the interview, read about the school where you are interviewing.

MANY APPLICANTS FIND that interviews are the toughest part of the application process. However, this apprehension need not be a problem. Approximately 10% to 20% of medical school applicants are offered interviews. If you have been offered one, you have already crossed a major hurdle. Once again, preparation is the key. During the early part of the summer, even before you have been offered an interview, begin preparing. Videotape yourself during a mock interview with a counselor or a friend; you may be surprised by what you see, both good and bad. A few days before the interview, read about the school where you are interviewing, and learn its past, present, and future objectives. These objectives can be obtained from brochures or from students attending that school. Before the interview, review what is written on your personal statement. Many questions will come from that page.

PART VI

keyword index

Page numbers in *italics* designate figures; "t" designates tables; *see also* refers to related topics.